THIRD EDITION

Men's Hairdressing

TRADITIONAL AND MODERN BARBERING

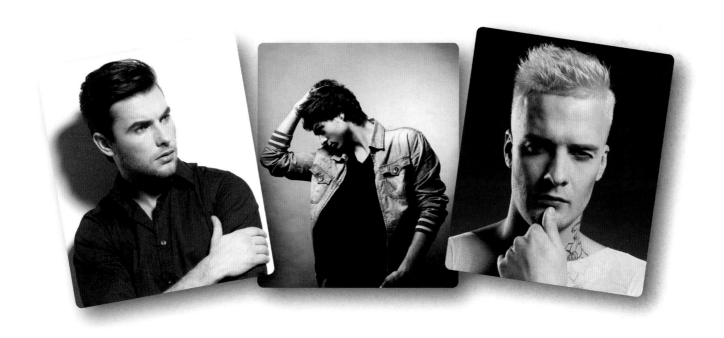

MAURICE LISTER

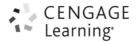
CENGAGE
Learning·

Australia • Brazil • Japan • Korea • Mexico • Singapore • Spain • United Kingdom • United States

HABIA SERIES LIST

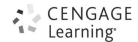

Men's Hairdressing Traditional and Modern Barbering, 3rd Edition
Maurice Lister

Publisher: Andrew Ashwin

Development Editor: Lauren Darby

Content Project Manager: Susan Povey

Manufacturing Manager: Eyvett Davis

Marketing Manager: Angela Lewis

Typesetter: MPS Limited

Cover design: HCT Creative

For product information and technology assistance,
contact **emea.info@cengage.com**
For permission to use material from this text or product,
and for permission queries,
email **emea.permissions@cengage.com**

British Library Cataloguing-in-Publication Data
A catalogue record for this book is available from the British Library.

ISBN: 978-1-4080-7742-9

Cengage Learning EMEA
Cheriton House, North Way, Andover
Hampshire, SP10 5BE. United Kingdom

Cengage Learning products are represented in Canada by Nelson Education Ltd.

For your lifelong learning solutions, visit
www.cengage.co.uk

Printed in China by RR Donnelley
Print Number: 01   Print Year: 2014

Contents

PART ONE Working in the Barber's Shop

PART TWO Menswork

PART THREE Advanced Menswork

Foreword from Habia

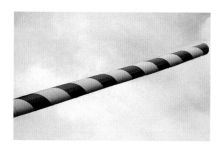

Men's Hairdressing has come a long way since the conventional 'short back and sides' and similarly Maurice Lister has taken *Men's Hairdressing: Traditional and Modern Barbering* through a particularly interesting journey. Now into its third edition, Maurice has packed this study guide with new and exciting content.

Maurice is never one for holding back, and his in-depth understanding of the industry shows through his ability to write in an engaging style; keeping the content simple yet making you feel that his considerable knowledge and experience are at your fingertips, firing you up for the next challenge.

It is therefore no surprise that the number one Barbering author, Maurice Lister, produces a superb book that moves with the times, techniques and developments within the industry. This third edition is the best yet.

I have known Maurice for a long time, working with him on many projects and so I'm delighted that Maurice continues to reflect the standards and ethos of Habia.

Jane Goldsbro
Director of Standards & Qualifications
Habia

About our partners

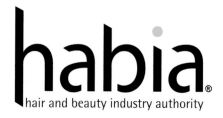

Habia, the Hair and Beauty Industry Authority is appointed by government to represent employers in the Hair and Beauty Sector. Habia's main role is to manage the development of the National Occupational Standards (NOS) for hairdressing, barbering, beauty therapy, nails and spa. They are developed by industry for industry and represent best practice to achieving skills and knowledge for a particular job role. The NOS are used as the building blocks for the development of all qualfications that are developed by Awarding Organizations and by Cengage to develop text books and support products for learners.

Habia is also responsible for the development and implementation of Apprenticeship Frame-works and issuing the apprenticeship certificates. Alongside providing information to employers on Government initiatives that may affect the hair and beauty industry be it educational, environmental or financial. A central point of contact for information, Habia provides guidance on careers, business development, legislation, salon health and safety.

Habia is part of SkillsActive, the Sector Skills Council that covers Hair & Beauty, Sports and the Active Leisure Sector.

City & Guilds are the leading Awarding Organization for Hairdressing, Barbering and Beauty related Industries.

Endorsed by

About the author

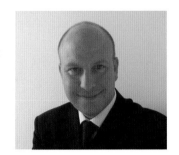

Maurice Lister started his career in the family business as a barber before going on to gain far-reaching expertise in education, training, assessment and quality assurance of hairdressing, barbering and other qualifications. Maurice has worked throughout the UK and Europe and in Pakistan, India, and the Gulf States. He has worked extensively as a development consultant for City & Guilds and HABIA, developing a range of qualifications, educational resources and assessment materials.

Maurice has been a City & Guilds external quality assurer for over 25 years and was previously the City & Guilds Chief Verifier for hair and beauty and one of only three Strategic Quality Advisors at City & Guilds. Maurice is a City & Guilds Chief Examiner and currently leads the City & Guilds hair and beauty external quality assurance team as Group Portfolio Consultant and is the lead consultant for all barbering qualifications.

Acknowledgements

On a personal note, I would like to thank my wife, Dawn for her continuing support and encouragement. I would also like to note special thanks to my uncle, Bill Morris who taught me the importance of traditional barbering principles and gave me the opportunity to develop these skills. I also note my special thanks to publishing consultant Claire Hart for her consistent patience and support whilst compiling this new edition. I wish to thank Lucy Mills, Claire Napoli, Lauren Darby, picture researcher Sarah Smithies and all at Cengage Learning for their patience, encouragement and support during the development of this third edition – thank you! My thanks also go to the staff at City & Guilds and at Habia for their continued friendship, support and endorsement.

Maurice Lister

The author would also like to thank the following: Adam Sloan at Big Yin Salons and the Men's Hairdressing Federation, Tracy Booton at Seagraves Gentleman's Barbers, Mike Taylor at the British Barbering Association, Gary Machin at Rogers Barber shops Ltd., Edward Hemmings at Alan d Hairdressing, Ebru Alkaya at Alan d Hairdressing, Nigel Sillis, Guy Kremer, Dr John Gray (Procter & Gamble), Redken, Wella, Dr A.L. Wright (Consultant Dermatologist, Bradford Royal Infirmary), Dr M.H. Beck (Consultant Dermatologist, Salford Royal Hospital), S. Lewis, Martin Turner, Helena Royle (Regis International Ltd), L'Oréal, Salon Ambience, Saks: Premier Collection, Claudia Woolley, Hair and Beauty Industry Authority, City & Guilds, Forfex Professional, Exit Hairdressing, Patrick Cameron, Charlie Miller, Simon Shaw, WAHL, Lee Stafford, MK Hair Studio, Daniel Hill, Charles Worthington, Ralph Kleeli, Goldwell Professional Haircare, Fudge, Comby, BaByliss Pro, Olymp, Regis International Ltd, Patricia Livingston, Paul Stafford, Clynol, David Adams, John J. Dibbons, Joico, Sorisa, Depilex, Chris Foster, Joshua Lomotey (Soft Sheen Carson), Sandra Gittens, Thornton Howdle Photography, Chris Mullen – Flanigans, Adam Young.

An additional special thanks to MK at Andis and MK Hair Studio & Academy, Erik Lander at Habia and Top Spot, Simon Shaw at Wahl, who were all involved in some of the various techniques photographs taken for this book; Wahl for sponsoring many of the photos for this new edition; Andis for sponsoring some of the photos for this new edition; Erik Lander at Top Spot, Corby for the loan of a barber's chair; Ian Lea Photography for his continuing involvement in most of the step-by-steps Andrew Eathorne for the videography of most of the QR code clips; Adrenaline Alley™ Studio, Corby for supplying studio facilities for the photo-shoot of new step-by-steps.

Thank you Frontier Medical Products (www.sharpsafe.co.uk) for the image of the sharps container. Special thanks to Barrie Carter for the offer of a photograph of his grandfather's barber's shop and to Nigel Sillis for supplying photographs of his father, Henry Sillis's barber's shop. Thanks also to Christopher Selleck for the offer of photographs of his high-frequency equipment. Thank you Adam Young for providing facial hair illustrations.

With great appreciation to the following for providing industry insight quotes:
Adam Sloan at Big Yin Salons and the Men's Hairdressing Federation, Tracy Booton at Seagraves Gentleman's Barbers, MK at Andis and MK Hair Studio & Academy, Mike Taylor at the British Barbering Association, Gary Machin at Rogers Barbershops Ltd., Edward Hemmings at Alan d Hairdressing, Ebru Alkaya at Alan d Hairdressing, Simon Shaw at Wahl, Lee Stafford at Staffords Salons and Erik Lander at Habia and Top Spot.

Finally, thanks to all those kind people who have allowed us to use photographs of their hair in this book.

The publisher would like to thank the many copyright holders who have kindly granted us permission to reproduce material throughout this text. Every effort has been made to contact all rights holders but in the unlikely event that anything has been overlooked please contact the publisher directly and we will happily make the necessary arrangements at the earliest opportunity.

Credits

Adam Sloan – 10 bl, 10 br, 43 c, 84 tl, 210 cla, 214 bl, 225 tr; **Alamy** – 72 tl (BSIP SA), 72 cb (Medical-on-Line), 225 cra (AF archive), 225 clb (AF archive), 287 bc (James Boardman); **American Crew, Inc.** – 79 crb, 95 cra, 156 bl; **Andis** – 191 cra; **British Barbers Association** – 42 tl; **Cengage** – 7 bl, 7 crb, 9 bl, 9 bc, 12, 1618 tr, 18 bc, 21 bl, 23 tr, 23 bl, 28, 33 b, 35 b, 39 b, 41 c, 42 tc, 46 c, 55, 55 br, 56 clb, 57 bc, 59 cr, 62 cl, 62 br, 63 bc, 64 bc, 65 bl, 66 tr, 70 tr, 74 tl, 76, 79 cra, 80 clb, 80 crb, 80 bc, 81 bl, 82 br, 86 cl, 90 tl, 95 crb, 96 bc, 98 cla, 98 clb, 101 clb, 101 c, 101 crb, 101 bl, 101 bc, 101 br, 102 tl, 102 tc, 102 tr, 106 bl, 110 bc, 112 tl, 112 br, 113 crb, 113 br, 115 cra, 115 crb, 118 bl, 120 tr, 120 bl, 121 tr, 125 tr, 125 br, 127 tr, 128 tl, 128 bl, 129 tl, 129 tc, 129 tr, 129 cra, 130 tl, 130 cl, 138 bl, 138 bc, 138 br, 139 tl, 139 tc, 139 tr, 139 cl, 139 c, 143 clb, 143 cb, 143 crb, 143 bl, 143 bc, 143 br, 144 tl, 144 tc, 144 tr, 144 cl, 145 bl, 145 bc, 145 br, 146 tl, 146 tc, 146 tr, 149 bc, 154 cla, 154 ca, 157 cra, 157 crb, 158 tl, 159 clb, 159 cb, 159 crb, 159 bl, 159 bc, 162 tl, 162 tcl, 162 tcr, 162 tr, 163 l, 163 cl, 163 cr, 163 r, 164 cla, 164 clb, 166 c, 170 clb, 172 bl, 173 tr, 173 cra, 173 bl, 175 cra, 176 ca, 185 bl, 192 ca, 192 cb, 192 cb, 193 tr, 193 cra, 193 bl, 194, 202 tl, 210 tc, 210 bc, 212 clb, 212 bc, 214 tl, 219 cla, 219 ca, 219 cra, 219 clb, 219 cb, 229 bc, 232, 238 clb, 239 tr, 240 br, 240 clb, 240 bl, 241 tr, 241 cra, 243 tl, 243 tc, 243 tr, 243 cla, 243 c, 243 cra, 244 tl, 244 bl, 244 bc, 244 br, 245 tl, 245 tc, 245 tr, 246 tl, 246 cl, 247 tc, 247 tr, 247 cra, 247 cr, 248 tc, 248 tr, 248 cla, 248 clb, 248 bl, 249 tl, 249 tc, 249 tr, 249 cla, 249 ca, 249 cra, 249 clb, 249 cb, 249 crb, 249 bl, 249 bc, 250 cl, 250 bl, 251 tr, 255 c, 259, 260 clb, 267 br, 268 cla, 268 clb, 269 tr, 269 cra, 269 crb, 269 br, 271 tr, 271 cla, 271 ca, 271 cra, 271 clb, 271 cb, 271 crb, 271 bl, 271 bc, 271 br, 271 tl, 271 tc, 271 tr, 271 l, 271 c, 271 r, 276, 281 clb, 281 bl, 282 tc, 282 ca, 282 cb, 282 bc, 284 cl, 284 clb, 284 bl, 285 tl, 285 tc, 285 tr, 285 cla, 285 ca, 285 cra, 285 crb, 285 bl, 285 bc, 285 br, 286 tl, 286 tc, 286 tr, 286 cla, 286 ca, 286 cra, 286 clb, 287 tc, 288 tc, 288 tr, 288 cl, 288 ca, 288 cr, 289 tl, 289 tc, 289 tr, 289 cl, 289 c, 289 cr, 292 bl, 298 c, 311, 18 tc, 19 br, 21 cr, 22 bl, 24 bl, 25 tr, 25 cra, 25 crb, 43 crb, 44 tl, 46 tl, 56 tl, 58 tl, 78 tl, 79 tr, 85 cra, 86 cb, 86 cbr, 86 bc, 86 bcr, 87 cra, 87 crb, 88 cla, 88 clb, 9297 br, 98 tc, 99 tr, 99 clb, 99 cb, 99 crb, 99 bl, 99 bc, 99 br, 100 tl, 100 tc, 100 tr, 104 cla, 104 ca, 104 cra, 111 cr, 111 crb, 111 br, 119 crb, 122 cl, 124 cla, 124 cl, 125 cr, 125 crb, 126 tr, 126 bc, 127 tl, 127 tc, 127 cr, 127 br, 129 crb, 130 bl, 130 bc, 130 br, 131 tl, 131 tc, 131 tr, 131 cla, 131 ca, 131 cra, 131 clb, 131 cb, 131 crb, 131 bl, 131 bc, 132 cl, 132 c, 132 cr, 132 clb, 132 cb, 132 crb, 132 bl, 132 bc, 132 br, 133 tl, 136 tl, 136 tc, 136 tr, 136 cla, 136 ca, 136 cra, 136 clb, 136 cb, 136 crb, 136 bl, 136 bc, 136 br, 137 clb, 137 cb, 137 crb, 137 bl, 137 bc, 137 br, 138 tl, 138 tc, 138 tr, 156 bc, 156 br, 160 br, 165 br, 188189 br, 192 tl, 192 bl, 195 tr, 195 bl, 196 clb, 198 cla, 198 ca, 198 cra, 198 clb, 198 cb, 198 crb, 198 bl, 200 cb, 201 clb, 208 clb, 210 cl, 210 br, 213 tr, 213 bl, 217 bl, 217 bc, 217 br, 218 tl, 218 tc, 218 tr, 218 cla, 218 ca, 218 cra, 218 clb, 218 cb, 218 crb, 220 clb, 220 cb, 220 crb, 220 bl, 220 bc, 220 br, 221 tl, 221 tc, 222 tl, 222 tc, 222 tr, 222 cla, 222 ca, 222 cra, 222 clb, 222 cb, 222 crb, 225 bl, 225 bc, 225 br, 226 tl, 226 tc, 226 tr, 226 cla, 226 ca, 226 cra, 226 clb, 226 cb, 226 crb, 228 bl, 238 bl, 241 cr, 241 crb, #1241 crb, #2267 tr, 273 bl, 283 cra, 283 br, 290 tl, 290 tc, 290 tr, 290 cl, 290 c, 290 cr, 294296 br, 298 cl, 299 tr, 299 cra, 300 bl, 301 br, 302 cra, 302 cl, 303 tl, 303 tc, 303 tr, 303 cla, 303 ca, 303 cra, 303 clb, 303 cb,

Signposting of Level 1, Level 2 and Level 3 barbering related NVQ/SVQ units covered in this book

Units/Chapters () = previous NVQ unit numbers	CHB1 (G7,G21, GH24)	CHB2 CHB3 (G3,G8)	CHB4 (G11)	CHB5 (GH3)	CHB7 CHB8 (G2,G4)	CHB9 CHB10 (GH1, GH8)	CHB14 (GH21)	CB2 AH42 (GB3)	CB3 (GB8)	CB4 (GB4)	CB5 (GB7)	CB6 (GB5)	CB7 (AH21)	CB8 (AH 35)	CB9 CH6 CHB11 (GB10, GH26 GH27)	CB1 CB10 (GB1, GB6)	CH12 CHB15 (GH5, GH14)	CB17 (GH25)
1. Origins of barbering		✓#	✓#				✓#											
2. Health & safety in the barber's shop	✓*	✓*		✓*												✓*		
3. Working effectively in the barber's shop		✓	✓#	✓*														
4. Client care for men	✓	✓*				✓*	✓*	✓*	✓*	✓*	✓*	✓*	✓*	✓*	✓*	✓*	✓*	✓*
5. Shampoo, condition and treat hair and scalp conditions	✓*	✓*		✓*		✓												
6. Cut facial hair using basic techniques	✓*	✓*		✓*						✓			✓*					
7. Cut men's hair using basic techniques	✓*	✓*		✓*				✓ (AH42 = ✓*)					✓*					
8. Dry and finish men's hair	✓*	✓*		✓*			✓*					✓						
9. Colour men's hair	✓*	✓*		✓*			✓*								✓#			
10. Create basic patterns in hair	✓*	✓*		✓*			✓*						✓					
11. Advanced men's hair cutting	✓*	✓*		✓*			✓*							✓*				
12. Shaving services	✓*	✓*		✓*			✓*									✓		
13. Face massage services	✓*	✓*		✓*			✓*											
14. Design and create facial hair shapes	✓*	✓*		✓*			✓*				✓			✓*				
15. Design and create patterns in hair	✓*	✓*		✓*			✓*							✓				
A Reception in the barber's shop	✓*	✓*		✓*	✓													
B Perm men's hair	✓*	✓*		✓*			✓*										✓#	
C Specialist hair and scalp treatments	✓*	✓*		✓*			✓*											✓

A, B, C = additional online chapters   ✓ = all covered by chapter   ✓* = relevant aspects covered by chapter   ✓# = basic aspects covered by chapter

Signposting of Level 1, Level 2 and Level 3 barbering related VRQ units covered in this book

Units/Chapters Red = City & Guilds Blue = ITEC Orange = VTCT (UV then #)	104 312 30337	001 002 101 102 115 201 313 612 629 20484 10478 21456	006 007 113 202 302 6911-02 600 638 613 20483 30491	203 240 303 601 614 20386 30506	003 204 230 305 602 20488	205 627 20492 30435	111 207 214 217 232 306 605 10480 20486	208 238 308 607 20512	210 604 20504	211 224 610 20505	005 212 316 405 908 920 20499 30498	215 235 406 606 20513 40519	114 216 611 639 20489	312 616 30507	313 626 30508
1. Origins of barbering		✓*				✓#					✓#				
2. Health & safety in the barber's shop		✓*?	✓	✓*											
3. Working effectively in the barber's shop		✓													
4. Client care for men	✓*	✓*	✓*	✓	✓*		✓*	✓*	✓*	✓*	✓*	✓*		✓*	✓*
5. Shampoo, condition and treat hair and scalp conditions		✓*	✓*	✓*	✓	✓*					✓*				
6. Cut facial hair using basic techniques		✓*	✓*	✓*		✓*				✓					
7. Cut men's hair using basic techniques		✓*	✓*	✓*		✓*			✓		✓*				
8. Dry and finish men's hair	✓	✓*	✓*	✓*		✓*					✓*				
9. Colour men's hair		✓*	✓*	✓*		✓*	✓#				✓*				
10. Create basic patterns in hair		✓*	✓*	✓*		✓*					✓*				
11. Advanced men's hair cutting		✓*	✓*	✓*		✓*					✓*	✓		✓	
12. Shaving services		✓*	✓*	✓*		✓*					✓*				
13. Face massage services		✓*	✓*	✓*		✓*					✓*				
14. Design and create facial hair shapes		✓*	✓*	✓*		✓*					✓*				✓
15. Design and create patterns in hair		✓*	✓*	✓*		✓*					✓*	✓			
A Reception in the barber's shop		✓*	✓*	✓*		✓*							✓		
B Perm men's hair		✓*	✓*	✓*		✓*		✓#			✓*				
C Specialist hair and scalp treatments		✓*	✓*	✓*		✓*					✓*				

A, B, C = additional online chapters   ✓ = all covered by chapter   ✓* = relevant aspects covered by chapter   ✓# = basic aspects covered by chapter

About this book

Throughout this textbook you will find many colourful text boxes designed to aid your learning and understanding as well as highlight key points. Here are examples and descriptions of each:

> " Gives you an inspirational glance into the knowledge and experience of a trusted industry expert, helping to motivate and instruct you in your own career. "

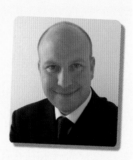

TIP ✓

Shares the author's experience and provides positive suggestions to improve knowledge and skills in each unit.

DON'T BE TEMPTED ✗

Don't be Tempted boxes warn you against bad practice in the salon.

HEALTH & SAFETY

Draws your attention to related health and safety information essential for each technical skill.

KEY DEFINITION

The definitions of key terms throughout each chapter are highlighted clearly in the margin to aid understanding.

ACTIVITY - FIND OUT

'Case Studies' and 'Find Out' activity boxes are featured in the book to provide additional tasks for you to further your understanding.

Directional arrows point you to other parts of the book that explore similar or related topics, so you can expand your learning.

Web boxes recommend certain supplementary sites that can be viewed online. Including indicators to material that might be waiting for you on the book's accompanying website.

BRINGING IT ALL TOGETHER

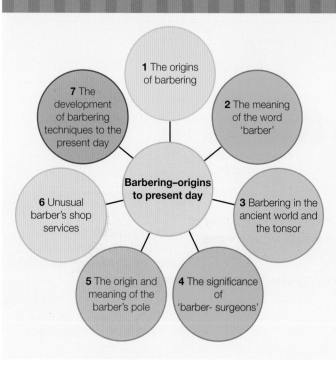

Barbering–origins to present day

1 The origins of barbering

2 The meaning of the word 'barber'

3 Barbering in the ancient world and the tonsor

4 The significance of 'barber- surgeons'

5 The origin and meaning of the barber's pole

6 Unusual barber's shop services

7 The development of barbering techniques to the present day

At the end of each chapter there is a useful revision section which has been specially devised to help you check your learning and prepare for your oral and written assessments.

Use these revision sections to test your knowledge as you progress through the course and seek guidance from your supervisor or assessor if you come across any areas that you're unsure of.

All the answers for these questions can be found online, on the textbook's accompanying website.

About the website

Use the *Men's Hairdressing: Traditional and Modern Barbering* 3rd Edition's accompanying website alongside this textbook for a complete blended learning solution!

The website contains:

- – Three online bonus chapters
- – Image galleries
- – Worksheets (linked to activities in the textbook) to download and complete
- – Answers to questions from 'Bringing it all together' feature

In order to access the learning resources on this website please search for *Men's Hairdressing* 3rd Edition on **www.cengagebrain.co.uk**

Videos

There are also many useful videos available online to accompany the step-by-step techniques featured in this book. Look out for the QR codes in the margin, scan them on your smartphone using a QR code app and watch the video content available online!

Image Galleries

Towards the end of some of the chapters in this book you will also find an image gallery box, these are to point you towards mood boards of further online images that will inspire your creative work for each subject area.

Accompanying video available for Effleurage, Rotary, Petrissage and Friction massage movements 'Shampoo and Condition Massage Movements'.

IMAGE GALLERY

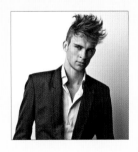

Visit the online image gallery on this book's accompanying website to see other contemporary barbers' shops and marketing ideas for barbering services.

Introduction by the author

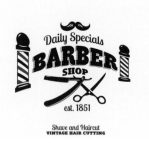

Men make up about 50 per cent of the population, yet until recent times few hairdressers specialized in the barbering skills required to develop their men's business. Many used a 'unisex' approach to 'menswork', often resulting in less satisfactory looks for men and the real danger that traditional barbering skills would be lost. Increasing interest in male grooming provided the required stimulus; the result, additional business opportunities for the skilled barber, which along with the frequent use of barbering techniques in women's hairdressing meant that barbering skills were again increasing in demand.

I originally wrote this book to help ensure that traditional barbering skills were not lost. The second edition sought to build on this aim and help the reader develop their barbering skills to meet these growing demands. I am, therefore, delighted this third edition that finds the barbering industry is revitalized. Barbering creativity is thriving, as seen in advanced and hair pattern work and dedicated barber's shops have a growing presence on the high street, mirrored by barbering's increasing recognition and importance in the world of hairdressing. Barbering is now represented through the British Barbering Association and Men's Hairdressing Federation, and menswork is fully recognized at all levels of the Barbering NVQs/SVQs and Vocationally Related Qualifications (VRQs). I am pleased to conclude that traditional barbering skills are now safely in the modern barbers' hands.

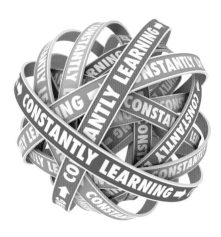

Whether you are an experienced hairdresser seeking to include menswork in your repertoire or just starting out on your barbering career, the book and additional online material is designed to provide you with all the information necessary to help you develop your potential in barbering. I have included simple step-by-steps and QR code links to video clips to help you understand the essential techniques and quotes from some colleagues in the barbering industry to guide and inspire your progress. For those undertaking the qualifications I have included key definitions, activities, case studies, revision notes and questions to help you more easily understand and prepare for examinations. For experienced barbers, I have included information to help you consolidate your knowledge and skills and have included inspiring advanced work that I hope will in turn provide inspiration for you to develop new services and increase the men's business. I hope you enjoy reading the book as much as I have enjoyed writing it!

Maurice Lister
August 2014

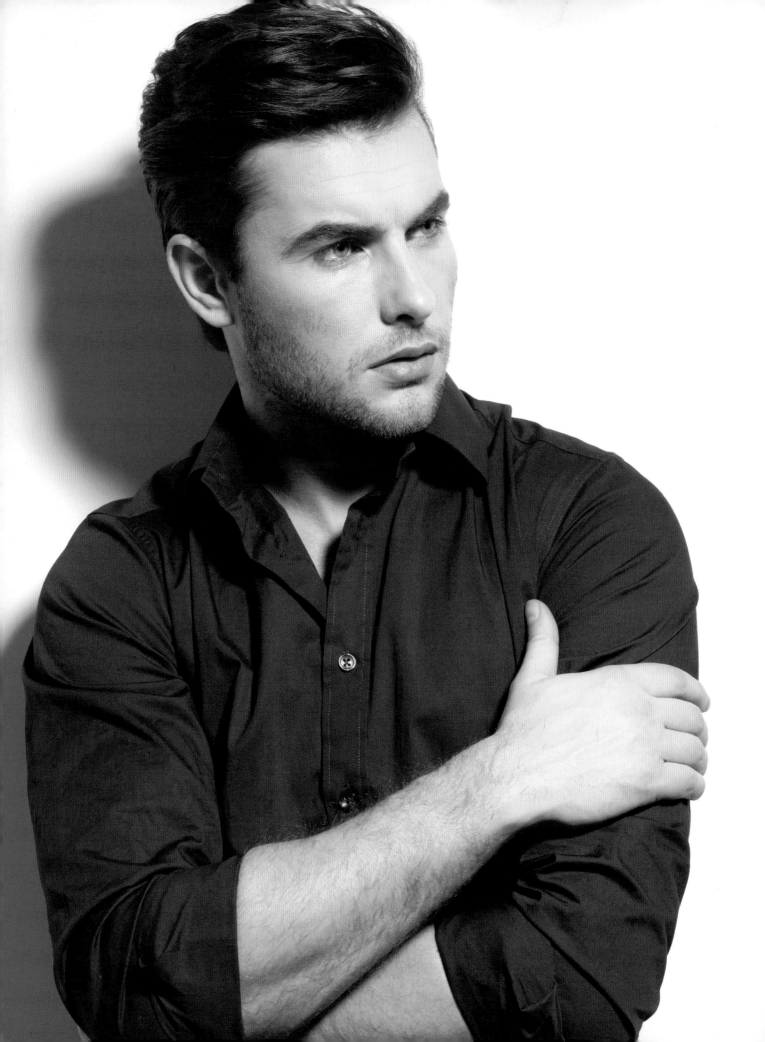

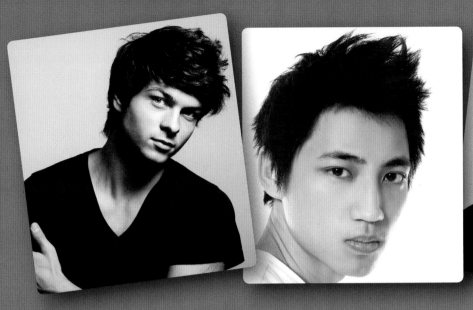

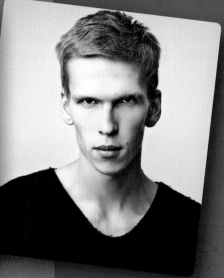

PART ONE

Working in the Barber's Shop

Part 1 introduces you to the barbering industry and the skills and knowledge you need to work safely and effectively in the barber's shop. You will cover the proud origins of barbering, the common hazards and risks in the barber's shop, the importance of working effectively with your clients and colleagues and the benefits of developing your skills and knowledge.

There is also an additional online chapter covering fulfilling reception duties in the barber's shop, including dealing with people at reception and making appointments in the barber's shop.

1 Barbering–from its origins to the present day

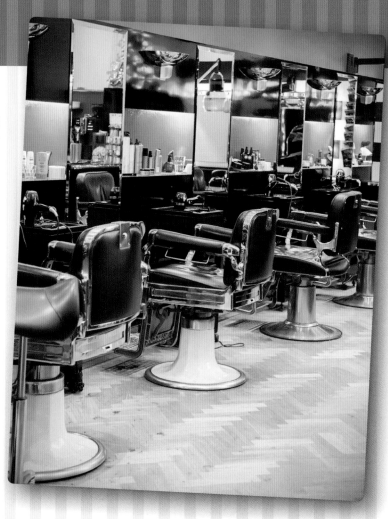

QUALIFICATION SIGNPOSTING

This chapter will help your studies of the following qualifications:

❖ Levels 1, 2 and 3 NVQ Diplomas in Barbering.
❖ City & Guilds VRQ Levels 1, 2 and 3 Awards, Certifications and Diplomas in Barbering, Barbering Techniques and Women's and Men's Hairdressing.
❖ ITEC VRQ Levels 1 and 2 Certificates and Diplomas in Barbering.
❖ VTCT VRQ Level 2 Certificates and Diplomas in Barbering and Barbering Studies.

For further information on the qualifications covered by this chapter see the qualification mapping grid at the front of the book.

LEARNING OBJECTIVES

This chapter discusses the evolution of barbering to the present day.

In this chapter you will learn:

◆ The origins of barbering.

◆ The meaning of the word 'barber'.

◆ Barbering in the ancient world and the meaning of tonsor.

◆ The significance of 'barber-surgeons'.

◆ The origin and meaning of the barber's pole.

◆ Unusual barber's shop services.

◆ The development of barbering principles and techniques to the present day.

INTRODUCTION

Barbering is the professional craft of cutting, styling, grooming and shaving men's hair. Barbers have a long, proud and varied past and present-day barbering techniques owe much to the methods developed by these early barbers. Many of the principles they established still apply today and the history of their development should be considered by anyone who has an interest in the work of the barber.

This chapter discusses the evolution of barbering to the present day and covers the following topics:

❖ The origins of barbering and barbering in the ancient world.

❖ The meaning of the word 'barber' and significance of beards in barbering.

❖ The meaning of tonsor.

❖ The significance of 'barber-surgeons'.

❖ The origin and meaning of the barber's pole.

❖ The unusual services that have been provided in barbers' shops.

❖ The development of barbering principles and how these established the techniques to the present day.

The origins of barbering

Barbering may accurately be described as one of the oldest professions in the world. Archaeologists have found simple cutting implements made from sharpened flints and bones, which show that haircutting was practised as long ago as 30 000 years BC. The Egyptians were the first to develop techniques and tools that we might recognize in barbering and hairdressing today. Excavation of Egyptian pyramids has unearthed many combs and cutting tools, including razors made of tempered copper and bronze that were used by Egyptians nearly 6000 years ago.

The word 'barber' is derived from the Latin word **barba**, meaning 'beard'. Many barbering skills developed because of the importance of the beard in past times. A beard was often considered to be a sign of wisdom and strength and, not surprisingly, also of manhood. The beard has been important in many religions throughout the ages and in some is still seen as important today.

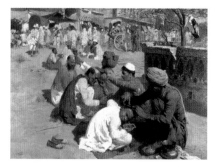
Street barbering in ancient times

Barbering in ancient times

Organized barbering services were offered as long ago as 1500 BC. In ancient Egypt many men had their beard and their head shaved as a sign of their status in society and for the easy maintenance that such styles provided. Egyptian barbers often preferred to work outdoors because of the hot climate. The barber would meet their clients in the street, where the client would kneel while the barber casually went about their work in full view of passers-by.

ACTIVITY – FIND OUT

Find out where street barbering might still be seen today.

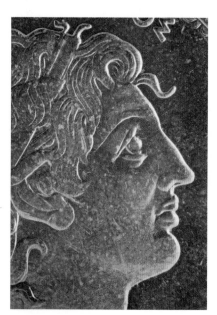
Alexander the Great

Street barbering

Although popular in ancient Egypt, shaving did not become commonplace in most other countries until around 400 BC, by which time hairstyling and barbering had evolved into highly developed crafts.

In ancient Greece wealthy men regularly had their hair cut and styled, often by their servants, but most members of the poorer classes still wore long hair and beards. In about 335 BC Alexander the Great, ruler of Greece at the time, prompted widespread shaving when he ordered his army, the Macedonians to remove their beards. This was a strategy to overcome his enemies', the Persians, tactic of grasping the Greek soldiers' beards during battle. Alexander himself was clean-shaven, which was unusual at that time as most rulers wore beards. This too encouraged shaving as men who admired Alexander copied his example.

In Rome by about 300 BC barbering services had become available to the general population. Slaves were still forced to wear their beards and hair long, as a sign of their lower status, but most other men visited the barber's shop. Roman men were usually clean-shaven so the barbers' shops were much frequented. They were used as meeting places,

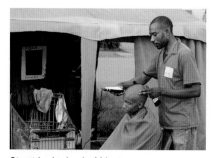
Street barbering in Africa

and were known to be good places to catch up with the local gossip. At the time Roman barbers were known as a **tonsor**, from the Latin, *Tondeo* meaning to shear or shave. Reflecting this history, barbers are sometimes today also referred to as tonsorial artists. Many Roman barbers enjoyed considerable wealth and status in Roman society because of the success of these early barbers' shops.

Barber-surgeons

By the Middle Ages barbering services were well established in England and across most of Europe, but barbers were no longer only shaving and haircutting. These early barbers were also the pioneers of many medical treatments. Known as barber-surgeons, because they performed both barbering and surgery, they frequently carried out bloodletting, simple surgery and wound dressing, and also pulled teeth – a simple form of dentistry.

The barber's pole

The familiar red-and-white striped pattern of the traditional barber's pole originated as the symbol of the barber-surgeons and their work in bloodletting.

Bloodletting involved cutting a vein on the patient's arm, in order to let out 'bad blood'. Many ailments were thought to be caused by 'bad blood', which was sometimes said to have been affected by evil spirits. Others, such as the ancient Greeks believed that the human body required a fine balance of all the fluids contained within, referred to as 'humours' and where there was an imbalance poor health would be the result. Although it was widely believed that removing this bad or imbalanced blood would bring about a speedy recovery, the treatment is not known to have been very successful. On the contrary, poor understanding of the cause of infection and the need for hygiene would often result in infection developing at the site of the cut, which would lead to other serious illnesses. **Leeches** were also used widely for early medical purposes and were also used by some barbers.

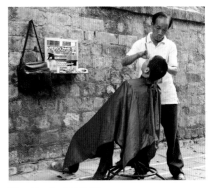

Street barbering today

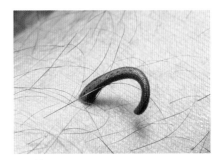

Leeching

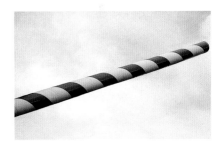

Barber's pole

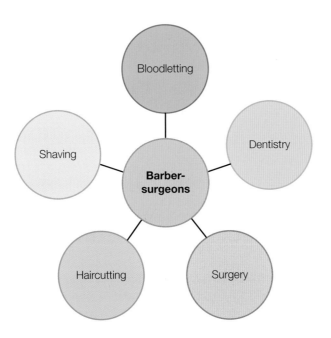

HEALTH & SAFETY

Bloodletting and the use of leeches is potentially very dangerous and should only be practiced by qualified medical professionals.

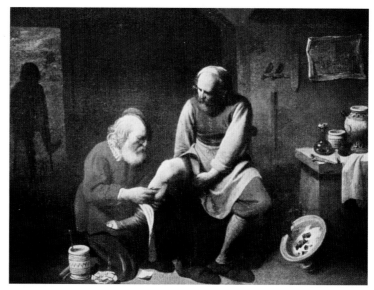

Historical image of bloodletting

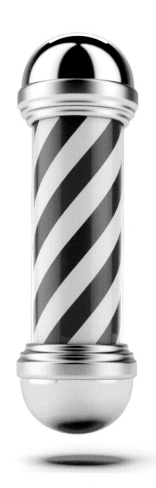

More recently it was discovered that some medical conditions can be improved by removing blood and during the twentieth century medical professionals started using leeches to help stimulate the movement of blood through the veins where it was sluggish. Perhaps the modern use of leeching indicates that those early barbers were not so wrong after all!

In bloodletting wounds were dressed with cloth bandages. In those days, before the risks of infection and blood-borne diseases were understood, the bandages were used over and over again: although they were white at first, with repeated use they became stained. Whilst hanging outside the barbers' shop to dry, they would twist together in the breeze with the newer, whiter bandages, forming the red-and-white striped pattern familiar to us now as the barber's pole.

Some barbers' poles also have a blue stripe, and others have a small bowl hanging beneath.

In this instance the pole is said to represent the post that the patient held onto whilst undergoing treatment. The blue stripe represents the blood from the veins, the red stripe the blood from the arteries. The arteries should not have been cut at all, but sometimes they were, by mistake; this illustrates how hazardous the treatment was. The bowl hanging beneath is often said to represent the bowl used to collect the patient's blood. In reality, it is more likely to have been the bowl used to collect lather during shaving.

During the thirteenth century the 'Barbers Company of London' was established, to help regulate and protect the developing barbering profession. Within a few years some of the barber-surgeons began to favour surgery and formed a 'Surgeons' Company' or 'Guild'. In the middle of the 1500s, after many years of disagreement, Henry VIII of England created an Act that united barbers and surgeons under one corporation. Under this Act barbers were prohibited from performing surgery, although they could continue bloodletting and teeth pulling; and the surgeons were prohibited from performing barbering and shaving services.

The barber and surgeon had been united in one profession for over 500 years when they were finally separated in 1745. George II of England passed an Act that divided barbers and surgeons into two distinct corporations. The 'Worshipful Company of Barbers' was formed and barbers dropped their use of the name 'barber-surgeons'. Since then barbers have not performed any medical services, indeed it may be unlawful for them to do so, but in many high streets today you will still see the red-and-white striped pole as a symbol of barbers' long, varied and significant past.

Unusual barber's shop services

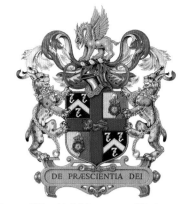

Crest of Worshipful Company of Barbers

In times past barbers also became known for performing other unusual services, such as servicing umbrellas and singeing hair, and more recently some barbers have offered threading services.

Umbrella services were less commonly offered and most often based in barbers' shops near busy transport hubs, such as bus and train stations where a traveller might urgently need an umbrella. Conversely, many traditional barbers' shops at one time offered hair singeing services.

Singeing involved the barber using either a lighted wax taper or electrical singeing equipment to singe the ends of the hair after cutting (most barbers preferred the wax taper). At the time, singeing was commonly thought to 'stop the hair bleeding', as it was believed that the goodness or life of the hair would run out through the cut open end of the hair shaft, but we now know this is not correct. However, it was found to sometimes help reduce *fragilitas crinium* (split ends), as the cells that make up the hair were fused together by the heat of the flame or heated appliance and so were less able to split apart. The flame also had antiseptic properties and singeing with this method could be useful in the removal of parasites that attach themselves to the hair. Stray hairs left after cutting could also be removed easily to create a smoother finish, especially on shorter styles.

Singeing services demanded that great care was taken to avoid damage to the hair or the barber or client being burnt. A thorough check was always made before starting the service to ensure that the client was not wearing any flammable hair dressings, such as hairspray as such substances could quickly ignite and cause serious harm. The barber, too, had to ensure they were not wearing such dressings on their hair. Other flammable substances were also kept well clear of the area during the service, e.g. hairspray could not be used by an adjacent barber.

The singeing process resembled the sectioning system used in cutting. At the end of the haircut the barber would retake the sections of hair as in cutting a uniform layer, e.g. at 90° to the head. A tail comb or sometimes the bottom of the taper was used to lift the section, which was transferred to and held in the other hand whilst the flame would be

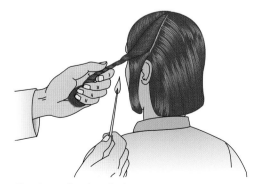

Singeing–twisted method

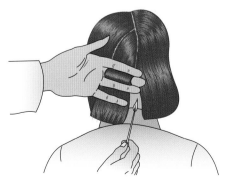

Singeing–flat method

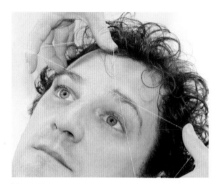

Threading

quickly run along the ends of the hair. This was continued around the head and when completed the hair would be dressed and finished with products, as required by the client. On longer hair, stray or frayed hairs further up the hair shaft were removed by either a twisting or a flat method.

Singeing has also been used in barbers' shops to remove hair growing in the clients' noses and on their ears, as the flame could quickly reach inside these areas. In some countries, e.g. Turkey, barbers can still be seen using singeing for this purpose, but in most barbers' shops singeing with a lighted taper is no longer performed because of the risks involved. Over the past few years electrically heated scissors have become available to allow some of the benefits of singeing to be obtained without the need to use an open flame. The scissors are insulated except for their cutting edges in order to protect the client's and barber's skin, and a computer is used to maintain the correct temperature for different hair thicknesses.

More recently **threading** has gained some popularity. Threading is a technique used to remove hair, similar to plucking hair with tweezers. Threading originates from Asia where it is performed on both men and women as part of a regular grooming and beauty treatment within families. Threading then became available more widely as a treatment offered by some beauty therapists. It is performed by crossing over and twisting a length of cotton between the thumb and first finger on each hand.

Tension in these threads at the point they cross over is created by twisting the cotton. This tension produces a gripping effect between the threads, which grips and plucks out individual hairs as the crossover point is passed over the hair to be removed. The technique allows for easy removal of fine hairs with minimal discomfort and may be used to remove hair outside any outline shape but is particularly used around eyebrows, sideburns, on the ears and in the nape.

ACTIVITY: CASE STUDY

You work in a modern barber's shop and the owner wants to promote the barbering services on offer. You have been specifically asked to suggest how designing facial hair shapes and shaving services should be included in this promotion. The owner is particularly keen to show contemporary work but equally wants you to emphasize the traditional aspects of these barbering services. Your ideas should be illustrated in a labelled image board.

Barbering today

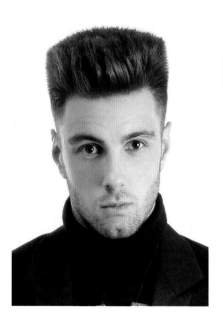

ADAM SLOAN Art Director BigYin Academy

" The barbering business is an exciting and important part of the hairdressing industry. Men are about half of the population so make sure you are skilled in barbering techniques and able to grow your barbering business! "

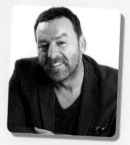

Today the term barbering is usually used to describe the work carried out by men's hairdressers, gents' hairdressers and men's hair stylists – all of whom might be described more simply as 'barbers'.

Of necessity there are many similarities between the work of men's hairdressers and women's hairdressers, but differences do remain between the work each carries out and by their use of different techniques, particularly where the client's hair is shorter. At one time it was very fashionable to have unisex salons, where both men and women could have their hair cut and styled. Unisex salons used barbering techniques but often did not specialize in men's hairdressing and as a result produced looks that were often less effective for men. A barber is someone who specializes in men's hairdressing, and who has developed high-level skills in using barbering techniques, especially for haircutting. These techniques follow 'barbering principles' that have evolved over time as being particularly suitable for dealing with the factors that typically affect men's hair and for creating the most suitable men's hairstyles and beard and moustache shapes. You will learn these principles in detail and understand how they are used to cut and style men's hair throughout the other chapters in this book. You will soon see that the central difference and indeed **essence** of being a barber is to incorporate these **barbering principles** into all of your work in the barber's shop!

Interest in male grooming continues to increase, as can be seen from the number of hair and skin care products now available specifically for men. Many barbers' shops now provide an important retail service for men seeking grooming and other male orientated products. Many more men are wearing fashion haircuts and the popularity of beards and moustaches continues, particularly with young men. This interest has led to many more barbers' shops opening and to an increase in the different services available to men. It has been shown that barbers' shops have been resourceful in meeting the changing demands and opportunities that have affected them over time. They have continually found additional ways to meet their clients' needs and maintain profits. Today the barber must continue to be highly skilled and creative in most aspects of hairdressing if they are to meet the needs of their clients and create the varied range of styles that are required. As will become evident through this book, modern men's hairdressing is not just about a 'dry trim' or a 'short back and sides'!

KEY DEFINITION

Essence: The most important quality, feature or nature of something that identifies it, defines it or simply makes it what it is.

KEY DEFINITION

Barbering principles: A system of rules that should be followed when cutting and styling men's hair to incorporate typical male features, such as head and face shape, facial hair and neck hair and produce the most suitable masculine looks.

Go to the website to access additional content on the importance of the barbering principles in men's hairdressing.

IMAGE GALLERY

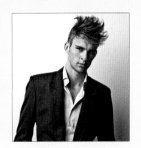

Visit the online image gallery on this book's accompanying website to see other contemporary barbers' shops and marketing ideas for barbering services.

BRINGING IT ALL TOGETHER

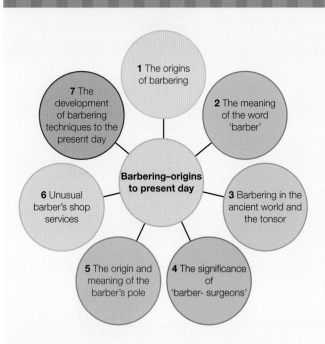

7 Modern barbering uses traditional barbering techniques to create both traditional and contemporary looks. Unlike unisex methods barbering techniques are designed to deal with men's hair and create men's hairstyles and beard and moustache shapes.

8 The 'essence' of being a barber is to incorporate barbering principles into all of your work in the barber's shop.

ACTIVITY – FIND OUT

Visit local barbers' shops and use the Internet to research the different types of barbers' shops that operate in different places. Find out if their decor and image is traditional or modern and which services are offered. Work out whether their location affects the image and services they offer.

Check your knowledge

1 Which civilization developed the first organized hairdressing tools and techniques?

2 Describe the origin of the word 'barber'.

3 Which one of the following is the correct definition of the Latin word 'barba':

   a. Hairdresser
   b. Barber
   c. Beard
   d. Head

4 Describe the earliest known haircutting tools.

5 How did Alexander the Great influence men's styling at the time?

6 Describe the main services offered by barber-surgeons.

7 Outline the meaning of the striped pattern on the barber's pole.

8 Describe the main benefits of singeing.

9 What is threading?

10 Which of the following statements are correct:

   i. Barbering principles describe how the factors that typically affect male clients should be incorporated into their haircut.

Summary

1 Origins – The Egyptians were the first to develop techniques and tools that we might recognize in barbering today.

2 'Barber' is derived from the Latin word *barba* meaning beard. A barber is someone who specializes in men's hairdressing.

3 Alexander the Great encouraged barbering services by requiring his army to be clean shaven. The Romans established organized barbers' shops. Barbers were wealthy and respected members of society. The Romans referred to barbers as *tonsors*.

4 Barber-surgeons provided bloodletting, surgery and dentistry in addition to haircutting and shaving services.

5 The barber's pole represents the different level of bloodstained bandages used by barber-surgeons in bloodletting. Today the pole is used to advertise the presence of a barber's shop even though bloodletting is no longer offered.

6 In the past some barbers' shops have offered unusual services, including umbrella servicing and hair singeing. More recently some barbers have taken to offering threading services.

ii. Barbering principles help establish the looks that are most suitable for male clients.

   a. Statement i is correct

   b. Statement ii is correct

   c. Statements i and ii are correct

   d. Statements i and ii are incorrect

11 What unusual service offered by some barbers' shops is related to the weather?

12 Describe the key differences between a unisex salon and a barber's shop.

13 What look have more young men been wearing over recent years?

14 What is a tonsor?

15 Describe threading.

2 Health and safety in the barber's shop

QUALIFICATION SIGNPOSTING

This chapter will help your studies of the following qualifications:

- ❖ Levels 1, 2 and 3 NVQ Diplomas in Barbering.
- ❖ City and Guilds VRQ Levels 1, 2 and 3 Awards, Certifications and Diplomas in Barbering, Barbering Techniques and Women's and Men's Hairdressing.
- ❖ ITEC VRQ Levels 1 and 2 Certificates and Diplomas in Barbering.
- ❖ VTCT VRQ Level 2 Certificates and Diplomas in Barbering and Barbering Studies.

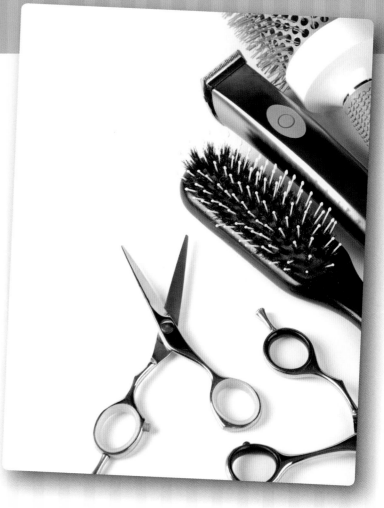

For further information on the qualifications covered by this chapter see the qualification mapping grid at the front of the book.

LEARNING OBJECTIVES

In this chapter you will learn:

◆ The health and safety legislation that affects the barber's shop.

◆ The common hazards and risks in the barber's shop.

◆ About contact dermatitis, its causes and how it can affect the barber.

◆ How to work safely in the barber's shop.

◆ The importance and maintenance of hygiene in the barber's shop.

INTRODUCTION

Barbering is an important and rewarding career and barbers' shops are often busy and fun places to work. You and your clients will often move between the reception and working areas whilst other barbers are busy using cutting and shaving tools and electrical equipment. At other times strong chemicals might be in use and often there will be hair clippings or products and water on the floor. You will work closely on many different people, who may have coughs and colds or other **contagious** conditions. You will spend long hours standing, working with arms raised and often in uncomfortable positions. These are just some of the hazards that the barber must consider.

Your career and health and the health of your clients and colleagues depends on you being aware of these and other **hazards** in the barber's shop. Your responsibility is to work carefully to minimize the chance of these hazards causing

harm. In later chapters you will cover the specific health and safety requirements of each barbering service. This chapter is about the general health and safety laws and rules from which these requirements and responsibilities are drawn.

The following are some of the important topics covered in this chapter:

❖ Health and safety legislation and its importance.

❖ The common hazards and risks in the barber's shop and how these should be minimized – including how to avoid contact dermatitis.

❖ General requirements for working safely in the barber's shop.

❖ The importance of maintaining high standards of hygiene in the barber's shop and how this is achieved.

Health and safety legislation

The Health and Safety at Work Act 1974 (HASAWA)

The Health and Safety at Work Act is known as an enabling act. This is because it creates the legal powers under which most other health and safety laws are made. These secondary laws are often known as 'Regulations', such as 'The Electricity at Work Regulations 1989'. The year shown after the name of the **legislation** or regulation indicates the year the law was passed. These laws must be followed and apply to everyone at work, whatever that work may be and whether they are the employee, employer or if self-employed.

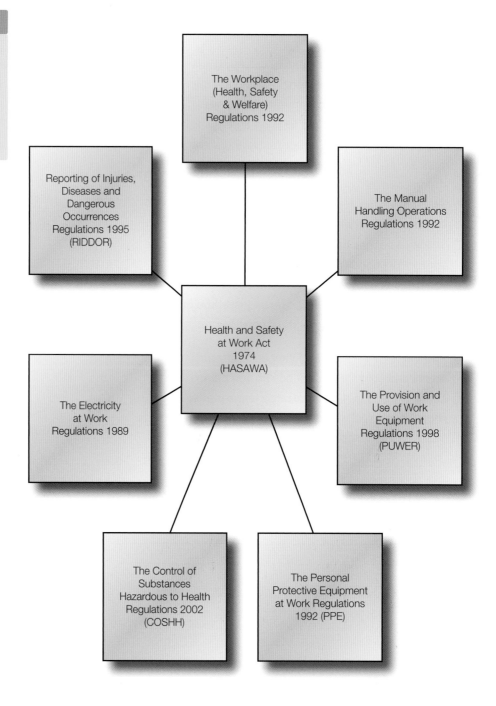

The Health and Safety at Work Act makes everyone in the barber's shop responsible for working in a safe and healthy way. The barber must take reasonable care for the health and safety of themselves and all others who may be affected by their action, or if a required action is not met. Employers and barber's shop owners must make sure their employees know how to work safely and follow the salon rules that are designed for this purpose. Under The Health and Safety at Work Act 1974 barbers must do what is necessary to help their employer to maintain health and safety policies within the barber's shop.

Health and Safety at Work etc. Act 1974

1974 CHAPTER 37

An Act to make further provision for securing the health, safety and welfare of persons at work, for protecting others against risks to health or safety in connection with the activities of persons at work, for controlling the keeping and use and preventing the unlawful acquisition, possession and use of dangerous substances, and for controlling certain emissions into the atmosphere; to make further provision with respect to the employment medical advisory service; to amend the law relating to building regulations, and the Building (Scotland) Act 1959; and for connected purposes. [31st July 1974]

KENYON YATES International Barbering Tutor

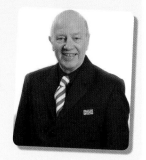

" The barber's shop is a busy environment with many potential hazards. Barbers must always follow high standards of safety and hygiene to reduce the **risk** of these hazards causing harm. Remember that a clean and safe barber's shop is not only required by law – it is something to be proud of and will help to ensure new and regular clients keep returning. "

There are many different factors that affect health and safety at work and as a result different hazards. These are covered by special regulations made under the powers of The Health and Safety at Work Act 1974. These are the main regulations that affect work in the barber's shop.

The Workplace (Health, Safety & Welfare) Regulations 1992

These are the main regulations requiring everyone at work to work in a way that helps to maintain a healthy and safe working environment. In the barber's shop the main requirements under these regulations include:

- ◆ Environment
  - ◆ Proper maintenance of equipment, fixtures and areas of glazing in the barber's shop.
  - ◆ Adequate ventilation and temperature.
  - ◆ Correct lighting for the work involved.
  - ◆ Safe flooring and entry/exit routes throughout the barber's shop.
- ◆ Hygiene
  - ◆ Maintaining standards of cleanliness, sanitization and sterilization during services.
  - ◆ General cleanliness throughout the barber's shop.
  - ◆ Suitable disposal of waste material, especially if **contaminated**.
- ◆ Facilities
  - ◆ Suitable workstations and seating areas.
  - ◆ Rest areas for staff refreshments and for changing to work clothes.

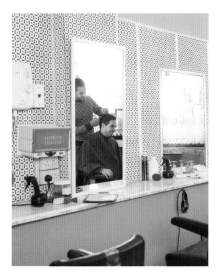

KEY DEFINITION

Risk: How likely it is that a hazard will cause harm.

KEY DEFINITION

Contamination: When an item or substance is polluted by some other potentially harmful substance.

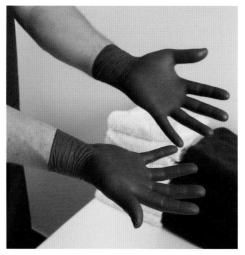

Gloves should be worn when handling contaminated items

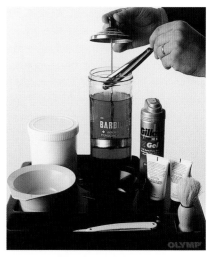

A clean and hygienic working area is good for client confidence

◆ Locations for staff to keep personal belongings.

◆ Safe drinking water.

◆ Suitable toilets and sanitation facilities.

The Manual Handling Operations Regulations 1992 Manual handling involves the lifting and handling of objects at work. In the barber's shop it is mostly relevant to the steps necessary when dealing with heavy or awkward shaped deliveries of stock. You need to ensure that you lift the delivery load in the correct way. Employers are required to carry out risk assessments on all employees for manual lifting and are responsible for ensuring employees follow these 'best practice' steps. Everyone must help to minimize the risks at work by placing heavy items in the correct place.

HSE Manual handling requirements

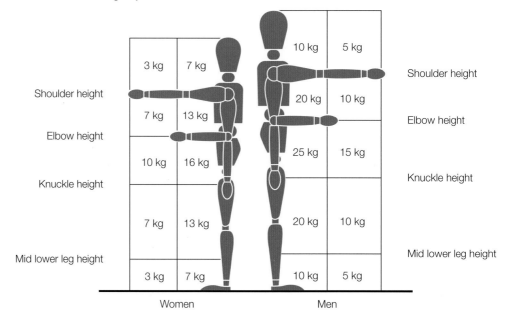

The following illustration compares how different items should be stored, handled and carried.

The Provision and Use of Work Equipment Regulations 1998 (PUWER)

These regulations require that all equipment used in the workplace is suitable for the purpose for which it is used. This means that the equipment must be maintained in accordance with the manufacturer's instructions that are supplied when the equipment is first purchased. The regulations also apply to older equipment so it is a good idea to retain the manufacturer's instructions. The Manual Handling Operations Regulations 1992 also require that all employees be trained in the use of the equipment. These are areas that will be covered in detail in the practical barbering chapters later in this book.

DON'T BE TEMPTED ✗

Remember that both new and old equipment must be properly maintained under PUWER. Don't be tempted to think that new equipment will not need maintenance! The manufacturer's instructions should be retained to make sure that the correct maintenance procedures are followed as the equipment gets older.

The Personal Protective Equipment at Work Regulations 1992 (PPE)

Employers are required under The Personal Protective Equipment at Work Regulations 1992 to provide suitable personal protective clothing and equipment (PPE) to all employees. The type of PPE must be suitable for the type of risk the employee is exposed to while working. In the barber's shop PPE is mostly supplied for services that involve a risk of blood contamination, through nicks to the skin during shaving services, and where potentially irritant products and chemicals are used, such as when shampooing, hair colouring and perming. For barbering PPE usually consists of:

◆ Gloves, which should be powder free non-latex gloves for single use, ideally vinyl and about 300 mm in length. Always select the correct size as it is important they fit properly, especially for shaving services.

◆ Barrier and skin creams – remember though, creams do not replace using gloves!

◆ Aprons and gowns.

Barbers must use the PPE supplied and report any damaged or shortages of suitable PPE to the manager.

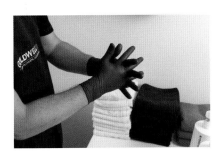

Protective gloves and apron

ACTIVITY – FIND OUT

Examine the available PPE in your barber's shop and note any items that are missing or where stocks are low. Make sure you know what the PPE is used for and how it should be used. Share your findings with your manager.

Go to the website to download a form where you can record your findings to share with others.

The correct use of PPE is particularly intended to help protect barbers from developing contact dermatitis, which can be a serious skin condition. The causes of contact dermatitis and how to prevent it are explained in the section 'Working safely in the barber's shop'.

The Control of Substances Hazardous to Health Regulations 2002 (COSHH)

The COSHH regulations cover the control of any substance likely to affect health and safety. This includes chemicals used for barber's shop services, such as shampoos, conditioners, sprays, wax, hair colourants, perms and shaving and massage creams. COSHH also covers general products used in the barber's shop for hygiene and cleaning. The regulations set out the requirements for the safe storage, handling, use and disposal of any substance and product, and particularly those products that could be potentially hazardous and able to cause harm to yourself or others.

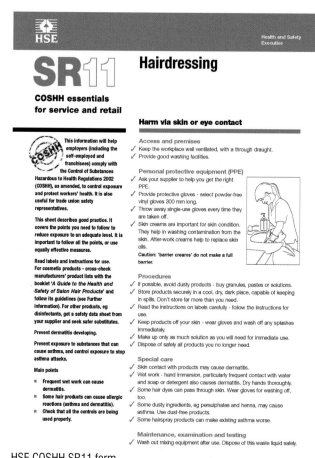

HSE COSHH SR11 form

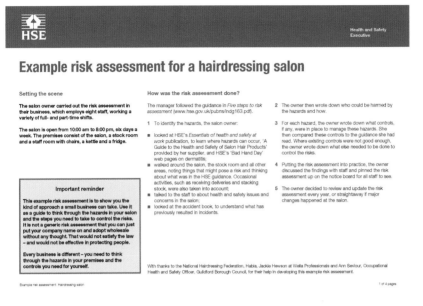

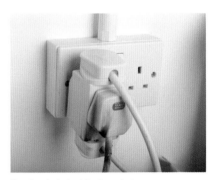

Example risk assessment for a hairdressing salon

COSHH risk assessment example

Employers are required to carry out a risk assessment of all products used and identify if the product is a low, medium or high risk. Manufacturers are required to provide information relating to COSHH on their products, which employers use to establish the risks involved. The employer must then ensure that all employees receive suitable training on how to safely handle the substances and products in their workplace. Remember: the product manufacturer's instructions provide the basis of this training and so should always be followed.

Overloaded electrical socket

The Electricity at Work Regulations 1989 The maintenance and use of all electrical equipment in the workplace is covered by these regulations. They require the employer to make sure that all electrical equipment is maintained and checked regularly

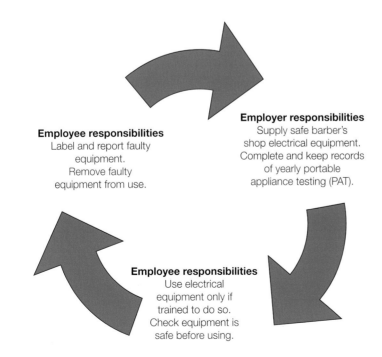

Employer responsibilities
Supply safe barber's shop electrical equipment. Complete and keep records of yearly portable appliance testing (PAT).

Employee responsibilities
Use electrical equipment only if trained to do so. Check equipment is safe before using.

Employee responsibilities
Label and report faulty equipment. Remove faulty equipment from use.

for safety through portable appliance testing, commonly known as PAT. Employers are also responsible for providing employees with training on the correct use of the equipment. The manufacturer's instructions form the basis of this training. The safe use of barbering equipment is covered in more detail in each of the chapters covering the barbering services later in this book.

Reporting of Injuries, Diseases and Dangerous Occurrences Regulations 1995 (RIDDOR)

Under these regulations employers are required to report certain accidents, diseases and dangerous occurrences that happen at work. The report is made to the Health and Safety Executive (HSE), who maintain records for statistical purposes and in case further investigation is required. The main reporting requirements are that if any of the following situations occur a telephone report is made to the HSE and followed up in writing within 10 days:

- An employee suffers a major injury in the workplace that prevents them from working for more than 3 days.
- An employee suffers a personal injury in the workplace and this results in more than 24 hours in hospital.
- An employee dies in the workplace.
- Someone is injured through violence in the workplace.
- A client or visitor to the salon is injured and taken to hospital.
- Certain industrial diseases are found to be present, such as asthma and occupational dermatitis – doctors would normally provide advice on whether a condition forms an occupational hazard.
- Dangerous situations, referred to as 'dangerous occurrences' have happened in the workplace, such as a fire, gas leak or explosion.

Employers and employees are also required to keep records of any accidents that happen in the salon. Accident records books are available for this purpose and are commonly used in barbers' shops. When an accident occurs the following details must be recorded:

- Name and contact details of all the people involved.
- The date, time and location.
- A clear description of any injury suffered, including the area of the body and whether the injury was bleeding.
- The name of the person responsible for any first aid.
- A summary of what action was taken and whether any treatment was provided.
- Whether the emergency services were called.

TIP ✓

Remember to make sure that any client details are kept confidential to comply with the Data Protection Act 1994. You must record clearly what happened in case the accident record is required later in any legal proceedings.

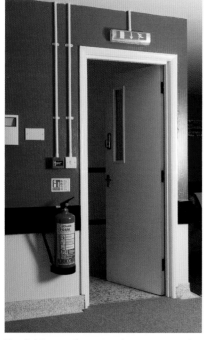

Fire fighting equipment and emergency exits should be easily seen

---

HEALTH & SAFETY

The person responsible for first aid must be informed whenever an accident happens in the barber's shop. If the first aider is not available and you suspect someone has suffered serious injury or harm, or has been taken unwell don't delay in calling the emergency services. The phone operator will talk you through the next steps and help you deal with the immediate situation.

The Fire Precautions Act 1971

This Act and the associated *Fire Precautions (Workplace) Regulations 1997* establish whether a workplace requires a fire certificate and what precautions must be taken to deal with fire risks. Local fire authorities inspect certain premises, such as those the public visit and issue fire certificates where the premises are selected as requiring a certificate and meet the certificate requirements. This process involves the fire officer checking that all required fire precautions have been taken. These precautions include the premises having the correct:

◆ Firefighting equipment – that must be serviced and maintained.

◆ Fire alarms – known as fire detection equipment.

◆ Fire exits – which must be kept unlocked and accessible whilst the premises are occupied.

Employers are responsible for training their employees in evacuation procedures that must be followed in the event of a fire or other emergency where it is safest to leave the building. The chosen assembly point must be clearly stated.

All employees must know these evacuation procedures and where the firefighting equipment is located. It is particularly important that the correct type of firefighting equipment to use on different types of fires is understood as fires can be made worse and other harm can arise from using the wrong extinguisher.

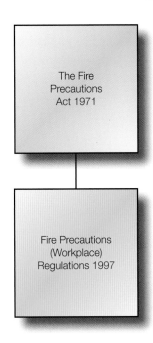

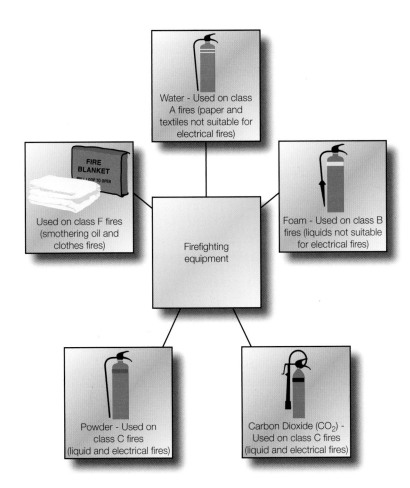

Water - Used on class A fires (paper and textiles not suitable for electrical fires)

Used on class F fires (smothering oil and clothes fires)

Foam - Used on class B fires (liquids not suitable for electrical fires)

Firefighting equipment

Powder - Used on class C fires (liquid and electrical fires)

Carbon Dioxide (CO_2) - Used on class C fires (liquid and electrical fires)

HEALTH & SAFETY

Remember that should you discover a fire:

◆ You must only fight the fire if it is blocking your exit, or if it is small and you have been trained in fighting fires.

◆ You should stay calm and raise the alarm.

◆ You should help to evacuate clients and colleagues.

◆ Contact the emergency services and follow the operator's instructions – you will need to give the full address of where the fire is located and who is involved.

◆ Remain at the chosen assembly point and watch for the fire services arriving. Assist the fire officers when they arrive.

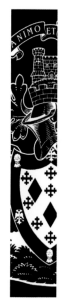

STOCKPORT
METROPOLITAN BOROUGH COUNCIL

LOCAL GOVERNMENT
(MISCELLANEOUS PROVISIONS)
ACT 1982

BYE-LAWS WITH RESPECT TO
HAIRDRESSERS AND BARBERS

Example of 'a local bye-law'

Bye-laws

Barbers must be particularly aware of the importance of bye-laws, which are laws made by local councils. They have legal status and must be followed. Some bye-laws set out in detail the minimum standards of hygiene and practices that barbers' shops must meet and in some cases the bye-law will prohibit certain services from being offered. This restriction is usually mostly applied to shaving services, where it can prohibit all professional shaving from being offered, or more often describe the type of razor and minimum standard of sterilization that must be used, for example some bye-laws prevent barbers' shops from using fixed-blade razors for shaving services.

Common hazards and risks in the barber's shop

Barber's must know the hazards and risks that they are likely to face in the barber's shop. The specific hazards and risks in different barbering services are covered in the relevant chapters later in this book. However, it is important to understand what is meant by a hazard and a risk to be able to deal with them correctly.

Hazards

Hazards are anything that has the potential to cause harm. The barber's shop has many specific hazards that are covered in later chapters, general examples include:

◆ Sharp tools, such as scissors and razors.

◆ Electricity and electrical equipment, especially hand tools.

◆ Trip hazards, such as spillages and damaged flooring.

◆ A range of chemicals – those for both professional use and cleaning purposes and the possibility of these causing contact dermatitis.

◆ Client position – proper seating and support for the client must be maintained throughout services. A barber's chair with headrest and reclining and height adjustments is essential, particularly to support the client's head during facial hair cutting, shaving and face massage services.

◆ Poor posture – the barber often stands for long hours whilst working and may need to adopt uncomfortable positions in order to reach the client and complete the

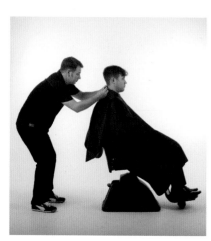

Poor posture

barbering service. Cutting stools should be used to help when the work requires bending low and the barber's chair will help when reaching.

Risks

The term risk refers to the likelihood that a hazard will actually cause harm. The likelihood changes under different conditions. This is best explained with a simple example of the hazard created if water is spilled on the floor. The spillage is the hazard; the risk of that hazard causing harm depends on:

◆ Where the water is spilt.

◆ The amount of water spilt.

◆ How long the water is left without a warning sign.

◆ How many people walk over the water and how often.

◆ How long the water is left before being mopped up.

It can be seen that such hazards should be removed as soon as possible. This would mean reporting the spillage so that a member of staff can warn people walking by until the water is mopped up. Even then the floor will still be wet but the risk can be reduced while the floor is drying by placing a sign by the wet floor.

Working safely in the barber's shop

Cutting services are the main activities of a busy barber. The risk of injury whilst using cutting tools and equipment must always be considered, as must the risks of working with electricity. Your responsibility is to follow all the barber's shop policies designed to maintain a healthy and safe environment. Remember – you have a legal duty to take reasonable care to avoid causing harm to yourself or anyone else through your work.

The specific chapters of barbering service cover what you must do to work safely in each area but, depending on your barber's shop policy, your general responsibilities might include:

◆ Comply with the barber's shop dress code and rules for smoking, drug use and drinking.

◆ Ensuring high standards of personal hygiene.

◆ Working in a clean and tidy and professional way at all times.

◆ Keeping tools and equipment clean, in good working order and sanitizing or sterilizing them as required.

◆ Using PPE when providing services involving possible contamination of blood and when handling chemicals stated as being hazardous in the COSHH assessment .

◆ Be aware of the risks of developing contact dermatitis – take care of your hands by washing them between services and always drying them thoroughly. Wear protective gloves when shampooing and handling chemicals. Regularly use a hand moisturiser.

◆ Following the manufacturers' instructions when using products, tools or equipment and only using those you have been trained to use. Remember that many products used in barbers' shops are potential irritants, for example shampoo, colour and perm lotion – make sure that you always follow guidelines for good hand care.

◆ Reporting, labelling and removing broken tools and equipment from the work area.

◆ Recognizing and then reporting any breaches of the barber's shop policies and health and safety requirements.

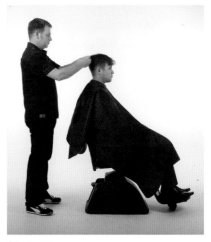

Good posture

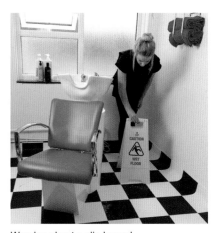

Warning about a slip hazard

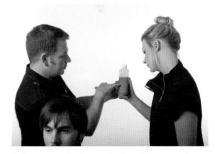

Follow manufacturers instructions - seek help if you are unsure

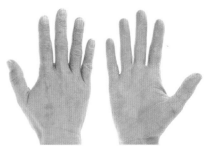

Contact dermatitis

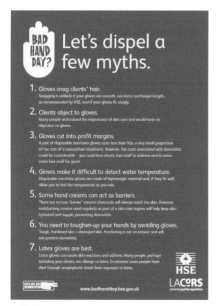

HSE Bad Hand Day Contact Dermatitis awareness leaflet

◆ Lifting heavy objects correctly in the way you have been trained to do and seeking help if any object is too heavy or awkward.

◆ Reporting any accidents and dangerous situations.

◆ Providing support to other members of staff to help them work safely.

Contact dermatitis

Hairdressers and barbers are at a greater risk of suffering from contact dermatitis at some point in their career than many other groups of workers. The condition is a rash and irritation of the skin caused by contact with irritant substances and frequent wet and damp conditions. It can be a serious condition and in the worst cases the sufferer may have to leave the barbering profession to prevent the condition recurring. The condition is reportable to the HSE under RIDDOR, (see p. 21). To minimise the risk of developing contact dermatitis you should always take care of your hands by wearing protective gloves when handling chemicals, and washing and drying your hands to remove any product in-between services. It is particularly important that the hands are dried thoroughly and for a hand moisturiser to be used regularly. This is especially important if you are often shampooing in the barber's shop. You should wear gloves during shampooing if shampooing is your main role, as your hands would otherwise be constantly wet and immersed in shampoo. The HSE has developed a range of guidance specifically for hairdressers and barbers to increase understanding of contact dermatitis and how to prevent it – make sure you protect your hands and barbering career by following this guidance! Go to HSE Hairdressing Contact Dermatitis pages at:

http://www.hse.gov.uk/hairdressing/dermatitis.htm

Contagious conditions

During their work barbers have physical contact with many different clients. These clients will often have coughs and colds and some may have other contagious or infectious conditions that the barber must consider to work safely. Barbers must be able to recognize the signs of possible infections and infestations of the skin and hair to avoid catching them and passing them from client to client or colleague. Barbers must be especially alert to the dangers of two serious conditions that may be contracted through open cuts and abrasions.

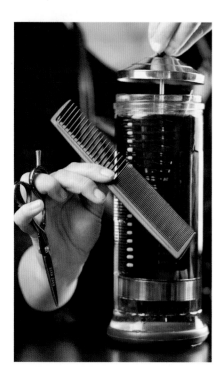

AIDS AIDS stands for acquired immunodeficiency syndrome. It is not a disease but a condition that makes the body more susceptible to diseases, and these may lead to death. To ensure that you protect your clients, your colleagues and yourself, you need to understand how AIDS is transmitted.

AIDS is caused by a virus known as the human immunodeficiency virus (HIV). People may carry the HIV virus – they are said to be 'HIV-positive' – without developing AIDS. However, a person who is HIV-positive could pass the virus to another person – but only if that person's infected body fluids, such as blood, come into contact with the other person's body fluids. Although this occurs most commonly through unprotected sex or when drug addicts share needles, the virus *can* be transferred through a cut or through broken skin.

However, medical experts have said that the virus cannot live for long outside the body – you cannot catch it from toilet seats, for example.

Hepatitis B Hepatitis B is a disease affecting the liver. This too is caused by a virus, the Hepatitis B virus (HBV). HBV is transmitted through infected body fluids such as blood, and also through infected water.

Hepatitis can affect the victim for a long time, and it can be fatal. Treatments are available, but the virus is known to be very resistant. It can survive a long time outside the body, so it is vital that you maintain a high standard of hygiene in all your work.

A vaccination is available to protect against Hepatitis B. As a barber you are at risk from this virus, so you should consider having this vaccination.

ACTIVITY – FIND OUT

Discuss your work as a barber with your doctor and ask for their advice regarding occupational health.

Hygiene in the barber's shop

Good hygiene is essential in the barber's shop. It will help prevent infection and **cross-infection**, which might happen if the tools used are dirty or if you or your client has an infectious condition or disease and looks professional. Cross-infection can happen through physical contact with another person, or through contact with a tool, such as a razor that has become infected.

The warm, humid atmosphere in the barber's shop is the type of environment that allows infectious organisms to multiply but good hygiene will limit their growth and may destroy them. Sterilization is the procedure used to destroy these organisms. It is achieved with physical heat or chemical agents and will destroy all the infectious and harmful micro-organisms. Sanitation will destroy some but not all microorganisms and is achieved through regular cleaning with bleach or disinfectant.

General rules for hygiene in the barber's shop

◆ Cover any cuts you may have, and ensure they remain covered. Wear gloves to ensure good infection control.

◆ Maintain a high standard of personal **hygiene**.

◆ Wash your hands regularly, but always remember to dry them thoroughly.

◆ Use a clean gown and clean towels for each client.

KEY DEFINITION

Cross-infection: The transmitting of an infectious condition or disease from one person to another.

HEALTH & SAFETY

Maintaining a hygienic barber's shop will ensure that the risk of infection and cross-infection is minimized.

KEY DEFINITION

Hygiene: Making sure that cleanliness is achieved in order to maintain good health.

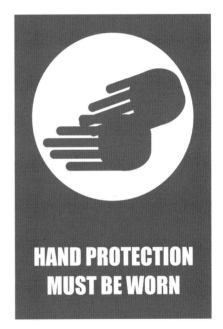

HAND PROTECTION MUST BE WORN

KEY DEFINITION

Unhygienic: Unclean and risking harm to health.

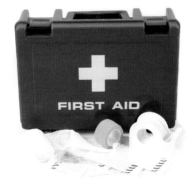

A sharps box

◆ Clean and sterilize or sanitize tools before using them on clients.

◆ Sanitize working surfaces regularly using bleach or disinfectant.

◆ Store dirty laundry in a sealed container.

◆ Put waste in suitable bags that can be sealed. Contaminated materials and sharps must be stored and disposed of as specified by the local environmental health authority.

DON'T BE TEMPTED

Good standards of hygiene are something to be proud of in both your personal life and professional life as a barber. Don't forget that your approach to meeting these standards affects how others see you. This is especially important in the barber's shop because you will be working closely with clients and they must have confidence in the cleanliness and safety of your work. Don't be tempted to fall casually into **unhygienic** practices – remember that the five second rule is a myth and that comb you drop on the floor must be sanitized before use!

BRINGING IT ALL TOGETHER

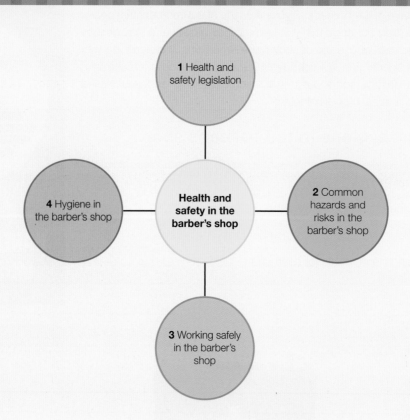

Summary

1   The Health and Safety at Work Act 1974 is the legislation that forms the regulations which govern health and safety in the workplace.

2   The Fire Precautions Act 1971 requires employers make sure that:

a. Firefighting equipment is available and maintained
b. Fire alarms are fitted
c. Fire exits are accessible whilst premises are occupied

3   Bye-laws are local council rules that might prevent barbers' shops from using fixed-blade razors for shaving services.

4   Risk refers to the likelihood that a hazard will actually cause harm.

5   Barbers must be aware of the risks of developing contact dermatitis and should take care of their hands by washing them between services and always drying them thoroughly.

6   Barbers must be especially alert to the dangers of HIV and Hepatitis B as these can be transmitted through open cuts and abrasions.

7   A barber's chair with headrest and reclining and height adjustments is essential to support the client's head during facial hair cutting, shaving and face massage services.

8   Barber's should adopt good posture during services to help prevent injuries.

9   Sterilization is the procedure used to destroy all the infectious and harmful micro-organisms.

10 If a barber drops a comb or tool on the floor it must be sterilized or sanitized before further use.

Activities

1   Draw and label a diagram of your barber's shop and include the locations of the following:

    a. Fire exits
    b. Firefighting equipment
    c. First aid box
    d. Accident book
    e. Sharps bin
    f. Chemicals storage cupboard
    g. Assembly point

2   FInd out

    Research the local bye-laws relating to your barber's shop, record your findings and check them with the manager.

3   FInd out

    Research contact dermatitis and gather together the guidance made available specifically for hairdressers and barbers. Create a file of this information for your barber's shop staff area to help raise awareness of the condition and how to prevent it. Show your manager the file before sharing it with your colleagues.

Check your knowledge

1   What does contagious mean?

2   What are the main hazards in the barber's shop?

3   What is meant by the PUWER?

4   What is the meaning of hazard?

5   What steps should a barber take to minimize the risk of contracting Hepatitis B whilst working in the barber's shop.

6   What is the difference between sterilization with sanitization?

7   What type of fire extinguisher should be used on a paper-based fire?

8   Which of the following fire extinguishers are suitable for use on an electrical fire?

    a. Powder Extinguisher
    b. CO_2 Extinguisher
    c. Foam Extinguisher
    d. Water Extinguisher

9   How does COSHH affect the barber's shop?

10 What must be reported under RIDDOR?

11 How might a fire blanket be used in the barber's shop?

12 What is contact dermatitis?

13 What steps should be taken to minimize the risk of developing contact dermatitis?

14 Which of the following statements are correct?

    a. Gloves must be worn to minimize the risk of cross-infection if the barber has a recent cut on their hand or if client's skin is ever broken during the service.
    b. Used gloves can be reused if they are washed in warm soapy water.

15 Which one of the following is the best method of PPE in the barber's shop?

    a. Latex gloves
    b. Barrier cream
    c. Vinyl gloves
    d. Moisturising cream

3 Working effectively in the barber's shop

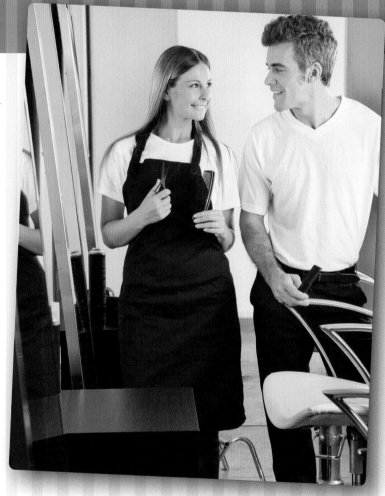

QUALIFICATION SIGNPOSTING

This chapter will help your studies of the following qualifications:

❖ Level 1 NVQ Certificate in Hairdressing and Barbering.

❖ Level 2 NVQ Awards and Diploma in Barbering.

❖ City & Guilds Level 2 VRQ Award, Certificate and Diploma in Barbering.

❖ ITEC Level 2 VRQ Certificate and Diplomas in Barbering and Men's Hairdressing.

❖ VTCT Level 2 VRQ Certificates and Diplomas in Barbering and Barbering Studies.

For further information on the qualifications covered by this chapter see the qualification mapping grid at the front of the book.

LEARNING OBJECTIVES

In this chapter you will learn:

◆ About working in the barbering industry.

◆ How to improve your personal performance at work in the barber's shop.

◆ How to work effectively as part of a team in the barber's shop.

INTRODUCTION

Barber's shops are often busy places where barbers work hard to provide the level of service and quality of work demanded by today's clients. **Top-notch** barbering skills, efficient working and effective teamwork are required to ensure that clients receive a great haircut, great customer service and the barber's shop business is maximized. This chapter is about these and other requirements for effective working and the responsibilities each barber has to meet them. The following are some of the topics covered:

❖ Working in the barbering industry.

❖ Improving your personal performance at work in the barber's shop.

❖ Working effectively as part of a team in the barber's shop.

Working in the barbering industry

Before reading this chapter it may help you to read CHAPTER 1, "Barbering – from its origins to the present day', as this will introduce you to the unique and proud position of the barbering industry.

The barbering industry comprises many different types of barbers and many different types of barber's shops. Some barbers' shops focus on modern and contemporary work and prefer to be known as 'men's hairdressers' and 'men's hair salons', whilst others specialize in traditional barbering skills and services and are very keen to be called 'barbers'. Conversely, some traditional barbers prefer to be called men's hairdressers and many specializing in contemporary work are keen to be called barbers. These contradictions may appear confusing. Nevertheless, what should be clear is that the terms 'barbering industry' and 'barber' may be used collectively for anyone whose work includes the specialist barbering principles and skills most suitable for men's hair.

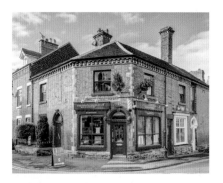

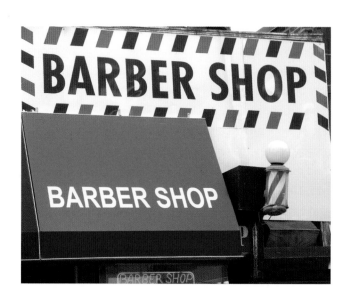

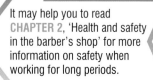

KEY DEFINITION

Top-notch: Something of the highest quality, sometimes called first-rate or excellent.

The barber's shop environment

It may help you to read CHAPTER 2, 'Health and safety in the barber's shop' for more information on safety when working for long periods.

Barbering can be a rewarding industry and barbers' shops are usually a great environment in which to work. The work can be tiring though, particularly at busy times such as immediately after normal 'office hours' when many clients call into the barber's shop on their way home. Many barbers' shops do not require appointments and at these times numerous clients often arrive at the same time. The barber must prepare for this, even if an appointment system is used as all appointments are likely to be taken and yet some clients may still wish to wait and see if they can be accommodated. The professional barber knows to plan for this time, taking adequate refreshment breaks during quieter periods so they are refreshed and ready to focus on meeting these work demands. On such occasions the barber will spend many hours standing, constantly moving their hands, raising and lowering their arms whilst concentrating on precise cutting movements. Yet again, the professional barber knows how to plan for this work, standing correctly and changing position to reduce fatigue and ensure the quality of their work is maintained.

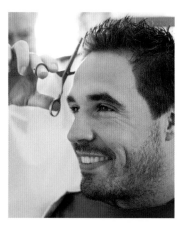

The quality of barbering work is always paramount but good customer service is important too. Remember that the client's whole visit should be a pleasant one – starting as they enter the barber's shop with the barber providing an enthusiastic greeting, continuing with the barber's polite and professional attitude throughout, and concluding with the barber thanking the client for their business.

TIP ✓

The professional barber knows when to 'chat' with their client and knows what is appropriate to discuss; always remembering that theirs is a professional relationship. Remember that barbers should also know when the client would prefer peace and quiet!

See CHAPTER 4, 'Client care for men' for more information about caring for your client.

DON'T BE TEMPTED ✗

Remember that as a professional barber your obligation is to ensure that your client receives a professional service. Don't be tempted to become overfriendly during the service, particularly with your loyal and regular clients, even if they are your friends outside of work. Remember that all your clients have the right to expect the same high standard of barbering and customer service.

TIP ✓

Remember that many barbers can provide a great haircut; it is often the customer service provided that differentiates the work and makes that new client a regular client!

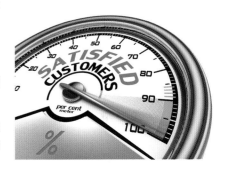

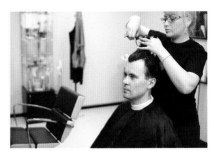

Like most businesses, barbers' shops also have quieter times, often during their main clients' normal working hours. This time should always be used effectively. Here are some examples:

◆ Make sure that the barber's shop is hygienically clean.

◆ Clean and maintain tools and equipment.

◆ Watch your colleagues at work – much can be learnt from considering the work of others!

◆ Practise your barbering techniques, particularly those that you know are not yet strengths – be your own honest guide and you will be best placed to become expert in such areas.

◆ Ensure that stock levels are maintained and reordered if required.

The barbering industry offers the barber and men's hairdresser an enjoyable and rewarding place to work. There are many different career routes available.

Barbering career choices

New entrants to the barbering industry usually start as a trainee barber or apprentice barber before progressing to more senior roles. In some barbers' shops these roles

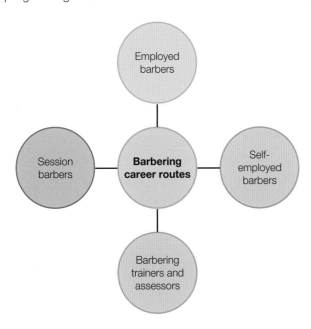

might include junior barber and senior barber, although often just the title 'barber' is used.

A barber's career success is ordinarily based on building a regular and loyal clientele; though there are some differences depending on whether they are working in employed or self-employed roles:

◆ Employed barbers – mostly work within one barber's shop or within a group of barber's shops. They often work with other employed barbers, or sometimes alongside barbers who are 'renting a chair' (see below). Their employment conditions and job role description differ according to the needs of each barber and barber's shop. Many include a basic salary and commission or bonus based system of payment, where over a certain number of client services or sales the barber earns a specific bonus or commission for each client and retail sale.

◆ Self-employed barbers – usually buy or lease premises to establish their own barber's shop or develop a freelance business providing barbering services to men at home and sometimes in hospitals and/or warden supported homes. Others rent space within an existing barber's shop, commonly known as 'renting a chair', where for example a weekly rent is paid to the barber's shop owner, to cover the space, heating, lighting and other costs used; the barber retaining the takings from their work. Though, sometimes the owner will also receive a percentage from the takings for a reduction in the upfront rental costs.

◆ Barbering trainers and assessors – usually work in colleges and private training providers, passing on their skills and experience to the next generation of barbers. Both full-time and part-time roles are held by those with the required training and assessment qualifications. They usually include attractive hourly rates of pay and opportunities for **continuous professional development** (CPD).

◆ Session barbers – work in photography or behind the scenes in stage, film and television, some also have women's hairdressing skills to be able to meet all the demands that these roles require. The financial and creative rewards for this freelance work can be significant.

Regardless of the eventual career choices, when establishing a barbering career the most important factor is whether the barber can work effectively in the barber's shop. This requires that the barber acquires and maintains updated, 'top-notch' barbering skills, known as CPD and is able to work effectively within the barber's shop team. These essential **attributes** will be considered in the next sections of this chapter.

> **KEY DEFINITION**
>
> Continuous Professional Development (CPD): Completing further training, qualifications and development activities to maintain up-to-date skills and knowledge, as identified in your personal work development plan.

> **KEY DEFINITION**
>
> Attributes: A quality or characteristic inherent in or ascribed to someone or something.

MIKE TAYLOR British Barbering Association

" The barbering industry offers the enthusiastic and skilled barber seemingly endless career opportunities. For some barbers working in one barber's shop, building a regular and loyal clientele, meets their personal, economic and professional ambitions. For others it is operating a group of busy barbers' shops, providing barbering services and employed and self-employed opportunities to many. Whilst for others, it is educating and training the next generation of barbers that provides the greatest satisfaction. Some barbers will even go on to work behind the scenes in stage, film and television. The common factor in the success of all these barbers is they maintain and provide first-rate barbering skills. Make sure you join them; get the training and the edge in your work. "

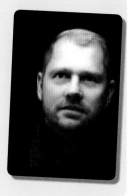

Improving your personal performance at work in the barber's shop

Most businesses rely on the role played by the people working within them for their success. Each person will have a job role, usually described in a written 'job description' and 'contract of employment' that sets out the part they are to play in meeting the business aims and objectives. The barber's shop is no different. To improve your personal performance at work in the barber's shop you must first understand what your role and responsibilities are, as defined in your **job description** and **contract of employment**.

> ## KEY DEFINITION
>
> Job description: A detailed written description of the duties and responsibilities for a given job agreed between the employer and employee.

> ## TIP ✔
>
> The successful functioning of the barber's shop requires that everyone works together to achieve its aims and objectives. Working together requires that each member of staff knows the job role of other members of staff, otherwise the staff will not know how their work fits together to make the barber's shop effective.

> ## KEY DEFINITION
>
> Contract of employment: A signed written agreement of the employment relations between an employer and an employee and their individual rights under law.

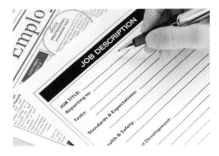

Job descriptions

Your job description will describe your role within the barber's shop and the responsibilities that this role includes. It will normally include your name and address and provide details on:

- Who you should report to for daily matters.
- Who to speak to if you have a problem or grievance at work.
- The name of anyone who is to report to you.
- The aims and objectives of the barber's shop.
- The requirements that you:
  - protect confidential information
  - follow the barber's shop health and safety policy
  - comply with the barber's shop equal opportunities policy and other policies.

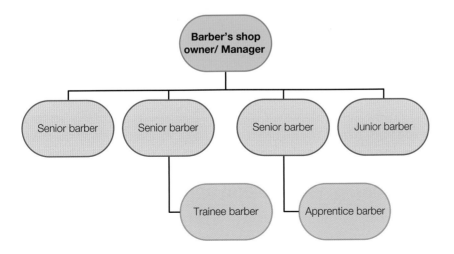

◆ The type and standard of work you must provide.

◆ The limits of your responsibility and who to speak to if faced with a situation that is outside of these limits.

> **TIP** ✔
>
> You should have received a job description and employment contract when you started work; they would have been signed and dated by you and the manager at that time. Make sure you keep them in a safe place as they are often used during performance appraisals and reviews. Ask your manager for a new copy if you have lost them.

Employment contracts

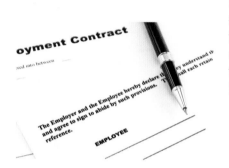

Employment contracts are similar to job descriptions in that they outline the barber's roles and responsibilities; indeed employment contracts often make specific reference to job descriptions. However, employment contracts go further to create a legally binding agreement between the barber and the employer, based on the employment conditions that were agreed when the barber first started work. Employment contracts will normally include your name, address and job title and details on:

◆ The normal working days and hours you are expected to work.

◆ The payment you will receive, including the amount per hour and how it will be paid.

◆ Your entitlement to paid annual holidays.

◆ Your entitlement to pay if you are unable to work through illness.

◆ Your entitlement to pay during maternity and paternity leave.

◆ Your entitlement and obligations to any pension payments.

◆ The procedures for your performance appraisal and reviews.

◆ The procedures for disciplinary matters, grievances and appeals.

◆ The period of notice required if you or the employer wishes you to leave.

> **ACTIVITY: CASE STUDY**
>
> **Job Descriptions**
> Compare your role in the barber's shop with that of your colleagues, as defined in their job descriptions. Think about how your role fits in with their work – are there any ways you could improve what you do to help make the barber's shop more effective?

Your job description and employment contract may be needed if you experience any problems at work and are likely to be discussed each year as part of your annual performance appraisal. They will also be necessary should you face a disciplinary matter, and if you have a grievance or need to appeal.

Disciplinary, grievance and appeal procedures

The disciplinary, grievance and associated appeals procedures used in your barber's shop should be provided in the staff handbooks or similar materials that were provided during your induction. Copies should also be freely available to staff, usually these are kept in the staff areas or on the staff intranet pages, if these are used.

It is a legal requirement that employers maintain specified procedures for dealing with any disciplinary actions that might arise. The employer must follow these procedures in each case or they might be liable to legal proceedings. Similar legal requirements apply to how any grievances are managed, and how any appeals following disciplinary and grievance hearings are handled. The main requirements for dealing with disciplinary, grievance and appeal matters include:

Disciplinary procedures

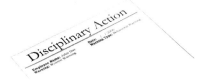

◆ You must be provided with clear written reasons for any disciplinary action against you.

◆ The disciplinary procedures and your rights must be clearly explained and be supplied in writing, including:

  ◆ who will be involved, particularly who will make the decisions and whether any hearing will be held

  ◆ the possible outcomes of the disciplinary action – typically including a verbal warning, a first written warning, a final written warning and in the worst cases the possibility of being dismissed

  ◆ your rights to be accompanied during any hearing

  ◆ your rights to appeal following the disciplinary hearing.

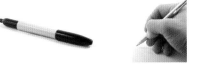

Grievance procedures   Should a situation arise that cannot be resolved informally a formal grievance may be submitted using the barber's shop grievance procedure. The procedure should include details of:

◆ To whom you should refer your grievance concerns.

◆ How the grievance should be made – sometimes verbally initially then confirmed by submitting a completed form supplied for this purpose.

◆ How any evidence you have to support your grievance should be handled and supplied to the grievance decision maker.

◆ The stages of the grievance procedure, including:

  ◆ when the grievance will be considered

  ◆ who will be involved

  ◆ when the results will be decided and communicated

  ◆ the types of outcome possible.

TIP ✔

Safety

Should you ever have any serious concerns at work, for example about harassment, bullying or unwanted advances you should speak to your manager, or if required another senior manager as soon as possible. You should record notes on any actions and conversations of concern, including the dates and names of those involved, as these will support your grievance submission. You should seek help and advice from outside the workplace if necessary.

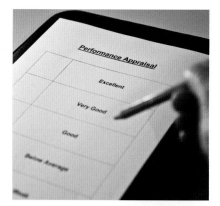

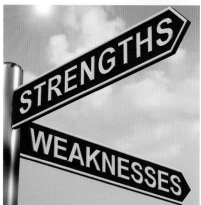

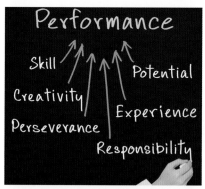

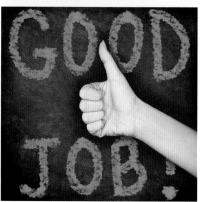

Appeals procedures The disciplinary and grievance procedures should include a right to appeal, particularly if more serious findings are decided, for example if the proceedings have resulted in you being dismissed. The full details of the procedure to follow will be provided in your barber's shop staff handbook or specific handbook of appeals procedures.

Performance appraisals and reviews

Performance appraisals, called performance reviews where they are completed more often, are intended to be a time where you and your manager can consider whether you have met the requirements stated in your job description and employment contract. They help to establish the strengths and weaknesses in your work, so that you can recognize them and make improvements where required. They also provide an opportunity for you to discuss the training and support provided by your employer to enable you to meet your role and responsibilities.

The period reviewed is normally the preceding year, based on the anniversary of when you commenced your employment. This is known as an 'annual performance appraisal'. Though, interim reviews can also be held, for example every 3 months where shorter term productivity targets might be discussed and agreed.

Performance appraisals and reviews should not be feared. Those who have worked hard should receive praise and recognition for the work, especially where they have met and/ or exceeded all the requirements in their job description.

Those who need help will have this identified as part of the appraisal process so that arrangements to provide training and support can be made. The appraisal will also identify where your roles and responsibilities can be enhanced as you gain experience and your skills and expertise develop.

> **TIP**
>
> Remember: appraisal is not just about your manager reviewing your progress, it is a two-way communication process where you should provide feedback on any problems affecting your role and highlight any training and support that you think would help you at work, particularly where this might benefit the business.

The appraisal and review process is often different but in most barbers' shops the key requirements will include the following:

◆ The appraiser (manager) will normally provide the appraisee (barber being appraised) a number of weeks' notice of the appraisal in order to provide time for the barber to prepare.

◆ The appraisal process might include you completing a self-appraisal form and making notes on any areas to discuss at the meeting, such as additional training requests.

◆ The progress of newer employees is usually reviewed more frequently to ensure they are making good progress and to identify any help that might be required.

◆ Established employees will normally have an annual appraisal unless a specific performance improvement plan and short or medium term **productivity** targets have been agreed.

Remember that performance appraisal should be seen as a continuous process intended to help you improve your performance over a period of time, involving improvement action plans where required. The process can be broken down into five key stages:

◆ Define – this stage is where the requirements and suggestions for improvement are established. It draws upon the job description, employment contract and agreed actions and targets from previous appraisals and reviews.

◆ Measure – this stage includes the barber performing against the defined requirements over a defined period of time. It also includes planning and preparation for the appraisal meeting, for example completing any self-appraisal, self-assessment form or skillscan document.

◆ Analyze – is an active stage of the appraisal meeting where the barber's performance and barber's shop support is considered and discussed in detail and any action plans and targets are agreed.

◆ Improve – follows the appraisal meeting and is where the barber and employer work to include and satisfy any agreed improvement plans and targets.

◆ Control – this stage is sometimes necessary where the required improvements are more serious, or where initially no improvements have been forthcoming. In the most serious cases this stage can involve disciplinary proceedings.

DON'T BE TEMPTED   X

You might be asked to meet specific short, medium or long term targets in your work. You must approach completing these targets seriously. Don't be tempted to think they are not important as they will usually have been set to meet specific objectives. Short term targets will usually need meeting within a few months, whilst long term targets may be over a year or more. Remember that failing to meet them might result in fewer profits for you, your colleagues and/or the barber's shop and in the worst cases could lead to disciplinary proceedings against you.

An important stage in preparing for the appraisal process, and likewise in improving your personal performance at work in the barber's shop, is the self-appraisal process. This should help you to identify those responsibilities where you have strengths and those areas that you need to develop. An example of a self-appraisal form is shown below and can be adapted to help you identify any area of your performance.

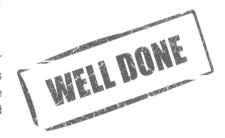

Self-appraisal form – general work 1 = Strength, 2 = Satisfactory, 3 = Weakness	
Work responsibilities	**Barber's self-appraisal**
Punctuality record	
Attendance record	
Dress code record	
Behaviour and attitude to work	

(continued)

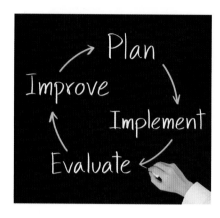

Self-appraisal form – general work 1 = Strength, 2 = Satisfactory, 3 = Weakness	
Quality of barbering work	
Quality of customer service	
Effective team working	
Problem-solving and using own initiative	
Sales activity	

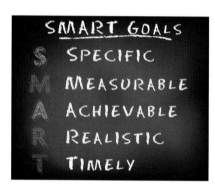

TIP ✓

Remember: your development is important, but your employer will want to see how this personal development contributes to the success of the barber's shop as a whole – it must help to achieve the aims of the barber's shop and ultimately make it more profitable!

Here are some important points to remember about appraisals and reviews:

◆ Before the appraisal or review check whether you have met all the previously agreed action plans and targets. Be prepared to discuss these, especially any that have not been achieved – remember: you must be able to explain the reason why you have not met them!

◆ Be prepared to discuss your current performance at work compared with your job description and employment contract. Prepare notes on any areas where you have performed well and on any that have caused you to have problems. Try to think of solutions to any problems, such as training or support that would help you overcome them.

◆ Be prepared to discuss how you think you are progressing and what your personal ambitions and goals are. Consider whether these goals are reasonable and achievable. Set out what you think is needed to help you achieve them. A 'SMART' – specific, measurable, achievable, realistic and targeted – personal development plan, with staged evaluations usually works best. This will help you and your employer decide what support is required and consequently whether your development plan is realistic.

◆ Listen carefully to what your manager has to say during the appraisal or review meeting. Make sure that you understand what is being said and ask questions if you are unsure, especially if the written copy of what has been agreed is unclear or does not appear to state what you agreed verbally.

◆ Remember to remain positive and think of the appraisal or review as an important opportunity that your employer has provided to think about you and your role in the barber's shop. Make the most of this opportunity and you will be best placed to realize your goals and be a valued member of the barber's shop team!

Using opportunities to develop your skills and knowledge – continuous professional development

Similar to other fashion based industries, the barbering industry often features fast-paced changes, frequently stimulated by the latest celebrity look or trend. The modern barber must maintain awareness of these trends and have the necessary skills to create them in order to meet their clients' needs; sometimes even before their clients realize they have these needs!

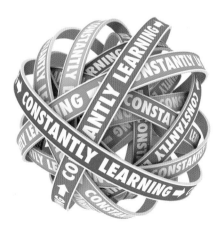

Only by being proactive and making best use of any opportunity to update and develop the barbering skills for these emerging looks can barbers stay ahead of such trends. Join them and you will be best placed to build your skills base and achieve your targets!

Maintaining CPD is the key, as this will ensure that you never stop learning, sometimes called 'lifelong learning'. This involves completing further training, qualifications and development activities determined by your personal development plan. Remember, your self-appraisal and personal skillscan review will help you to decide what areas to include in your development plan. You should use this to identify the areas that you need to develop during discussions with the manager to see how they can be supported through CPD.

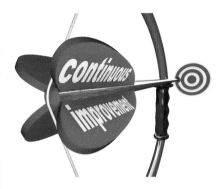

Skillscan review form 1 = Strength, 2 = Satisfactory, 3 = Weakness	
Skills and knowledge	**Barber's skillcan review**
Health and safety in the barber's shop	
Working effectively in the barber's shop	
Client care for men	
Shampooing, conditioning and treating hair and scalp conditions	
Cutting facial hair using basic techniques	
Cutting men's hair using basic techniques	
Drying and finishing men's hair	
Colouring men's hair	
Creating basic patterns in hair	
Advanced men's hair cutting	
Shaving services	
Face massage services	
Designing facial hair shapes	
Design and create patterns in hair	
Fulfil reception duties in the barber's shop	
Perming men's hair	
Specialist hair and scalp treatments	

TIP ✔

You can learn from watching others work; take every opportunity to analyze how your colleagues approach their work and where appropriate ask for clarification to help you understand their approach.

Awareness of current barbering and men's hairdressing trends

There are many ways to maintain your awareness of current barbering industry trends; here are just a few ideas.

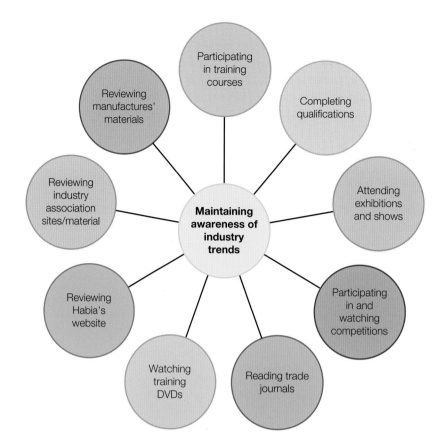

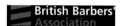

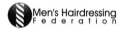

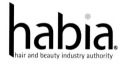

Barbering and men's hairdressing associations In times long past the barbering profession was represented by the 'Barbers Company of London', but more recently the barbering and men's hairdressing industry has not been specifically represented. Today, however, there are vibrant and growing professional communities representing the interests of barber's and men's hairdressers. These are the 'British Barbering Association' (BBA) and the 'Men's Hairdressing Federation' (MHFed). These associations offer their members a range of benefits and are a great source of ideas for barbering CPD and current barbering trend awareness. You should visit their websites and consider the benefits of joining them!

Habia If you are completing a National Vocational Qualification (NVQ) you will be working towards National Occupational Standards (NOS) developed by the body that represent the hairdressing and barbering industry, called the Hair and Beauty Industry Authority (Habia). It is Habia who work with industry experts to determine what is required in an NVQ for an individual to be called 'competent' and ready to work in industry. The NOS are also useful to those not taking the NVQ, as they provide structured routes for development from the Level 1 and 2 Trainee roles through to Level 3 and 4 advanced work and management roles. Information on Habia and the NOS is available via Habia's website.

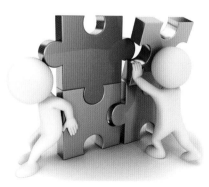

Working effectively as part of a team in the barber's shop

Working all day in a busy barber's shop can be tiring and sometimes stressful. This can lead to irritations and shorter tempers amongst you and your colleagues than usually experienced, but you must remain professional and should recognize that by working together in harmony the work and stress is shared and more easily handled.

Team harmony

Good teamwork in the barber's shop is essential. It will create a happy and professional working environment, enabling barbers to 'get the job done right'!

Good teamwork requires harmony, which is derived from everyone being polite, professional and respectful at all times, even if sometimes people do not get on so well. It is important that you show you trust and respect for your colleagues and that you value their work and help, remembering to thank them – just as they will when you offer to help them. Remain professional and keep private matters private, especially where a colleague has shared personal information with you. Be particularly careful not to gossip about such matters – imagine how you would feel if your trust was broken!

Such shared values will help develop and maintain team harmony. Remember that working as a team means everyone achieves more, as individual goals are more easily met when part of the overall team goal. The alternative is disharmony in the team and consequently the risk of an unhappy and ineffective barber's shop where clients might feel uncomfortable and their business may be lost.

Maintaining harmony requires that you are considerate. You should remain alert to the needs of your colleagues and offer support and assistance where required. Likewise, you should also speak up and ask for help whenever you are unsure about how to proceed in your work, or if you have made an error.

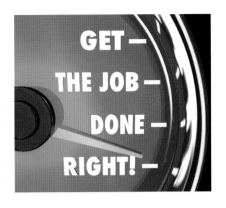

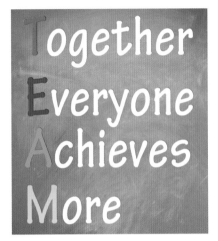

ADAM SLOAN Men's Hairdressing Federation

" Effective teamwork is the glue that binds the barber's shop team together. It enables consistent performance to the highest levels, even when under the extreme pressure of those busiest days. Good teamwork and team players are a 'must have' in all successful barber's shops! "

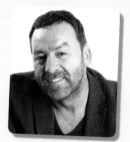

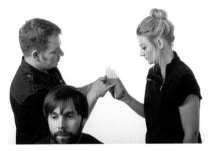

Teams are happy to assist each other!

Offering assistance

One of the main and enjoyable benefits of harmonious and effective teamwork is the opportunity to offer and receive assistance at work. You should be alert and **reactive** to sudden increases in the work demands of your colleagues; offering them help, especially if there is a problem and you are not busy. You should also be more **proactive**; anticipating where your help might be needed, such as when you can see that due to booked appointments help will be needed at a specific time or because you can anticipate a problem might arise and can offer your assistance to prevent the problem occurring.

Remember to show you are enthusiastic when helping others, but be careful to work within your capabilities and limits of responsibility, ask your manager if you are unsure.

KEY DEFINITION

Reactive: Responding to an event or problem after it has occurred and then making a change or offering help.

TIP ✓

Safety
Working outside the limits of your responsibility and capabilities can be dangerous and/or harmful to your barber's shop business. Remember you must follow the responsibilities defined in your job description and barber's shop policies at all times.

KEY DEFINITION

Proactive: Anticipating an event or problem then making a change or offering help before the event or problem occurs.

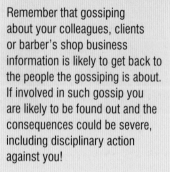

Teamwork

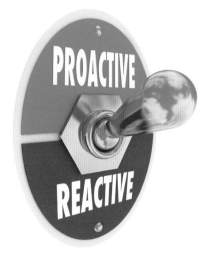

The professional barber knows when to react and how to be proactive

Behaviour at work

The barber's shop is a professional working environment where members of the public are present, hence you must ensure that you maintain a professional image at all times. This includes being polite and respectful to every client and all of your colleagues at all times. You should never shout or swear whilst at work, even in the staff areas as sound travels! Make sure you follow the barber's shop rules for eating and drinking; these activities are usually prohibited in the working areas. You should be **circumspect** in all of your work and dealings with your clients and others, keeping private all matters they have told you in confidence. This should include details relating to the services they have had and all other commercially sensitive information about your barber's shop business. Ask your manager if you are unsure.

KEY DEFINITION

Circumspect: Being discreet when dealing with people.

TIP ✓

Remember that gossiping about your colleagues, clients or barber's shop business information is likely to get back to the people the gossiping is about. If involved in such gossip you are likely to be found out and the consequences could be severe, including disciplinary action against you!

TIP ✓

Avoid discussing personal problems and difficult subjects with clients and colleagues. Remember that the barber's shop should be a professional environment; it is not suitable for personal issues unless they directly relate to the business. If your client or colleague raises a personal issue or makes comments indicating they have a strong opinion that might offend others remain tactful and respectful and try to move the conversation on. Be careful not to become involved and do not make similar comments, even if you agree. With colleagues you can suggest that they speak to their manager.

GARY MACHIN **Barber and director of Roger's Barber Shops**

❝ Always be mindful that you are a professional barber – be enthusiastic when talking with your clients and colleagues, but be careful to stay within professional boundaries whilst at work. Make sure that you cannot be accused of causing offence by something that you say or do! ❞

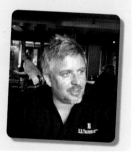

Misunderstandings

In a busy barber's shop misunderstandings and disagreements are bound to happen from time to time. The important thing is to see this in the context of the busy and sometimes stressful environment which can mean people say and do things they don't really mean. You should take care not to do this yourself but must be prepared to 'forgive and forget' so that the harmony of the team is not affected. Here are some important points to consider if you have had a misunderstanding or disagreement with a colleague in the barber's shop:

◆ Deal with the misunderstanding as quickly as possible so that it does not become aggravated and taken out of proper proportion.

◆ Show that you are eager to resolve the misunderstanding by the non-confrontational words and body language you use.

◆ Remain calm and positive at all times – do not raise your voice.

◆ Consider the details leading to the misunderstanding from your colleague's perspective – be ready to accept your part and apologize where required.

◆ Refer the misunderstanding to your manager for help if you cannot resolve it between yourselves.

Effective teamwork includes you making effective use of all your time at work. Remember that failing to do so can lead to your colleagues feeling 'put upon' especially if they have to deal with work that you could have completed.

Make effective use of your time at work

You must make effective use of your time throughout your working day in order to complete your daily work duties and support the barber's shop team and objectives. You should plan your day ahead, noting the client appointments if your barber's shop operates an appointments system. Where possible, work out your priorities for the day, for example if a stock delivery or sales representative is expected, or if a special client service, such as a wedding party is to be completed.

Focussing on the day's work at the start of the day will help you prioritize your work and remain effective throughout the day; thereby avoiding any problems.

You must work to the specified time allowed for each service, which will be set by your barber's shop; or by Habia if you are being assessed for an NVQ where maximum service times are specified.

Barber's shops also have quieter times, however and this time should also be used effectively. Here are some examples:

◆ Clean the barber's shop so that it is hygienically clean.

◆ Clean and maintain tools and equipment.

◆ Watch your other colleagues if still at work – offer to assist them where required – remember much can be learnt from considering the work of others!

◆ Practise your barbering techniques.

◆ Maintain stock levels and record the need for stock orders to be made.

IMAGE GALLERY

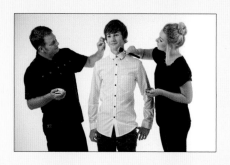

Visit the online gallery on this book's accompanying website to see other ideas for improving teamwork and other opportunities for learning in the barbering industry.

BRINGING IT ALL TOGETHER

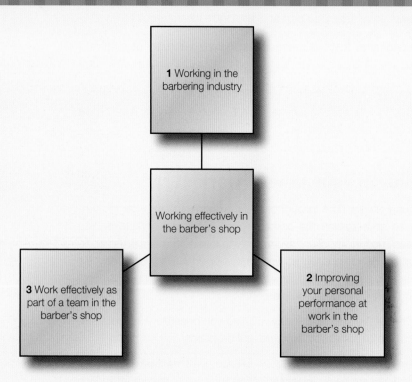

1 Working in the barbering industry

Working effectively in the barber's shop

3 Work effectively as part of a team in the barber's shop

2 Improving your personal performance at work in the barber's shop

Summary

1 The terms 'barbering industry' and 'barber' may be used collectively for anyone whose work includes the specialist barbering principles and skills most suitable for men's hair.

Barbers spend many hours standing, constantly moving their hands, raising and lowering their arms whilst concentrating on precise cutting movements. But the barber knows how to stand correctly and change position to reduce fatigue and ensure the quality of their work is maintained.

The professional barber knows when to 'chat' with their client and knows what is appropriate to discuss. Don't be tempted to become overfriendly during the service, particularly with your loyal and regular clients, even if they are your friend outside work.

Barbers have numerous career choices but most will start as either employed or self-employed barbers. Self-employed barbers may buy or lease premises to establish their own barber's shop or may develop a freelance business. Others may rent space within an existing barber's shop, commonly known as 'renting a chair'.

2   Job descriptions describe your role within the barber's shop and the responsibilities that this role includes. Employment contracts are similar but they go further to create a legally binding agreement between the barber and the employer, based on the employment conditions that were agreed when the barber first started work.

Your barber's shop must maintain procedures for dealing with disciplinary issues and grievances and an appeal system for appealing about findings from these procedures.

Performance appraisals and reviews help to establish the strengths and weaknesses in your work, so that you can recognize them and make improvements where required.

The barber must maintain awareness of trends and use CPD to ensure they have the necessary skills to create the looks involved in order to meet their clients' needs. The 'British Barbering Association' (BBA) and the 'Men's Hairdressing Federation' (MHFed) offer their members a range of benefits and are a great source of ideas for barbering CPD and current barbering trend awareness.

Habia work with industry experts to determine what is required in an NVQ for an individual to be called 'competent' and ready to work in the industry.

3   Good teamwork requires harmony, which is derived from everyone being polite, professional and respectful at all times, even if sometimes people do not get on so well. You should be alert and reactive to sudden increases in the work demands of your colleagues; offer them help, especially if there is a problem or if you are not busy. Consider any misunderstanding from your colleague's perspective – be ready to accept your part and apologize where required. You must make effective use of your time throughout your working day in order to complete your daily work duties and support the barber's shop team and objectives.

Activity

1   Research the current trends in barbering using the Internet, library and trade journals. Consider these trends against your current skills and experience.

Complete a skillscan (see page 41) and discuss your findings with your manager in order to update your personal development plan. Where possible arrange to complete the CPD required to enable you to maximize the potential of the identified trends.

Check your knowledge

1   What information might be obtained from Habia?

2   Which of the following documents must be issued to you at the start of your employment in the barber's shop?

   a. A style book showing the expected range of work
   b. A contract of employment
   c. A staff time sheet showing the expected hours of work
   d. A job description

3   Describe how to deal with a client that is making statements that could be deemed offensive.

4   Describe five methods of maintaining awareness of current barbering industry trends.

5   Explain why gossiping in the barber's shop should be avoided.

6   Where should food and drink be consumed by staff in the barber's shop?

7   Which of the following statements is correct?

   a. If you fail to meet productivity targets the barber's shop could lose revenue and disciplinary procedures might be taken against you.
   b. Short term targets are normally over 3 months' duration.

8   Describe the purpose of performance appraisals.

9   Explain how you could identify your strengths and areas to develop.

10 Describe the benefits of a barber maintaining CPD.

11 State the meaning of BBA and MHFed. What might these be useful for?

12 List three methods that should be used to resolve misunderstandings between colleagues in the barber's shop.

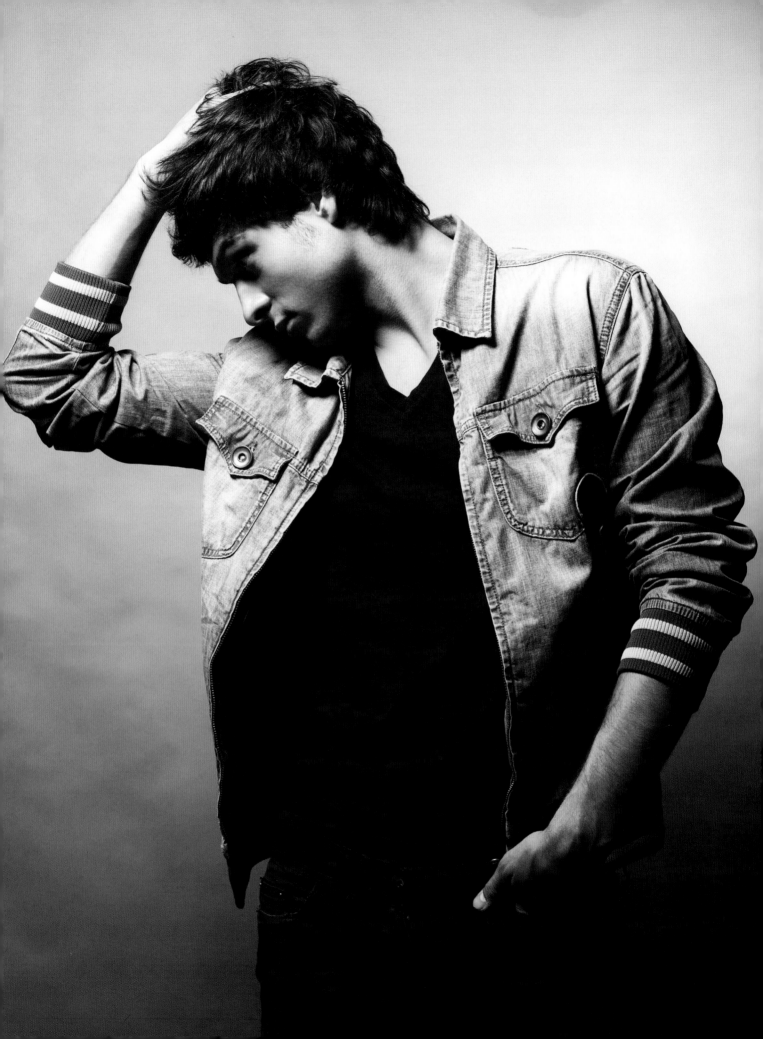

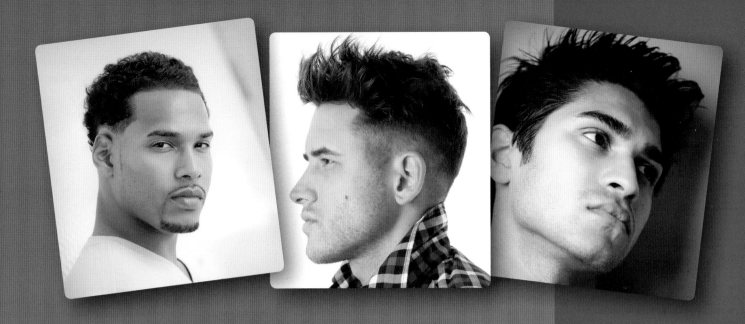

PART TWO
Menswork

In Part 2 of this book you will learn about the basic skills and knowledge required of the junior barber. These include client care, shampooing and conditioning, cutting facial hair, cutting hair, drying and styling hair, colouring hair and creating basic patterns in hair. You will cover important topics, such as the health and safety and consultation requirements for different services, and the fundamental barbering principles and skills of cutting and styling hair. There is also an additional online chapter covering the basic principles of perming and neutralizing men's hair.

4 Client care for men

QUALIFICATION SIGNPOSTING

This chapter will help your studies of the following qualifications:

❖ Level 2 NVQ Diploma in Barbering.
❖ Level 3 NVQ Diploma in Barbering.
❖ Level 2 NVQ Award Advise and Consult with Clients.
❖ Level 3 NVQ Award in Providing Hairdressing Consultation Services.
❖ City & Guilds Level 2 VRQ Certificate and Diploma in Barbering.
❖ City & Guilds Level 3 VRQ Diploma in Barbering.
❖ City & Guilds Level 2 VRQ Diploma in Women's and Men's Hairdressing.
❖ ITEC Level 1 VRQ Certificate in Barbering.
❖ ITEC Level 2 and 3 VRQ Awards, Certificates and Diplomas in Barbering and Men's Hairdressing.
❖ VTCT Level 2 and 3 VRQ Certificates and Diplomas in Barbering.
❖ VTCT Level 2 and 3 VRQ Diplomas in Barbering Studies.

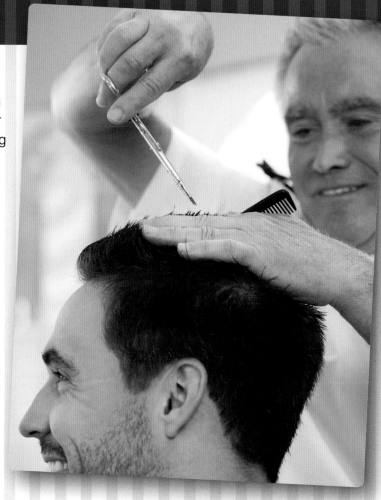

For further information on the qualifications covered by this chapter see the qualification mapping grid at the front of the book.

LEARNING OBJECTIVES

In this chapter you will learn:

◆ About effective communication with your client.

◆ How to recognize the needs of your client.

◆ How to prepare your client for different services.

◆ When to refer your client to others.

◆ How to care for your client.

◆ How to offer aftercare advice.

◆ About the hair and the skin.

◆ How to identify hair and skin conditions and disorders.

◆ How to determine when services should or should not be carried out.

◆ The importance of salon hygiene.

INTRODUCTION

Client care is an essential part of any hairdressing service: it forms an important part of all barbers' work. Providing care involves you working to meet your clients' needs, so that they are satisfied with every aspect of the service you offer. Good client care is a sign of professional standards of work, which all clients should be able to expect.

Client care is achieved through many different skills, including good communication, technical ability and good manners. The following are some of the important topics covered in this chapter:

❖ Communicating with your client.

❖ Recognizing the needs of your client.

❖ Preparing your client for different services.

❖ Referring your client to others.

❖ Caring for your client.

❖ Offering aftercare advice.

❖ Knowing about the hair and the skin.

❖ Identifying hair and skin conditions and disorders.

❖ Determining when services should or should not be carried out.

❖ Salon hygiene.

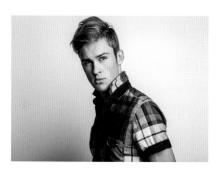

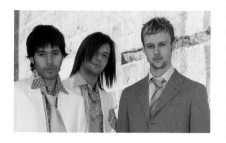

Client care for men

In essence, client care is the process of caring for your client, and it is the same for both men and women. It involves you looking after your client, ensuring that they are comfortable and safe throughout the service, and that ultimately they are satisfied with the end result.

Client care should begin when the client makes his appointment, which may be in person or over the telephone. It resumes when they enter the salon, and continues until they leave. Client care should also feature in the offer of **aftercare advice**. This involves you providing advice on aftercare products and tips on grooming and styling to help the client maintain their style at home.

In the salon, the first, and essential, stage of client care is the consultation. This must take place before any service is carried out, both for new and existing clients.

Consultation

Consultation is a two-way process between you and your client, whereby you identify the client's wishes, determine their suitability for the requested service, and provide advice on the most suitable course of action. It involves you both talking to the client and listening to them, so that you can accurately establish their needs. You will need to exchange ideas, and you may need to refer to photographs or sketches to help you clarify the ideas and reach an agreement.

Consultation is *always* necessary

In the barber's shop clients sometimes have their hair cut dry. Indeed, you have probably heard the request 'A dry trim, please' on many occasions. It may seem as if consultation is unnecessary for such clients, especially if they are regular customers at your salon. However, you must *always* carry out a consultation. This is an opportunity for you to find out about any problems the client has had with their hair which you could help correct. Many clients who change salons say it was because the new barber took the time to find out what they wanted, whereas the previous barber assumed he knew but was mistaken!

But more importantly, it is vital that you identify any **contraindications** to the requested service as the presence of such a condition will make proceeding with the requested service unwise. It is particularly important to establish the condition of the client's hair and skin and presence of any possible infections or infestations, so that you can select the best course of action and protect your other clients, your colleagues and yourself.

GARY MACHIN Barber and director of Roger's Barber Shops

"   Every client whether new to the barber's shop or a loyal customer deserves and should receive the best service available. The best service starts with the best consultation you can provide – it is simply the foundation of everything else. Forget this and you risk losing the client, your reputation and much more besides.   "

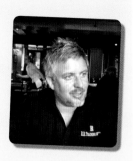

Talking with the client

Listen carefully to what your client says – after all, most clients usually know a lot about their own hair. Sometimes you may realize that a satisfactory result would not be likely: you will then need to advise your client to have a different service or a different style from the one they have requested. Remember to do this tactfully, and explain in simple and clear language the reasons for your recommendation.

As part of the consultation, you will need to examine the hair and scalp. The hair should always be *dry* when you do this, so that you can see any problems clearly. Proceed with the service only when you have accurately established what is to be done and have obtained the client's understanding and agreement.

Here are some important points to remember about **consultation**:

- Be **tactful**.

- Observe the client's confidentiality at all times.

- Accurately determine the client's wishes, both before and during the service.

- Use your skills of questioning and observation to gather all available information.

- Where necessary, perform tests to determine what services can be carried out: ensure throughout that you work safely and protect the client from harm.

- Ensure that you identify any adverse conditions of the hair or skin – if you suspect that an infection or infestation is present, you must not carry out the service.

- Before proceeding, ensure that the client understands and agrees with the service.

- Take into account any hairpieces that the client may be wearing – determine how these may affect the services to be provided.

- Record information about the client accurately, so that you can retrieve and review it easily on their subsequent visits to the salon.

Referring your client to others

Sometimes it is necessary to refer your client on to other specialists who are better able to deal with their particular requirements. Some examples of the conditions that should be referred and which specialists are appropriate are provided in the tables later in this chapter. At other times you may need to seek advice from specialists before you can

KEY DEFINITION

Consultation: An essential process before every service to identify the client's wishes, determine whether they are suitable for the requested service, establish the products and techniques to use and provide advice on suitable alternatives.

KEY DEFINITION

Tactful: Thinking about the rights and feelings of other people, maintaining their privacy and dealing with their needs sensitively.

HEALTH & SAFETY

Remember – if you are in doubt about conditions or disorders on a client always seek advice before commencing the service, especially if you suspect a condition may be **infectious**. Make sure that you know and follow your salon's policy for contraindications and referring clients on to others.

carry out the service requested. There are several different types of internal and external specialist advice available, relevant to the conditions you are likely to see when providing barbering services. It is important that you know what each specialist does and how they may be contacted. Here are some examples of the specialists and their areas of advice or work that are most often referred to in barbers' shops and hairdressing salons.

Specialist	Area of advice/work	Contact details
◆ Senior, experienced colleagues, e.g. those with Level 3 and above Barbering or Hairdressing Qualifications	◆ Clarification of simple recognizable conditions and disorders seen within the salon	◆ Your barber's shop should have a communication policy that sets out who you refer to in the salon with these types of problems
◆ Barber's shop/Salon manager	◆ Second technical opinion and advice on service requirements ◆ Confirmation of the need to refer clients on to external specialists	◆ Use the contact details specified by your barber's shop
◆ Manufacturers' information and advice lines	◆ Some general hair care advice ◆ Usually more specific advice about using the manufacturer's own products	◆ Telephone numbers, postal address and online address usually shown on products ◆ Details also in telephone directories
◆ GP or Doctor	◆ General medicine	◆ Clients should contact their own GP
◆ Trichologist (Clinical Trichology)	◆ Diseases and disorders of the hair and scalp	◆ Local telephone directories ◆ Institute of Trichologists (www.trichologists.org.uk)
◆ Dermatologist	◆ Skin diseases and disorders	◆ Referral usually through the client's own GP
◆ NHS 111 Advice and NHS Choices UK	◆ General medical advice and information within the UK over the telephone or online	◆ Urgent medical advice by calling 111 when it's not a 999 emergency. ◆ Visit NHS Choices at www.nhs.uk for more general healthcare information
◆ Chemist (Pharmacist)	◆ General health advice and the provision of medicines and treatments	◆ Local pharmacy details found in regional telephone directories

ACTIVITY – FIND OUT

Find out the contact details for your senior, experienced colleagues, the barber's shop manager, the manufacturers' information and advice lines, the local GP or Doctor, local Trichologist(s) and local Chemist(s).

Go to the website to download a form to record these useful contact details for your barber's shop.

Caring for your client

Throughout the service, you must take care of your client and ensure that he is comfortable. This can be achieved by following some simple rules:

1 *Security* Ensure that the client's coat and belongings are placed safely in the place specified by your barber's shop.

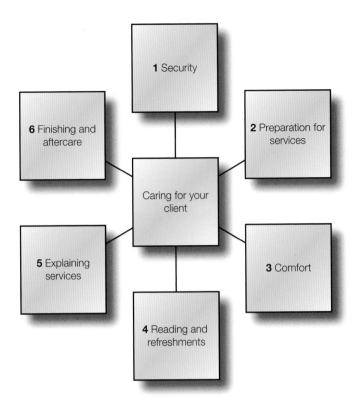

2 **Preparation** Gather together all the materials, products, tools and equipment you will require before you begin work.

3 **Comfort** Ensure that the protective gown, the cutting collar, towels, cotton wool pads and so on all remain in their correct places before and during services. During cutting services, remove excess hair cuttings from the client and the gown or cutting collar.

4 **Reading materials and refreshments** In accordance with your barber's shop policy, offer the client reading materials or refreshments, especially during lengthy processes such as colouring and perming.

5 **Explanation** Before you start make sure you explain how long the service might take, ask the client if they have any questions, and reassure them if necessary. As the service progresses, let the client know what you are doing – especially during perming, colouring or lightening.

6 **Finishing** Ensure that the client's clothes are not damp or stained, and that all loose hair clippings have been removed. Provide advice on aftercare products and style maintenance, including when the next appointment should be made. Return the client's coat and belongings to them. Remember to offer to make the next appointment for them, or ask the receptionist to do so.

TIP ✓

Never carry out a hairdressing service without a consultation. It is unprofessional and is likely to result in a dissatisfied client, or worse!

TIP ✓

Make sure you make a record of any staining or damage to the client's clothes and inform your manager or supervisor.

Preparing the client

Gowning and protecting the client

Following the consultation, and before you proceed with the services to be carried out, the client must be correctly gowned and protected. Which gowns, towels and so on are needed will depend on the service to be performed: this is explained in more detail in

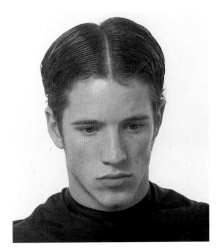

Basic gown and neck strip

the relevant chapters. Here are some *general* rules to follow when gowning and protecting clients.

◆ **The chair** Before seating the client, check that the chair is clean: remove any hairs that may have fallen on the seat or the back of the chair. Lock the chair so that it does not spin whilst the client sits down. Position the chair and the client in the correct position for the service to be carried out.

◆ **The gown** Place a tissue or neck strip around the client's collar, and then secure a clean gown into position. A range of modern gowns are available that include different fastening systems, some use buttons, pop studs and rubber/plastic/silicone collars. Remember that neck strips should always be used for hygiene and comfort reasons unless the gown has a rubber type collar, which should be sanitized before use on each new client.

◆ **Shampooing** If the client is to be shampooed, one or two towels will be required. For a back-wash basin, one towel should be placed over the back and shoulders. For a front-wash basin, one towel should be placed across their chest and tucked in at the neck, and a second towel placed over the shoulders and the first towel.

◆ **Cutting** If cutting, use a cutting collar and/or cutting cape. Make sure no hair can fall down between the client and the chair back.

◆ **Shaving** When shaving, place a clean towel around the front of the client. A paper towel should then be placed over the towel and across the client's shoulder (from their neck towards your body).

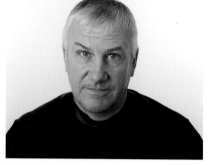

Modern gown with built in silicon cutting collar

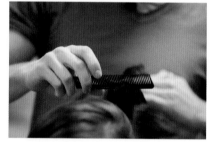

Detangling the hair

> **TIP** ✓
>
> Remember to lock chairs that swivel so that they will not spin around whilst the clients are sitting down.

Preparing the client's hair

The client's hair must be freed from any tangles before you can work with it effectively.

Begin by teasing the hair apart with your fingers. If the hair is long and very tangled, follow these simple steps.

1 Using a wide-toothed comb and beginning near the nape, take a section of hair and comb through the ends, removing any tangles. Gradually work up the section of hair until the comb will travel easily from the roots to the ends.

2 Continue taking sections in this way, working up the back and sides, until all the tangles are removed. Take care not to jerk the client's head whilst combing the hair.

Aftercare advice

You should provide advice on aftercare products, and tips on grooming and styling to help your client maintain their hair at home. This is also an opportunity for you to promote other beneficial salon services and products.

Gowned client with a plastic cutting collar

Here are some suggestions for you to consider:

◆ Always offer advice and tips on styling to clients who have had new styles.

◆ Encourage clients to ask about services, introduce them to new services.

◆ Suggest products that will benefit clients most and keep their hair in good condition.

The structure of the hair and skin

Anyone with an interest in providing barbering or hairdressing services must understand the basic properties of the hair and the skin, and the effects that certain services have on their structures. The location and function of the cuticles, cortex, hair follicles and blood supply must all be understood, as these often affect the choice of techniques and how they are applied. The different types of hair, the hair-growth cycle and the hair's chemical composition and physical properties should also be known.

The hair

Hairs are to be found covering all parts of the body, except for the palms of the hands, the soles of the feet and the eyelids.

Types of hair

◆ There are three different types of hair: **Lanugo, Vellus and Terminal**.

Lanugo hair Lanugo hair is a very fine downy hair that covers the body of unborn and newborn babies. It is usually lost either at birth or soon afterwards.

Vellus hair Vellus hair is very fine hair which occurs on most parts of the body. It can often be seen on the cheeks of women, and on the forehead and scalp of men with male-pattern alopecia (baldness), as the vellus hair is not usually lost.

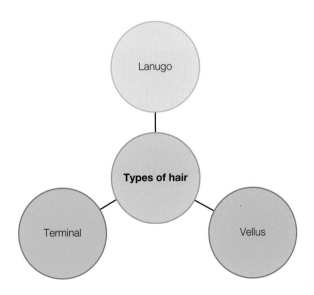

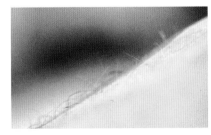

Vellus hair

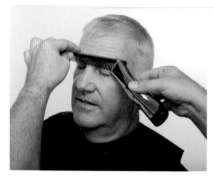

Trimming the eyebrows – a type of terminal hair

Terminal hair Terminal hair is the longer hair that occurs on the head, arms, legs, eyebrows and pubic areas, and on the face and chest in men.

Hair structure

Each individual hair shaft consists of three layers.

The cuticle The cuticle is the thin outer layer of the hair shaft, which is made up of colourless cells. The cells look like scales and overlap like tiles on a roof. The scales point away from the roots and *towards* the ends: the hair feels smooth if you rub your hand from the roots to the ends, but rough if you rub it from ends to the roots, especially if the cuticles are damaged.

The cuticle forms a protective surface to the hair and so helps to maintain its condition. Healthy hair shines because all the cuticle cells are lying flat and the light is reflected. Damaged and rough cuticles trap the light, making the hair appear dull and lifeless.

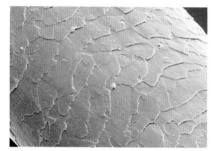

Hair cuticles, seen under an electron microscope

The cortex The cortex is the middle layer of the hair. It is by far the largest part of the hair and is the main source of the hair's strength. The cortex is where the changes take place during blow-drying, perming, relaxing, lightening and colouring. The cortex is made up of many long strands of fibres, which resemble springs twisted together. The largest strands are the cortical cells, which are themselves made of smaller bundles called macrofibrils. These in turn are made up of bundles of microfibrils, and these in turn of bundles of protofibrils. All these fibres and cells are held together by linkages and chains which determine the hair's elasticity, thickness, strength and curl pattern.

The colour of the hair is determined by the pigment, which is also found in the cortex.

The medulla The medulla is the very fine core of the hair. It does not have any real function and is not always present, particularly in fine blond hair.

The chemical composition of hair

The cortical cells are made from molecules of amino acids. These are combinations of the elements carbon, oxygen, nitrogen, hydrogen and sulphur.

Amino acids are joined together by peptide bonds, forming long chains called polypeptides. These in turn form proteins.

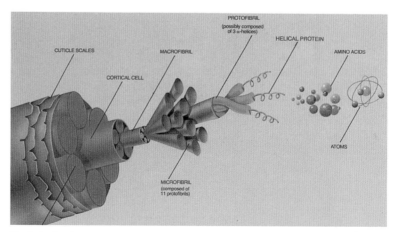

The hair structure

The principal protein in hair is called keratin, and it is also found in the nails and the skin. Keratin has elastic properties which make the hair flexible and allow it to be stretched and curled without breaking.

Keratin chains are combined in hair in a coiled, spring-like shape. They are held in this shape by linkages *within* chains and *between* chains. There are three different kinds of linkage:

- disulphide bridges or sulphur bonds

- salt links

- hydrogen bonds

The disulphide bridges are very strong linkages, but they can be broken and remade using chemicals during processes such as perming. It is this breaking and remaking of disulphide bridges that allows hair to be moulded to a new *permanent* shape.

The salt links and hydrogen bonds are much weaker, and are easily broken just with water. This allows the hair to be easily stretched and moulded, as when blow-waving. This change is only temporary, however, and the hair will return to its natural state when moisture enters. (See Chapter 11, Advanced men's hair cutting.)

The physical characteristics of hair

Hair is hygroscopic: it absorbs water from the atmosphere. The amount of water absorbed depends upon the humidity of the atmosphere – how dry or damp the air is – as well as how dry the *hair* is.

Hair naturally contains some moisture, which lubricates the fibres and allows the hair to stretch and recoil. Hair is also porous: it will absorb water like a sponge soaking up water. (This is called capillary action.)

Damaged hair is far more porous than healthy hair, and loses its natural moisture much more quickly. This is why it is more difficult to stretch and mould dry and damaged hair.

Hair is often categorized by other different physical characteristics, such as:

- Hair density – the number of individual hairs per square centimetre – defined as thin, medium and thick.

- Hair texture – how thick each individual strand of hair is – defined as fine, medium and coarse.

- Hair elasticity – how stretchy the hair is without breaking.

- Hair porosity – how easily the hair will absorb moisture.

- Hair condition – whether hair is normal, dry, oily or damaged.

- Hair growth patterns – the direction individual hairs grow as a result of the position and shape of the hair follicles – creating patterns such as the crown, double crown, nape whorl, calf lick and widow's peak.

These hair characteristics are important in most of the work in the barber's shop and will be covered in greater detail in the relevant chapters.

KEY DEFINITION

Keratin: The main protein from which the hair, nails and the skin are made. Keratin has elastic properties which allow it to stretch and return to its original length without damage. This makes the hair flexible and allows it to be stretched and curled without breaking.

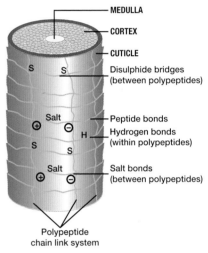

MEDULLA
CORTEX
CUTICLE
Disulphide bridges (between polypeptides)
Peptide bonds
Hydrogen bonds (within polypeptides)
Salt bonds (between polypeptides)
Polypeptide chain link system

Salt links

Hair types

Traditionally there were three different hair types, each of which can be of fine, medium or coarse textures:

- ◆ **Caucasian** or **European** hair is mainly straight or lightly waved.

- ◆ **Black** or **African-Caribbean** hair has tight curls or kinks.

- ◆ **Mongoloid** or **Asian** hair is usually very straight and coarse.

More recently, however, hair type has been classified according to the structure of the hair rather than by reference to racial or geographical features, and by hair characteristics. These new classifications more accurately describe the hair type, particularly in a multi-cultural society. The classifications are as follows:

Type 1 – Straight Hair

- ◆ S1a – is straight fine/ thin hair. This hair type usually hangs freely and is very soft and difficult to curl. It is often shiny and has a tendency to be oily. It is usually more resistant to damage. Caucasian or European hair is usually in this category.

- ◆ S1b – is straight hair that often has better volume and body. Caucasian or European hair is usually in this category.

- ◆ S1c – hair is coarse and usually very straight and extremely difficult to curl. Category 1c was previously called Mongoloid or Asian hair.

Type 2 – Wavy Hair (Caucasian or European hair is usually in this category.)

- ◆ W2a – hair is fine/ thin with a loose and stretched 'S' shaped wave pattern. Straight and curled styles are usually possible.

- ◆ W2b – is medium wavy hair that has a more defined wave pattern. It can be more difficult to style but once achieved the waves hold the look well.

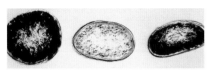

Cross-sections through hair: left, Mongoloid (usually type 1c); centre, Caucasian (usually type 1a/1b); right, African-Caribbean (usually type 4a/4b/4c)

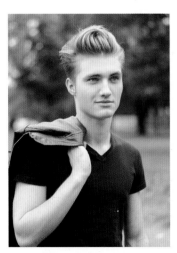

Type W2a-Caucasian or European hair

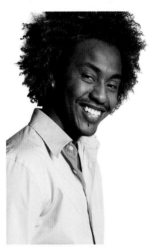

Type K4a-Black or African-Caribbean hair

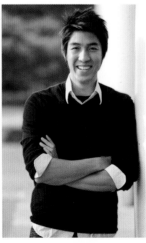

Type S1c-Mongoloid or Asian hair

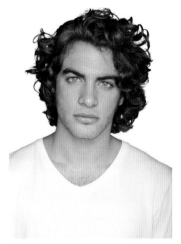

Type C3a-Caucasian or European hair

◆ W2c – hair is coarse with clearly defined waves. The hair tends to be frizzy, less shiny and more difficult to style.

Type 3 – Curly Hair (Caucasian, European and Black hair can all be found in this category.)

◆ C3a – hair has loose 'S' shaped curls that fall freely. It can be fine and thin or thicker and fuller. Type C3a hair has a tendency to be duller and frizzy particularly in humid conditions and is more prone to damage.

◆ C3b – hair is characterized by tighter well defined curls similar to ringlets. Again, it can be less shiny, fine and thin or thicker and fuller and tends to turn frizzy. It is usually more susceptible to damage.

◆ C3c – hair has strongly defined curls similar to a corkscrew curl pattern. It is often duller and frizzy, particularly in humid conditions. It is more easily damaged.

Type 4 – Very Curly Hair (Black or African-Caribbean hair would typically be in this category.)

◆ K4a – hair is soft but with a very tightly coiled 'S' curl pattern. It is often dull and more fragile.

◆ K4b – hair is wiry and very tightly coiled, sometimes referred to as a kinky or 'Z' shaped pattern. It is duller and more fragile that type K4a.

◆ K4c – hair is very wiry and kinky with a strong 'Z' pattern. It is often very fragile and easily damaged.

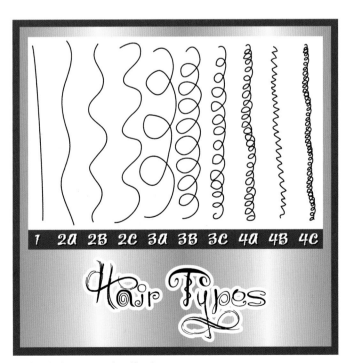

Modern hair types or classifications

> **TIP** ✔
>
> Hair classifications – the hair classifications are sometimes just known as 1, 2, 3 and 4 but you can add S to 1 to remember S1 = straight, add W to 2 for wavy, C to 3 for curly and K to 4 for kinky (or VC for very curly).

Hair growth

Hair grows continually for a period of between about 1 year and 6 years. Each individual hair grows following a cycle, which includes a period of growth, rest and loss. The duration of the growing stage determines the length to which a person can grow their hair. Normally hair grows at a rate of about 1.25 centimetres or 0.5 inches each month, or about 15 centimetres or 6 inches per year.

Eventually the hair falls out, but before it leaves the hair follicle a new hair is usually ready to replace it. If a new hair is not present an area of baldness will develop, as in male-pattern baldness. Normally, however, the cycle of growth is not really noticeable: because the hairs are all at different stages of growth, some are always in the growing stage.

Stages of growth There are three basic stages of growth:

◆ *Anagen* This is the active growing stage of the hair growth cycle, which may last from about 3 months to several years.

◆ *Catagen* This is the stage when the hair stops growing. It lasts for about 2 weeks. During this stage the hair separates from the papilla and begins to move up the follicle.

◆ *Telogen* This is the resting stage. During this stage the follicle shrinks and separates from the papilla. This stage lasts for only a short period, after which a new anagen stage begins.

Factors affecting hair growth The healthy growth of new hair can be affected by many different factors. Here are some of the most common and their effects:

◆ Poor health – hair may become thinner, sparse, or stop growing; elasticity, strength and gloss are likely to reduce.

◆ Poor diet – as poor health.

◆ Increasing age – as poor health.

◆ Gender – more men suffer hair loss through male pattern alopecia.

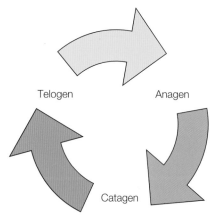

Stages of hair growth

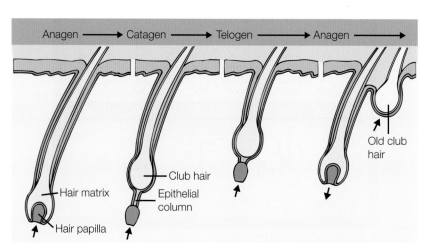

The hair growth cycle

◆ Heredity – male pattern alopecia is one type of **hereditary** condition.

◆ Hormones – fluctuating hormone levels affect hair growth rates: male hormones (androgens) speed up hair growth; female hormones. (oestrogens) slow it down.

◆ Climate and environment – hair may lose elasticity, strength and gloss and may become discoloured.

◆ Harsh physical treatment – hair is likely to lose elasticity, strength and gloss; hair breakage likely.

◆ Chemicals – over-processing leads to loss of elasticity, gloss and hair breakage.

◆ Disease – some diseases will cause hair loss; others affect growth rates and the composition of the hair.

KEY DEFINITION

Hereditary: A condition or feature, such as the colour of the eyes or hair that is naturally passed on from parents to their children.

The skin

The skin is a complex organ which covers the whole of the body. Indeed, it is the largest organ of the body. The skin across the head containing terminal hairs is known as the scalp. The skin has many different layers and it performs several important functions.

Protection The skin provides a tough, flexible, waterproof covering which protects the underlying tissues from injury. It prevents harmful substances from entering the body unless the skin is cut, and contains a pigment called melanin which absorbs harmful ultraviolet rays from the sun.

The surface of the skin is itself protected by its natural oil, called sebum. This is mildly acidic (about pH 5.6) and has anti-bacterial properties which help prevent the growth of

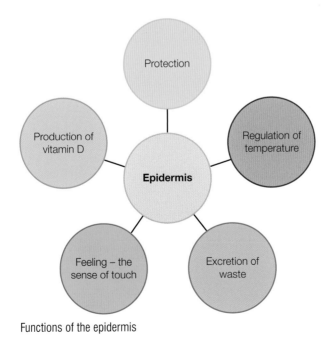

Functions of the epidermis

bacteria. Sebum also prevents the loss of water from the underlying layers of the skin, and so prevents the skin from drying out.

Regulation of body temperature The temperature of the body is regulated through sweating. Sweat evaporates and cools the surface of the skin.

Excretion of waste Waste products such as water and salt are removed from the body through sweating.

Feeling and sensation The skin contains nerves that allow the sensations of heat, cold, pain and touch to be experienced. These form a warning system that helps us to avoid harm and injury.

Production of vitamin D When exposed to sunlight, the skin produces vitamin D.

The epidermis

The epidermis is the layer of the skin nearest the surface. It is made up of five layers:

◆ *The horny layer* This forms the outermost part of the skin. It has a hard surface, which is constantly being worn away and renewed by new cells. It takes about 1 month for cells to move up from the bottom of the epidermis to the top.

◆ *The clear layer* This is a transparent layer, which contains the protein keratin.

◆ *The granular layer* This contains granular cells. It is situated between the living cells below and the hardened dead cells above.

◆ *The mixed layer* This contains a mixture of different live cells, including prickle cells, which lie just below the granular layer. The skin's colour pigment, melanin, is also to be found in this layer.

◆ *The germinating layer* This lies at the bottom of the epidermis and is connected to the basement membrane, which is attached to the dermis (see below). It is the most active layer, where new epidermal cells are produced.

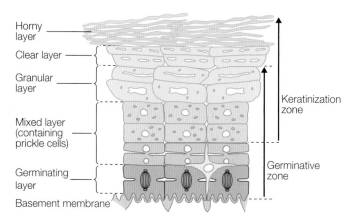

The epidermis

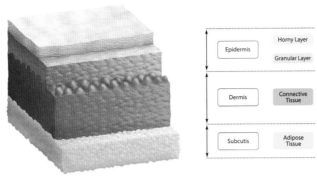

Layers of human skin

The dermis

The dermis lies in the middle part of the skin and is much thicker than the epidermis. It comprises **connective tissue** and has a good supply of blood and is the source of nutrients for the skin.

◆ *The reticular layer* The lower area of the dermis is composed of protein fibres which allow the skin to expand and contract.

◆ *The papillary layer* The upper part of the dermis contains tiny projections called papillae, which contain the nerve endings.

The subcutaneous layer

The subcutaneous layer lies below the dermis. It contains **adipose tissue** – it is where the body stores fat.

The hair follicle

The hair follicle is the source of the hair's growth. Follicles are found all over the body, except on the lips, the palms of the hands and the soles of the feet.

At the bottom of the follicle is the hair papilla and a tiny group of cells called the germinal matrix. These are supplied with nerves and a good supply of blood to nourish cell growth. Hair is formed when the cells grow and move up the hair follicle. Gradually the cells

> **KEY DEFINITION**
>
> Connective tissue: Tissues in the body that provide structure and support.

> **KEY DEFINITION**
>
> Adipose tissue: Body fat or loose connective tissue.

The hair in skin

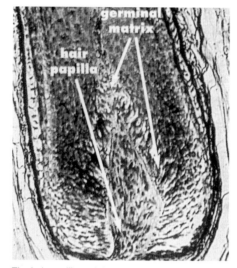

The hair papilla and the germinal matrix

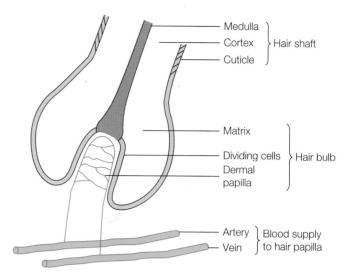

The hair bulb

harden and die, and the hair is formed. First the hair bulb is formed, then more cells are produced, and sooner or later they appear above the skin surface.

The sweat gland

The sweat glands are found all over the body. They lie alongside each hair follicle and produce sweat which passes up onto the surface of the skin.

The sebaceous gland

Sebaceous glands or oil glands are found all over the body, except on the palms of the hands and the soles of the feet. They are usually situated alongside the hair follicle, which they open into: this allows their oil, sebum, to be secreted onto the hair and skin.

The arrector pili muscle

The arrector pili muscle is attached at one end to the hair follicle and at the other to the epidermis: when the muscle contracts, the hair stands erect. Together the erect hairs trap a layer of warm air around the body.

Conditions of the hair and skin

Client consultation will seek to establish the condition of the client's hair and skin. Barbers need to know these conditions in order to choose the most suitable products and techniques to use and most importantly some conditions are contraindications that prevent the service being carried out. The following table covers the conditions mostly likely to occur in the barber's shop.

Bacterial diseases

Condition	Infectious?	Cause	Symptoms	Service/Treatment/ advice
Furunculosis (boils and abscesses)	Yes	Infection of the hair follicles by staphylococcal bacteria	Inflamed pus-filled spots with swelling and pain	Possible contraindication; service may be possible if area is avoided. Ensure good hygiene. By a doctor or NHS Advice
Sycosis barbae (barber's itch)	Yes	A bacterial infection of the hairy parts of the face by staphylococcal bacteria. Similar to *folliculitis*	Small, yellow spots around the follicle, with irritation and inflammation	Possible contraindication; service may be possible if area is avoided. Ensure good hygiene. By a doctor or NHS Advice
Impetigo	Yes (highly)	A bacterial (staphylococcal or streptococcal) infection of the upper layers of the skin. Sometimes caused by shaving too close, which allows ingrown hairs to develop, which can become infected	Burning irritation with spots appearing, which become dry and crusted. The spots merge to form larger patches	Contraindication; service not possible. By a doctor or NHS Advice
Folliculitis (inflammation of the hair follicles)	Yes	A bacterial infection by staphylococcal bacteria, or sometimes chemical or physical damage	Inflamed follicles	Possible contraindication; service may be possible if area is avoided. Ensure good hygiene. By a doctor or NHS Advice

TIP ✓

African-Caribbean men can be more susceptible to ingrowing hairs because their tight curly K4 type hair more easily grows into the skin. Regular exfoliation to remove the top layers of dead skin cells can help the hair grow out through the follicles and so prevent ingrowing hairs.

KEY DEFINITION

Infectious: A condition that is capable of being transmitted or passed to another person so that they then become affected by the same condition. Sometimes such conditions are also said to be contagious.

ACTIVITY: CASE STUDY – STEVE

Steve is a new client in your salon. He requests a shampoo, haircut, with tapered neckline and a facial hair design service. During the consultation you notice he has several small yellow spots around the facial hairs near his mouth. The skin here also appears to be reddened and inflamed. Steve also has an inflamed area of skin near the nape. What action should be taken regarding Steve's requests?

Viral diseases

Condition	Infectious?	Cause	Symptoms	Service/Treatment/advice
Herpes simplex (cold sore)	Yes	A viral infection of the skin, possibly following exposure to extreme heat or cold, or reaction to food or drugs. The skin may carry the virus for many years	Irritation and swelling with inflammation, followed by the appearance of fluid-filled blisters, usually on and around the lips	Possible contraindication; service may be possible if area is avoided. Ensure good hygiene. By a doctor or NHS Advice
Warts	Yes	A viral infection at the bottom of the epidermis, which causes the skin to harden and the skin cells to multiply	Raised, roughened skin, often brown or discoloured	Possible contraindication; service may be possible if area is avoided. Ensure good hygiene. By a doctor or products available from a pharmacist or NHS Direct

ACTIVITY: CASE STUDY – AADI

Aadi is a regular client in your salon, although it is the first time you will provide the service. He requests a grade 1 fade haircut and a full face shaving service. During the consultation you notice he has greyish-white flakes of skin on his jacket collar and an area of red skin with silvery-yellow scales behind each ear. Aadi also has a similar area of skin on his top lip. What action should be taken regarding Aadi's requests?

Fungal diseases

Condition	Infectious?	Cause	Symptoms	Service/Treatment/advice
Tinea capitis (ringworm of the head)	Yes (highly)	A fungal parasite, which infects the skin or hair	Circular areas of greyish white skin, each surrounded by a red ring. The hair is often broken close to the skin and it looks dull	Contraindication; service not possible. By a doctor or NHS Advice

Infestations by parasites (infectious)

Condition	Infectious?	Cause	Symptoms	Service/Treatment/advice
Scabies	Yes (highly)	An allergic skin reaction to the presence of the itch mite, a small animal about the size of a pinhead, which burrows into the skin, where it lays its eggs	A red rash, usually found in the folds of the skin between the fingers and on the wrists. It is very itchy	Contraindication, service not possible. By a doctor or with products available from a pharmacist or NHS Advice

Condition	Infectious?	Cause	Symptoms	Service/Treatment/advice
Pediculosis capitis (head lice)	Yes	An infestation of the head by head lice	The lice can be seen by parting the hair, but more commonly the eggs (nits), or the empty egg cases, can be seen stuck to the hairs	Contraindication; service not possible. By a doctor or with products available from a pharmacist or NHS Advice

ACTIVITY: CASE STUDY – ADAM

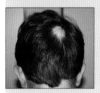

Adam is a regular client who has arrived for his monthly haircut. During the consultation you see this condition in his hair:

What action should be taken regarding Adam's request?

HEALTH & SAFETY

The presence of an identified infectious condition or infestation is known as a contraindication, which normally prevents all barbering services from being carried out. Services might, however, be possible where an infectious condition is localized and the risk of cross-infection is very minimal, e.g. where the client has a regular spot or abscess and this would not be touched during the service and good standards of hygiene will be followed.

Remember: You should always check with an experienced colleague or the manager before carrying out any service if you suspect an infectious condition is present.

Disorders of the hair and skin

Condition	Infectious?	Cause	Symptoms	Service/Treatment/ advice
Acne (a condition affecting the hair follicles and sebaceous glands)	No	Not known	Spots or bumps, often seen on the face and forehead, which cause soreness, irritation and inflammation	Possible contraindication; service may be possible if area is avoided. Ensure good hygiene. By a doctor or NHS Advice

(Continued)

Condition	Infectious?	Cause	Symptoms	Service/Treatment/ advice
Alopecia (baldness or thin hair growth)	No	The hair follicles are not able to produce new hairs. The causes of alopecia are not fully understood but some forms, such as *alopecia areata*, may be brought on by stress. *Male-pattern alopecia* is hereditary. Pulling, such as when the hair is left in tight plaits for a long period, causes *alopecia traction*. *Cicatrical alopecia* is the result of scarring arising from physical or chemical damage to the follicles	Areas of baldness or thinning hair growth. Male-pattern alopecia often follows the Hamilton pattern (see image below)	Style should be adapted to ensure hair loss affected areas are best covered by remaining hair, otherwise where large areas are affected shorter styles should usually be advised. By a doctor, trichologist or NHS Advice
Canities	No	The colour pigment does not form in new hair growth – often associated with increasing age	White hairs are visible	Services are possible. Tinting might be recommended
Dandruff (pityriasis capitis)	No	A fungal infection, or through physical or chemical irritation	Small greyish-white flakes of skin	Shampoo and condition using suitable anti-dandruff products. Other medicines and shampoos are available from doctors and pharmacists
Eczema and dermatitis	No	Physical irritation or an allergic reaction	The skin may be inflamed and split with weeping areas. There may be some irritation and pain	Possible contraindication; service may be possible if area is avoided. Ensure good hygiene. By a doctor or NHS Advice

Condition	Infectious?	Cause	Symptoms	Service/Treatment/ advice
Seborrhea	No	Over-production of sebum, which may be due to physical or chemical irritants	Greasy, lank hair and greasy skin	Shampoo regularly using suitable products, gentle massage movements and warm (not hot) water. A trichologist or doctor should treat extreme cases
Psoriasis	No	Unknown	Patches of raised thickened skin, which may be red with silvery or yellow scales. The skin may be sore and/or itchy	Possible contraindication; service may be possible if area is avoided. Ensure good hygiene. By a doctor or a dermatologist or NHS Advice

Adverse conditions of the hair and skin

Condition	Infectious?	Cause	Symptoms	Service/Treatment/advice
Fragilitas crinium (split ends)	No	Physical or chemical damage	The ends of the hairs are dry and split	Remove the hair ends by cutting. Use a conditioner
Monilethrix (beaded hair)	No	The hair develops irregularly while in the follicle	Bead-like swellings of the hair shafts, which often cause the hair to break close to the skin	By a doctor or trichologist. Chemical services should be avoided. Handle with care and use conditioner regularly. NHS Advice
Trichorrhexis nodosa	No	Physical or chemical damage	Patches of swelling and splitting on the hair shaft	Avoid chemical services. Cutting and conditioning

(Continued)

Condition	Infectious?	Cause	Symptoms	Service/Treatment/advice
Sebaceous cyst 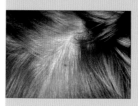	No	A blocked sebaceous gland	Bumps or lumps, about 10–50 mm across, on the scalp or nape	Possible contraindication; service may be possible if area is avoided. Ensure good hygiene. Removal of the cyst by a doctor. NHS Advice
Damaged cuticle	No	Physical or chemical damage	Rough areas of cuticle. The hair is dry and porous	Apply conditioners, thickeners or restructurants

ACTIVITY: CASE STUDY – WALK-IN CLIENT

A new walk-in client is requesting a dry cut grade 3. During the consultation you see this condition in his hair – you note that the skin appears grey in the centre but pink around the edges. Some hair has broken off from the area:

What action should be taken regarding the client?

Working safely

The barber must be able to recognize probable infections and infestations of the skin and hair in order to avoid catching them or passing them from one client to another. You must be especially alert to the dangers of two serious conditions that may be contracted through open cuts and abrasions.

AIDS AIDS stands for acquired immunodeficiency syndrome. It is not a disease but a condition that makes the body more susceptible to diseases, and these may lead to death. To ensure that you protect your clients, your colleagues and yourself, you need to understand how AIDS is transmitted.

AIDS is caused by a virus known as the human immunodeficiency virus (HIV). People may carry the HIV virus – they are said to be 'HIV-positive' – without developing AIDS. However, a person who is HIV-positive could pass the virus to another person – but only if that person's infected body fluids, such as blood, come into contact with the other person's body fluids. Although this occurs most commonly through unprotected sex or when drug addicts share needles, the virus *can* be transferred through a cut or through broken skin.

The virus cannot live for long outside the body – you cannot catch it from toilet seats, for example.

Hepatitis B Hepatitis B is a disease affecting the liver. This too is caused by a virus, the Hepatitis B virus (HBV). HBV is transmitted through infected body fluids such as blood, and also through infected water.

Hepatitis can affect the victim for a long time, and it can be fatal. Treatments are available, but the virus is known to be very resistant. It can survive a long time outside the body, so it is vital that you maintain a high standard of hygiene.

A vaccination is available to protect against Hepatitis B. As a barber you are at risk from this virus, so you should consider having this vaccination.

HEALTH & SAFETY

If you suspect that an infectious condition is present, you must not proceed with the service. Seek advice from your manager or supervisor if necessary, and tactfully suggest that your client go to his doctor.

Health and safety

The need for hygiene

Effective hygiene is necessary in the salon to prevent infection and cross-infection, which may occur if the salon is dirty or if you or your client has an infectious condition or disease. Cross-infection usually occurs through physical contact with another person or via a tool, such as a razor, which has become infected.

The warm, humid atmosphere in the salon can be the perfect home for infectious organisms. Sterilization with physical or chemical agents will destroy all the infectious and harmful micro-organisms, however, and sanitation will destroy some but not all microorganisms. Regular cleaning with bleach or disinfectant will ensure that the risk of infection and cross-infection in the salon is minimized.

General salon hygiene rules

Always follow your salon's health and safety procedures.

◆ Cover any cuts or open wounds you may have, and ensure they remain covered. Wear gloves to ensure the highest level of protection.

◆ Maintain a high standard of personal hygiene. Wash your hands regularly.

◆ Use a clean gown and clean towels for each client.

◆ Be sure to clean and sterilize tools before using them on clients.

◆ Keep working surfaces clean. Sanitize them regularly using bleach or disinfectant.

◆ Store dirty laundry in a sealed container.

◆ Put waste in suitable bags that can be sealed. Contaminated materials and sharps must be stored and disposed of as specified by the local environmental health authority.

See CHAPTER 2 for further information on 'Health and safety in the barber's shop'.

BRINGING IT ALL TOGETHER

Summary

1   Be tactful when asking questions and providing advice.

2   Consultation is always necessary.

3   Make sure the client is properly gowned, seated and protected before commencing services – take care preparing their hair, especially when detangling.

4   Know who to go to for advice on how to ensure client care – keep contact details to hand just in case.

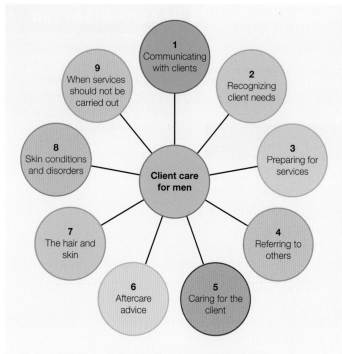

9   The presence of an identified infectious condition or infestation normally prevents all barbering services from being carried out. Disorders and adverse conditions of the hair and skin are not normally contagious and services can normally be carried out, although they must be adapted to meet the disorder or condition present.

Activities

1   Draw and label a diagram of a hair follicle in the skin.

2   Effective communication is an essential part of the consultation process. Take turns role playing the part of clients who are happy, confused and angry and practise these verbal and non-verbal communication skills with your colleagues:

◆   verbal: open questions, probing questions, closed questions.

◆   non-verbal:

   ◆   written – a telephone message to a client or colleague

   ◆   body language – posture, gestures, nearness and eye contact.

   Check your work with your manager or tutor.

3   Visit local chemists and use the Internet to find out what products are available over the counter for treating different conditions of the hair and scalp. Check the prices and compare the products with those in your own salon. Are there any available that you would recommend your manager to keep in stock? Make a list of the products that you stock, noting their key features and benefits. With your manager's permission, share this with your colleagues for use when promoting the products to clients.

4   Part of the barber's role is to sell products and services to clients so that the barber's shop is profitable. Visit the library or use the Internet to research the Consumer and Retail Legislation for promoting and selling products and services. Compare these rules with those in your salon and make a list of the key things that must be adhered to when selling.

5   Practise your selling skills with your colleagues. Make sure that you know your salon's policy for referring

5   Make sure that the client is comfortable throughout the service and has reading material and refreshments, as required. Make sure their belongings are safe and keep them informed on progress with the service.

6   Aftercare advice should always be provided to ensure that the client can maintain the style in-between visits to the barber's shop.

7   Hair type can now mainly be categorized as S1 – Straight Hair, W2 – Wavy Hair, C3 – Curly Hair and VC4 or K4 – Very Curly Hair or Kinky Hair. Further categories are defined as a, b or c. Hair, nails and skin are made of a protein called Keratin. The hair structure comprises the cuticles, cortex and medulla. Hair grows in a cycle of Anagen, Categen, Telogen before returning to Anagen. Normally hair grows at a rate of about 1.25 centimetres or 0.5 inches each month, or about 15 centimetres or 6 inches per year. The skin has three main layers the uppermost epidermis, the dermis in the middle and the subcutaneous layer below. Hair grows from the papilla located at the bottom of the hair follicles in the skin.

8   Bacterial diseases, viral diseases, fungal diseases and infestation by parasites are all infectious conditions that a barber must be aware of to protect his clients, his colleagues and his own health and well-being.

clients to other salons or retail outlets when you do not offer requested services or products.

Remember when selling you should:

◆ look for buying signals – is the client asking about the product or service to show they are interested or changing the subject because they are not?

◆ provide honest and accurate information about the most suitable product or service for the client:

  ◆ highlight the features – how it works, what it costs

  ◆ highlight the benefits – how it will enhance the client's hair

  ◆ use the product as an aid – let the client handle it, or use pictures to promote the service.

◆ close the sale or offer alternatives:

  ◆ allow the client time to make up his mind – don't push them or you may lose the sale and maybe even the client!

  ◆ confirm the sale when the client is happy with the chosen product or service

  ◆ offer suitable alternatives if the client is unsure

  ◆ if specified by your salon you may refer the client to other salons or outlets if you do not offer the service or product.

6   Use the Internet to find out more about bacteria, viruses, fungi and parasites that are the cause of many diseases and disorders. Try to obtain pictures that will help you identify them. Find out how each is contracted and treated. Check your findings with your manager or tutor.

7   Working efficiently so as not to keep clients waiting is an important part of client care. Check your NVQ/SVQ logbook or use the Internet to visit HABIA's website to find out the maximum service times specified for each service offered in barbers' shops. Compare these times with the times required by your own salon. Discuss these with your manager to make sure that you understand the reason for any differences.

Check your knowledge

1   State when good client care should begin.

2   Which clients should be consulted before services are carried out?

3   Describe nine points that should be remembered when carrying out a consultation.

4   Outline six rules of caring for your client.

5   What must be removed from the hair before commencing work?

6   State two reasons for providing aftercare advice.

7   Describe vellus hair.

8   Describe the middle layer of the hair.

9   Hair is said to be 'hygroscopic'. Describe what this means.

10 When viewed as a cross section, what shape is African-Caribbean hair?

11 Name the hair growth stage where the hair separates from the papilla.

12 List five functions of the skin.

13 Name the two main layers of skin that the hair follicle passes through.

14 Why do we have an arrector pili muscle?

15 Describe the cause and symptoms of sycosis barbae.

16 Describe two different types of infestation that may be seen in a barber's shop.

17 What is meant by the 'Hamilton pattern'?

18 Describe two methods of treatment for fragilitas crinium.

19 Describe how to protect yourself, clients and colleagues from contracting HIV whilst working in the barber's shop.

20 Compare sterilization with sanitation and outline the key differences.

5 Shampooing and conditioning men's hair

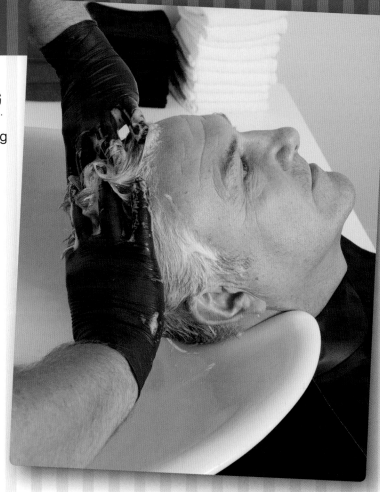

QUALIFICATION SIGNPOSTING

This chapter will help your studies of the following qualifications:

❖ Level 1 NVQ Diploma in Barbering.

❖ Level 2 NVQ Diploma in Barbering.

❖ City & Guilds Level 2 VRQ Award, Certificate and Diploma in Barbering.

❖ City & Guilds Level 2 VRQ Diploma in Women's and Men's Hairdressing.

❖ City & Guilds Level 2 VRQ Diploma in Women's and Men's Hairdressing.

❖ ITEC Level 1 VRQ Certificate in Barbering.

❖ ITEC Level 2 VRQ Awards, Certificates and Diplomas in Barbering and Men's Hairdressing.

❖ VTCT Level 2 VRQ Certificates and Diplomas in Barbering.

❖ VTCT Level 2 VRQ Diploma in Barbering Studies.

For further information on the qualifications covered by this chapter see the qualification mapping grid at the front of the book.

LEARNING OBJECTIVES

In this chapter you will learn:

◆ About shampooing in the barber's shop.

◆ The reasons for shampooing and conditioning the hair and scalp.

◆ How shampoos and conditioners work.

◆ How to select the correct shampooing and conditioning product.

◆ How to prepare for shampooing and conditioning.

◆ The shampooing and conditioning techniques used.

◆ A shampooing and conditioning procedure.

◆ What aftercare advice to provide.

◆ How to maintain health and safety when shampooing and conditioning.

INTRODUCTION

Shampooing and conditioning prepares the hair and scalp for other barber's shop services. The correct use of shampoos and conditioners forms the basis of all good hair care regimes. They help to keep the hair clean and healthy and have an effect on most other hairdressing services – maximizing the potential of the finished look. Both at home and in the barber's shop, shampooing and conditioning requires careful thought to make sure that the correct type of product is used. Many different shampoos and conditioners have been developed. The science behind them can be complex but the basic functions are simple and must be understood if the barber is to provide accurate services and advice.

In this chapter we will be looking at the techniques used for shampooing and conditioning men's hair and will be covering the following learning objectives:

❖ Shampooing in the barber's shop.

❖ Reasons for shampooing and conditioning.

❖ How shampoos and conditioners work.

❖ Selecting the correct product.

❖ Preparation for shampooing and conditioning.

❖ Shampooing and conditioning techniques.

❖ A shampooing and conditioning procedure.

❖ Aftercare advice.

❖ Notes on health and safety.

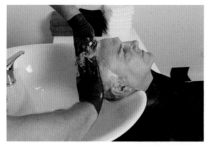
Effleurage movement

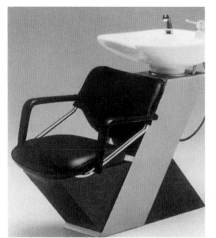
Back wash basin

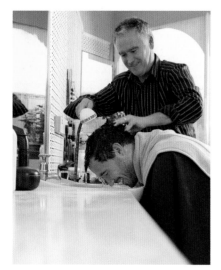
Using a front wash basin

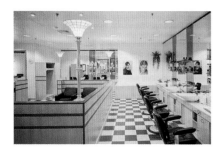

Shampooing in the barber's shop

Shampooing and conditioning services have often been carried out in barbers' shops, but the popularity of dry cutting and the fact most men did not have weekly appointments for setting or blow-drying meant that these services were not always used. Dry shampooing, using spirit based lotions or dry powders like talcum powder was also once popular, but these methods are less effective than wet shampooing and are rarely, if ever, used in barbers' shops today.

Many more men now have their hair cut wet and it is usually shampooed first. Sometimes the hair is shampooed after cutting, particularly on very short haircuts to remove the tiny excess hairs, to make the client feel more comfortable and to obtain the best finish. Other men just enjoy the refreshing and relaxing sensation of the scalp massage provided during shampooing.

TIP

When cutting grade 1 to 4 looks with a clipper and comb attachment it is best to shampoo the hair to make sure that any missed longer hairs stand proud of the new cut length. This will obtain the best finish and prevent you having an unhappy client, who might otherwise find these longer hairs when they next shampoo their hair!

The process of shampooing and conditioning is mostly the same for men and women. Some products do differ, usually in their perfume and packaging. Women tend to have hairdressing services that use chemicals more often and so, usually, more women than men need conditioning treatments. One main difference is that in barbers' shops the clients often have their hair shampooed at front wash basins rather than at back wash basins. This situation developed mostly because each barber's working station had its own basin installed so that clients did not have to leave the chair to be shampooed.

TIP

Before commencing the shampoo ask your client if he has back or neck problems that might affect how he can position his head against the basin. Remember that the client may be reclined or bent forward for several minutes and this action could be uncomfortable. In some cases the client might prefer the front wash rather than back wash. Always make sure that your client is comfortable throughout the process.

TRACY BOOTON SSRB, co-owner of Seagraves Gentleman's Barbers

" Shampooing and conditioning is an important service in the barber's shop as it helps improve the client's hair and scalp condition and prepare the hair so you can provide the best cut. "

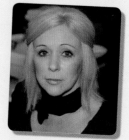

Reasons for shampooing and conditioning

Shampooing

The main purpose of shampooing is to clean the hair and scalp. A thorough shampoo will remove dirt, sweat, grease, hairspray and other substances that coat the hair and scalp. The removal of such substances is an essential part of the preparation for other hairdressing services, such as perming where any deposits of grease left on the hair shaft could block the perming chemicals and result in an unsuccessful perm. Shampooing is also used to remove the products used in other hairdressing services, including colouring and bleaching. At other times, the shampoo itself may include colouring ingredients that add colour to the hair. Whatever the purpose, a good shampoo should also be relaxing and enjoyable for the client.

Conditioning

Conditioning is used to restore the hair and scalp to a healthier state than previously. It is used to improve damage to the hair and scalp caused by both external factors, such as excessive use of heat when drying the hair, and internal factors, including poor diet and illness. Here are some of the factors that affect the condition of the hair and scalp and which can be improved by conditioning treatments:

External factors

- Physical damage – for example caused by harsh brushing or exposure to the sun and wind, etc.
- Chemical damage – for example caused by over-processing when perming hair, relaxing hair or bleaching hair, etc.

Internal factors

- General health and lifestyle – for example poor diet, the effects of medication, genetic conditions, pregnancy and stress.

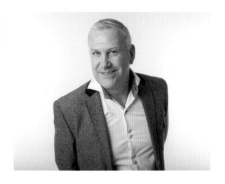

Cuticle Deposits

Cortex

Dirt on hair cuticle

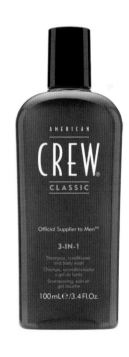

How shampoos and conditioners work

Shampoos

On its own, water cannot dissolve the substances that become attached to the hair and scalp. Shampoo is added and rubbed into the head and hair so that its cleaning ingredients and the dirt are agitated. The cleaners surround the particles of dirt, which are then rinsed away with water to leave the hair and scalp clean. Modern shampoos are very effective and only a little is required to clean the hair and scalp. A small amount, about 2–3 cm diameter, in the palm of your hand will usually be sufficient if thoroughly spread around the head and massaged effectively.

There are many different types of shampoo, but they can all be divided into four main groups:

- *Soap shampoos* – are not usually used in barbers' shops today, as the soap content leaves deposits of scum on the hair and scalp when they are used with hard water.
- *Soapless shampoos* – are used in most barbers' shops because they work well with both hard and soft water and do not leave deposits of scum.

KEY DEFINITION

Detergent: A substance that is able to attract and hold onto dirt particles so that they become suspended within a liquid.

KEY DEFINITION

Hydrophilic: A substance that is attracted to water and is easily dissolved in water.

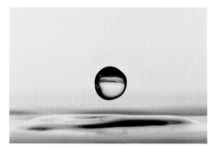

A magnified water droplet – the droplet is formed through surface tension

◆ *Synthetic detergents* – the main ingredient in most soapless shampoos used today.

◆ *'2 in 1'* – products that act as a shampoo and as a frequent use conditioner; often popular with male clients as they are quick and easy to use.

Detergents

Water alone will not spread out thoroughly over the hair because weak electrical forces make the water molecules stick together to form water droplets. This electrical force is strongest at the surface of the water and is known as surface tension – the effects of surface tension can be seen when a water droplet forms.

Modern shampoos contain **detergents** that help to reduce the effect of these electrical forces, thereby reducing surface tension and allowing the water molecules to spread out and wet the hair. This means that you will also see detergents referred to as wetting agents.

A detergent molecule has two ends. One end is hydrophobic, meaning it repels water molecules (it attracts grease molecules instead), and the other end is **hydrophilic**, meaning it attracts water molecules. When the hair is shampooed, the **hydrophobic** ends of the detergent molecules are attracted to and surround each grease molecule (sebum). The grease molecules are then lifted away from the hair and scalp and suspended in the shampoo. This suspension is called an emulsion. Any dirt is held on the hair and scalp by the grease that is present, so when the grease lifts from the hair and scalp the dirt is removed too.

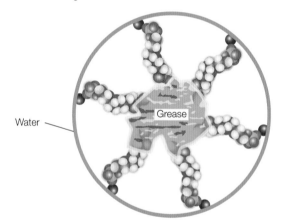

Water
Grease

Detergent molecules surrounding grease

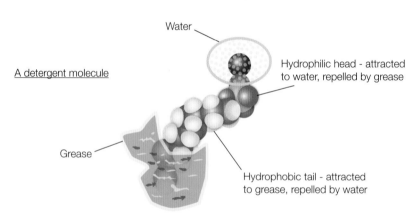

Water

A detergent molecule

Hydrophilic head - attracted to water, repelled by grease

Grease

Hydrophobic tail - attracted to grease, repelled by water

Simplified view of a detergent molecule

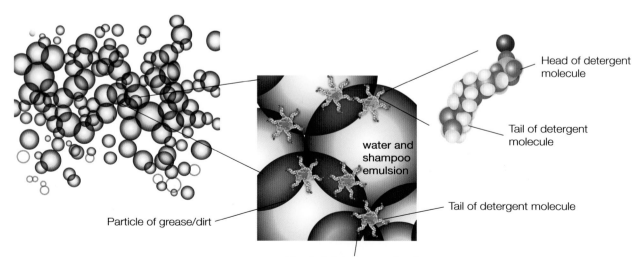

Head of detergent molecule

Tail of detergent molecule

water and shampoo emulsion

Tail of detergent molecule

Particle of grease/dirt

Head of detergent molecule

A shampoo emulsion with suspended grease and dirt molecules

'2 in 1' shampoos

'2 in 1' shampoos – so-called because they act as a shampoo and as a frequent use conditioner – usually contain conditioner particles as well as detergent. The conditioner particles are a form of silicone, e.g. dimethicone, or positive electrically charged molecules. Hair has a slightly negative charge, which is greater where hair is damaged. Positive and negative electrical charges are attracted to each other, so when the hair is rinsed after shampooing the conditioning particles are released and attracted to the hair where they smooth the cuticle, especially where the hair is damaged. The conditioning particles are prevented from building up because shampooing removes the conditioning particles that were deposited previously.

Conditioners

As can be seen from the list of shampoo products above, many shampoos now contain some conditioning ingredients to provide for the conditioning required by most people. But other conditioners have been developed to meet clients' requirements when more specific or intensive conditioning is needed, such as after chemical processing.

Like '2 in 1' shampoos, most modern conditioners have positive electrically charged molecules that are attracted to the negatively charged hair. This provides what might be called an 'automatic' application of the conditioning molecules, as more are attracted to areas of damage where the negative charge in the hair is greater. These substances are called substantive conditioners. An additional benefit of applying positively charged conditioning molecules is that they cancel out the negative charge in the hair when they become attached and so reduce the static electricity that makes hair difficult to style and dress.

Other conditioners contain thickeners, restructurants and protein hydrolysates that combine with the polypeptide chains within the hair to create additional temporary linkages that help the hair regain strength and elasticity. Essentially conditioners re-balance the chemicals in the hair, support the structure and coat the cuticle to counteract the effects of physical and chemical damage.

Dimethicone molecules

KEY DEFINITION

Hydrophobic: A substance that is repelled by water and is difficult or impossible to dissolve in water.

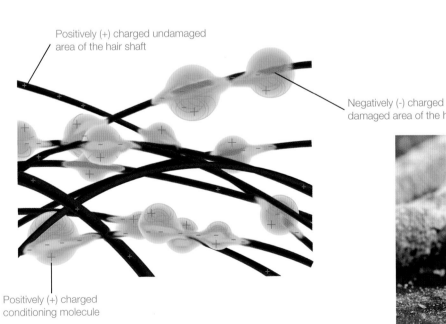

Positively (+) charged undamaged area of the hair shaft

Negatively (-) charged damaged area of the hair shaft

Positively (+) charged conditioning molecule

Substantive conditioning molecules: the + conditioning molecules are attracted to the - (damaged) areas of the hair shaft

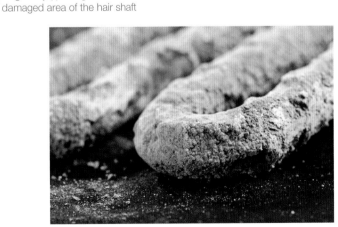

Limescale deposits on the heating element of a steamer

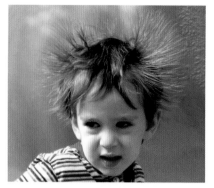

Static electricity in the hair

The importance of water quality in shampooing and conditioning

Hard water contains more calcium and/or magnesium salts than soft water. These substances react with sodium stearate in soap to form scum, or calcium magnesium stearate (soapless shampoos should be used in barbers' shops to avoid such problems). Whether an area has hard or soft water is a natural phenomenon of the geology of the local land. You might see mineral deposits form in kettles or around spray heads in barbers' shops in hard water areas. **Distilled water** should be used in steamers to avoid hard water deposits damaging the equipment.

The pH scale

The pH scale measures acidity and alkalinity ranging from pH1 to pH14. A pH of 1 indicates the strongest acid whilst a pH of 14 indicates the strongest alkaline; a pH of 7 is considered neutral. Understanding the pH scale is important in hairdressing because of the effects that some hairdressing chemicals have on the body's natural pH levels. The normal pH of the hair is pH 4.5–5.5 and the pH of the surface of the skin is pH 5–6, mildly acidic, caused by an oil produced in the skin called sebum. This acidic coating is called the skin's acid mantle. This mantle acts as a barrier to infection, slowing down the growth of bacteria and keeping the skin healthy. Raising the pH level above 5–6, which may happen if it is not re-balanced after certain hairdressing services that use alkaline products, e.g. perming, would reduce the effectiveness of this barrier and make infections more likely to occur. Some conditioning products are designed specifically to re-balance the natural pH of the hair and scalp after chemical services and are known as pH balanced conditioners.

Approximate pH Values of Various Substances

Acid	0.1–6.9
Alkali	7.1–14.0
Neutral solution	7.0
Normal hair/scalp	4.5–5.5
Pre-perm shampoo	7.0
pH-balanced shampoo/conditioner	4.5–5.5

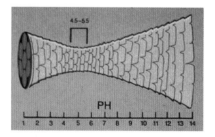

How pH affects the hair

Hair is also affected by the level of acidity and alkalinity. When it is slightly alkaline the cuticles lift and the hair shaft swells, however if it is mildly acidic the cuticles close up. Very strong readings towards either acid or alkaline will cause the hair to break down. The pH of a substance can be measured using pH papers, or Litmus papers that change colour to indicate pH value.

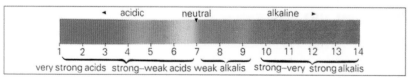

The pH scale

Selecting the correct product

Shampooing and conditioning is very similar for men and women. The same process is used and the same products are usually equally suitable, but some differences do occur. Men tend to want products that contain less perfume and the packaging of retail products for men is designed specifically to attract them. However, the choice of product is really made on the basis of more scientific factors, such as the needs of the hair and scalp.

Selecting shampoo products

The choice of the correct shampoo depends on several factors.

◆ *Water quality* – as we have seen earlier the minerals in hard water will react with sodium stearate in soap to form scum. Soapless shampoos that do not produce scum should therefore be used in barber's shops.

◆ *Services planned* – the services that will follow the shampooing process must be considered to make sure that the shampoo used is compatible with the forthcoming service, e.g. pre-perm shampoos should be used before a perm.

◆ *The reason for the shampoo* – why is the shampoo being performed? Is it to clean, remove colour products, add colour products or condition?

◆ *The frequency of the shampoo* – hair that is washed more often is usually less dirty and greasy, so milder shampoos designed for frequent use should be used.

◆ *The hair type and texture* – coarse and thick hair needs a shampoo that will make it more pliable, while fine hair benefits from a shampoo that adds body.

◆ *Hair condition* – a list of common hair conditions and examples of their treatment is provided in Chapter 4, 'Client care for men'.

Here are some popular shampoos, their ingredients and uses:

◆ *Medicated* – to maintain healthy hair and scalp.

◆ *Treatment* – many different shampoos are developed to treat different problems, like over-greasy hair and scalp or dandruff. Ingredients include selenium sulphide or zinc for dandruff.

◆ *Pre-perm* – used before a perm to remove substances that could affect the perming process.

◆ *'2 in 1'* – acts as a shampoo and as a frequent use conditioner. Contains conditioner particles that are positively electrically charged to be attracted to the hair, especially where the hair is damaged.

◆ *Egg* – egg white is used to improve over-greasy conditions and egg yolk is used for dry hair.

◆ *Camomile* – used to brighten blond hair. Can be effective against greasy conditions.

◆ *Coconut* – used for dry hair. Helps to smooth the hair and improve its elasticity.

◆ *Lemon* – used for over-greasy hair. The citrus ingredients cut through the grease and the slightly acidic pH closes the hair cuticle and makes the hair shine.

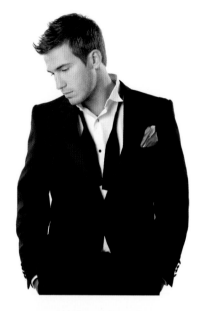

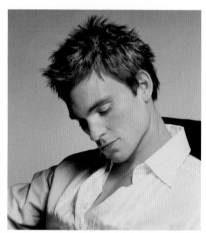

See **CHAPTER 4**, 'Client care for men' for more information of common hair conditions and examples of their treatment.

HEALTH & SAFETY

You must carry out a thorough consultation to ensure that you identify any adverse conditions of the hair or skin that may be present. It is particularly important to establish whether a suspected infection or infestation is present, as this would prevent you from shampooing or conditioning the hair.

Selecting conditioning products

There are two main types of conditioner:

- *Surface conditioners* – these add gloss and shine to the hair by smoothing the cuticle, which also makes the hair more manageable. They remain on the surface of the hair and do not enter the cortex. They include reconditioning creams and oils and dressing creams and lotions and contain ingredients such as vegetable and mineral oils, lanolin, lecithin and acetic acid.

- *Penetrating conditioners* – these enter the cortex through capillary action, i.e. the conditioner is drawn into the hair shaft through the tiny spaces in the hair structure. These conditioners can repair the cortical fibres, introduce moisture and smooth the cuticle. They contain ingredients such as protein hydrolysates, humectants (substances that hold water) and moisturisers.

The choice of correct conditioner also depends on several factors:

- *Services planned and carried out* – the services that will follow the conditioning process must be considered to make sure that the conditioner used is compatible with the forthcoming service, e.g. only use conditioners designed for use before perming or the chemicals in the perm will not be able to enter the hair shaft. Some conditioners are used after other hairdressing services, for example anti-oxidants to stop chemicals processing and pH balancers to re-balance pH levels.

- *The reason for the conditioner* – why is it being performed? Is it to protect the hair before chemical services, add moisture or help reconstruct the cortical fibres?

- *The frequency of the conditioner* – hair that is washed and conditioned more often is usually less dry, so conditioners for frequent use should be used.

- *The hair type and texture* – coarse and thick hair needs a conditioner that will make it more pliable. Fine hair is improved by conditioners that contain catatonic polymers that add body.

- *Hair condition* – a list of common hair conditions and examples of their treatment is provided in Chapter 4, 'Client care for men'.

Here are some popular conditioners, their ingredients and uses:

- *Anti-oxidants* – conditioners used after chemical processing to stop oxidation and neutralize alkaline.

- *pH balancers* – used after chemical processing to restore pH levels.

- *Pre-perm conditioners* – used before a perm to even out porosity and improve the perming process.

- *'2 in 1'* – acts as a shampoo and as a frequent use conditioner. Contains conditioner particles that are positively electrically charged that are attracted to the hair, especially where the hair is damaged. Easy and quick for clients to use at home.

- *Lacquer* – help resist the ingress of moisture and to shape the hair. Can smooth the cuticle and enhance the glossy appearance.

- *Restructurants* – these penetrate the hair shaft and help repair and support damaged cortical fibres, making the hair more pliable and able to be styled.

- *Other dressings* – help add and retain moisture and smooth the cuticles.

ACTIVITY – Find Out

Find out what shampooing and conditioning products are used for different purposes within your barber's shop. Go to the website to download a form where you can record your findings to share with your colleagues.

Consultation prior to shampooing and conditioning

It is important to consider the client's hair type, texture and condition and the other hairdressing services required when choosing the product, water temperature and shampoo massage techniques to be used. You must give careful consideration to each of the following factors before you start work:

◆ Why does the client want the shampoo or conditioning treatment?

◆ Look for signs of broken skin, abnormalities on the skin or any unusual facial features or beard growth patterns.

◆ Is the hair fine, medium or coarse?

◆ Is the hair growth dense or sparse – does the density of growth vary around the head?

◆ Determine which other hairdressing services are to be provided following the shampooing or conditioning.

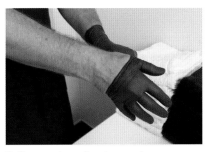

See **CHAPTER 4**, 'Client care for men' for more information on hair condition, suspected infections and suspected infestations.

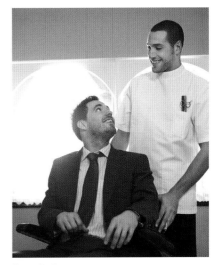
Putting on gloves for shampooing

ACTIVITY: CASE STUDY – MARK

Mark is a new client in your barber's shop. He requests a shampoo, cut and blow-dry and informs you that his fine hair is often very greasy by the evening after shampooing that morning. During the consultation you notice he has small greyish white flakes on his jacket collar, scalp and within his hair roots. What action should be taken regarding Mark's request?

See **CHAPTER 2**, 'Health and safety in the barber's shop' for more information on contact dermatitis and working safely in the barber's shop.

Preparation for shampooing and conditioning

◆ Carry out your consultation with the client. Look for signs of broken skin, and any abnormalities on the skin.

◆ Determine the client's wishes and confirm what is to be done.

◆ Gather together all the products, towels, tools and equipment you will require before you begin work.

◆ You should wear gloves whilst shampooing to help protect your hands from developing contact dermatitis.

◆ The client should be gowned correctly for the type of basin you are using. A back wash basin requires a gown and then a clean towel placed across the client's back, a front wash basin requires a gown and a towel across the client's chest with a second towel across his back and over the first towel. Make sure the towels are tucked in at the neck to prevent them from falling when the client leans forward.

Consultation

◆ Position the client in the chair correctly so that his head can be positioned comfortably over the basin. Ensure his head is correctly supported by the back wash basin when using this method and make sure their neck and head remain comfortable without undue pressure – stop the service and allow the client to raise and reposition their neck and head if they experience any discomfort.

◆ Carefully comb the hair through before commencing. Look out for areas of sparse growth, scarring or other unusual features you may not have seen earlier.

Accompanying video available for Effleurage, Rotary, Petrissage and Friction massage movements

HEALTH & SAFETY

Make sure that your fingernails are not too long before performing manual scalp massage, as long fingernails could dig into the skin, even though wearing gloves!

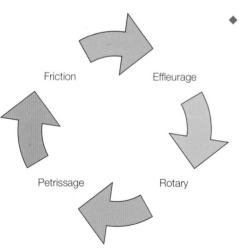

Manual massage techniques

Shampooing and conditioning techniques

The following manual massage techniques are commonly used when shampooing and conditioning hair.

◆ **Effleurage** is a gentle, gliding, stroking movement where the fingers and palms of the hands move freely around the head. It is the foundation of all good massage and is used to distribute the shampoo product, induce relaxation, particularly at the start and the completion of the shampooing procedure.

◆ **Rotary** movements are made with the fingers which make small circular, or rotary movements on the head. Rotary has similarities with petrissage, however the fingers move less across the scalp during each movement. Rotary is good for cleaning the scalp during shampooing and it creates an invigorating sensation for the client.

◆ **Petrissage** is performed through a mixture of pinching, kneading and rolling movements across the scalp. It is applied with both hands, which often work together to gently lift the skin between the fingers and thumbs, where it is squeezed, rolled and pinched with a gentle but firm pressure. Petrissage is similar to rotary movements but the slower and rhythmical pressure is better suited to conditioning treatments.

◆ **Friction**, or vibration, is a rubbing movement often used with friction hair tonics in scalp massage. It has a stimulating affect on the scalp and produces an invigorating sensation for the client.

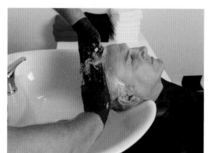

Effleurage hand position

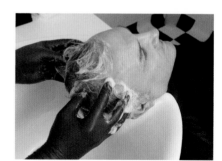

Rotary hand position

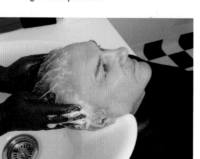

Petrissage hand position

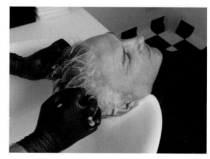

Friction hand position

The effleurage, petrissage and friction massage techniques are also commonly used when providing scalp massage as part of conditioning services. This form of scalp massage is explained fully in the additional online Chapter, 'Specialist hair and scalp treatments'.

ACTIVITY: CASE STUDY – CHENG

Cheng is a new client in your barber's shop. During the consultation for a shampoo, cut and blow-dry you notice his hair is unusually dry and some *fragilitas crinium* is apparent. Cheng informs you he works in construction and regularly wears a hard hat and is in dusty conditions. What action should be recommended for shampooing and conditioning Cheng's hair?

A shampooing and conditioning procedure

1 Ensure that your client is correctly gowned and protected.

2 Wear the PPE required in your barber's shop. This should include an apron and gloves.

3 Prepare the hair, as required.

4 Check that the client is comfortable.

5 Be careful not to scald your client's head or your own hand – turn on the cold water first and then add the hot water until the correct temperature is achieved. Test the temperature on the back of your hand or wrist before applying the flow of water to the client's head.

6 Check that the flow of water is not too strong or water will splash off the client's head and wet their clothes and the barber's shop.

7 Maintain your hand in the flow of water during rinsing to check that the water temperature remains stable.

8 Thoroughly wet the hair, controlling the flow to keep the client's clothes, and your own clothes and the rest of the barber's shop dry. Turn off the water.

9 Apply sufficient shampoo for the length and density of hair into the palm of your hand (a 2–3 cm diameter amount is usually sufficient). Spread the shampoo over the palms of both hands and then distribute it throughout the hair and scalp using effleurage.

10 Use light effleurage movements to relax the client, each hand moving in alternate directions (imagine you are drawing a zigzag pattern across the head). Work slowly and carefully to let the client become accustomed to the sensation.

11 Move the fingers back towards the temples then make small circular rotary movements working back across the head to the crown area. Repeat this series of movements several times working up to the top of the head.

12 Slide your fingers down the back of the head and make spiralling rotary movements with each hand down to the nape, moving back up towards the crown after each stroke.

HEALTH & SAFETY

Make sure that the water temperature is suitable when first applied to the client and that the client is comfortable throughout the shampoo service.

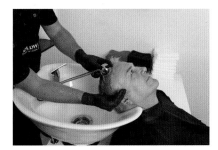
Control the water flow

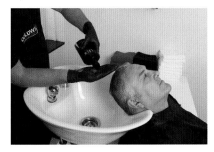
Correct amount of shampoo

TIP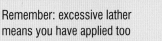

Remember: excessive lather means you have applied too much shampoo. Make sure you avoid waste and help protect the environment by using small amounts first; additional shampoo can be applied if the hair is particularly long, dense or greasy.

HEALTH & SAFETY

Always use clean gowns and towels for each client. Maintain high standards of hygiene in your work.

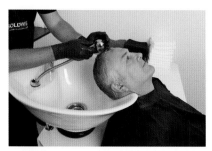

Wetting the hair

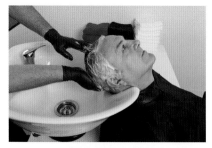

Distribute the shampoo across your hands and then across the head

HEALTH & SAFETY

Always make sure you remove shampoo and other hairdressing products from your hands and dry them carefully. Gently pat your hands when drying them. Failure to follow these steps can make your hands dry and sore and can lead to contact dermatitis.

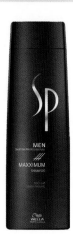

13 Place the fingers on the front hairline. Using light pinching and squeezing petrissage movements, work back along the head to the crown. Slide the fingers back down to the temples and then work back up towards the top of the crown, using the pinching movements as before. Make sure you cover all of the head.

14 Slide back down to the nape area. Using the middle fingers of each hand make two deep, rotating petrissage movements then continue this movement up across the head and to the temples. Repeat this movement several times.

15 Slide your fingers back to the front hairline. Using your fingertips apply a light friction movement and work back across the head to the crown and down the back to the nape. Repeat these movements from the sides to the nape. You should develop a gentle rhythm to make the movement enjoyable for the client.

16 Complete the massage routine with gentle sweeping effleurage movements across the head.

17 Repeat steps 4 and 5 and rinse the hair thoroughly.

18 Apply more shampoo and repeat steps 8–16 if required.

19 A surface conditioner can now be applied, if required.

20 After the final rinsing, turn off the water and replace the spray head. Wrap the hair in a towel and gently remove any surplus water. Reposition the client, check that dirt, grease and any products have been removed from the hair and scalp and that all shampoo has been rinsed out.

21 Comb the client's hair back away from his face using a wide toothed comb to avoid pulling the hair.

TIP

Commercial service times for shampooing and conditioning
You must work efficiently when carrying out any barber's shop service, working to commercially acceptable times. This means making sufficient time for the service to be completed correctly but within the maximum time allowed. Other barber's shop services and your colleagues often rely on you meeting these times, especially when shampooing and conditioning – make sure you don't overrun but be mindful of the client's needs – never appear to be rushing!

Aftercare advice

Remember to advise your client on how to maintain and improve their hair in-between visits to the barber's shop. Here are some ways you can help them achieve good results:

◆ Products to use – suggest which shampooing and conditioning products will help them achieve good hair and scalp condition. This is particularly important if you identified that a treatment shampoo is necessary, such as for dry hair or dandruff. This is a good opportunity to highlight the benefits of the products you have used to shampoo and condition their hair and to recommend they buy these from your barber's shop.

◆ How to use products – explain how the product should be used to achieve the best effects (you can highlight this to them as you shampoo and condition their hair). Help them find and understand the manufacturer's instructions.

Health and safety

Everyone in the barber's shop has a duty to work safely and keep his or her environment safe. When shampooing and conditioning it is important to consider health and safety because of the risks associated with using hot water and electricity. Here are some important health and safety factors that you must consider when providing shampooing and conditioning services:

◆ If the client has any cuts or abrasions on his face, or you suspect that an infection or infestation is present, the work must not be carried out.

◆ Always make sure you remove shampoo and other hairdressing products from your hands and dry them carefully. Gently pat your hands when drying them. Failure to follow these steps can make your hands dry and sore and can lead to contact dermatitis (see Chapter 2 for more detailed information on this condition and how it can affect your career).

◆ Always turn on the cold water first and add the hot water afterwards. Check the temperature of the water on you own hand and keep checking it to prevent scalding.

◆ Electrical equipment must always be handled and used with care in accordance with the manufacturer's instructions.

◆ *Never* use or place electrical equipment near water.

◆ *Do not* go near electrical equipment that is lying in water – isolate the mains power first.

◆ Visually check that electrical equipment is safe to use before commencing work – check that the cable has not frayed or been pulled and that the plug is not loose.

◆ Pay attention to the position of cables when using and storing electrical equipment.

◆ Only use clean tools and equipment.

◆ Make sure that you know the whereabouts of your barber's shop's first-aid kit. Keep yourself up-to-date with your barber's shop's first-aid and accident procedures.

◆ Electrical equipment must be regularly tested and given a certificate of testing (PAT certificate) to confirm that it is safe for use. Your barber's shop owner will ensure that this is carried out, as required.

◆ Maintain spray heads and steamers correctly and keep them free from limescale by using distilled water and de-scaling products.

◆ Make sure you know where the mains water stopcock and mains electricity switch are so that you can turn off the supplies quickly if problems occur. Suggest these are labelled clearly to help others find them should an emergency arise.

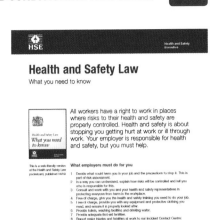

Health and Safety Law
What you need to know

HSE Health and Safety information leaflet

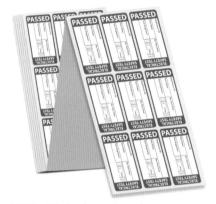

PAT Certificates for equipment

See **CHAPTER 2**, 'Health and safety in the barber's shop' for more information on working safely in the barber's shop.

BRINGING IT ALL TOGETHER

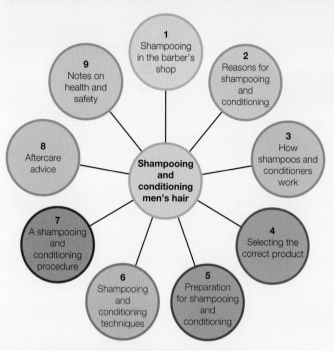

Summary

1   The process of shampooing and conditioning is mostly the same for men and women. Some products do differ, usually in their perfume and packaging.

2   The main purpose of shampooing is to clean the hair and scalp. Shampooing is essential preparation for many other hairdressing services, such as perming where any deposits of grease left on the hair shaft could block the perming chemicals. Shampooing is also used to remove the products used in other hairdressing services.

3   Modern shampoos contain detergents that act as wetting agents that help reduce surface tension, allowing the water molecules to spread out and wet the hair.

    ◆ Substantive conditioners have positive (+) electrically charged molecules that are attracted to the negatively (−) charged hair.

    ◆ Hard water contains more calcium and/or magnesium salts than soft water. Distilled water should be used in steamers to avoid these hard water deposits damaging the equipment.

    ◆ A detergent molecule has two ends. One end is hydrophobic, meaning it repels water molecules. The other end is hydrophilic, meaning it attracts water

molecules. During shampooing the hydrophobic ends are attracted to and surround grease molecules, which are then lifted away from the hair and scalp and suspended in the shampoo ready for rinsing.

    ◆ The normal pH of the hair is pH 4.5–5.5 and the pH of the surface of the skin is pH 5–6. Strong acid and alkaline is harmful to the hair and skin. pH-balanced shampoo/conditioner has a pH of 4.5-5.5.

    ◆ Weak alkaline substances cause the hair cuticles to lift up and the hair shaft to swell. Mildly acidic substances make the cuticles close up.

4   Surface conditioners lie within the cuticle scales. Penetrating conditioners enter the cortex through capillary action.

5   Ensure the client is comfortable throughout the shampooing and conditioning service – take particular care that their neck and head are positioned correctly when using back wash basins. Stop the service and allow the client to raise and reposition their neck and head if they experience any discomfort.

6   Effleurage is a circular, stroking movement used to distribute the shampoo product. Rotary is a massage movement used in shampooing. Petrissage is a similar movement to rotary but is better used in conditioning treatments.

7   When shampooing always turn on the cold water first and then add the hot water until the correct temperature is achieved. Test the temperature on the back of your hand before applying to the client's head, which is more sensitive. A 2–3 cm diameter amount of shampoo or conditioner is usually sufficient for men's hair.

8   Your aftercare advice is a good opportunity to highlight the benefits of the products you have used to shampoo and condition their hair and to recommend they buy these from your barber's shop.

9   Make sure you remove shampoo and other hairdressing products from your hands and dry them carefully to help prevent contact dermatitis.

    ◆ Always turn on the cold water first and add the hot water afterwards to avoid scalding your hands or the client's scalp.

    ◆ *Never* use or place electrical equipment near water.

Activities

Find out whether the water in your barber's shop is temporarily or permanently soft or hard. What steps are required to deal with the type of water in your barber's shop.

1   Find out where the water stopcock and main electricity switch are located in your barber's shop. Make sure you know how to turn them off in case of an emergency, such as a burst pipe or electrical fire. Suggest they are labelled to help others find them in an emergency.

2   Examine your colleagues' hair and let them examine yours to assess each others' hair and scalp condition. Write down your findings and check your results with your manager or tutor.

3   Find out the range of expected service times for shampooing and conditioning in your barber's shop. What are the minimum and maximum times allowed? What maximum times are specified by your qualification?

Check your knowledge:

1   Describe dry shampooing

2   What are the main differences in shampooing in barber's shops when compared with unisex or women's salons?

3   What is the main purpose of shampooing?

4   List two causes of physical damage to the hair.

5   List the four main types of shampoo.

6   Describe how a detergent works.

7   What is the meaning of the term 'hydrophobic'?

   a. A substance that attracts water
   b. A substance that repels water
   c. A substance that attracts particles of dirt
   d. A substance that repels grease molecules

8   What is one benefit of using a substantive conditioner?

9   Provide two reasons for the importance of considering the hardness of water in shampooing and conditioning.

10   What is the normal pH value of skin?

   a. 2.5 to 3.5
   b. 3.5 to 4.5
   c. 4.5 to 5.5
   d. 5.5 to 6.5

11   What is the correct type of shampoo to use on greasy hair?

   a. Coconut
   b. Lemon
   c. Egg yolk
   d. Almond

12   To make sure the cold water is running really cold.

13   Describe the type of hair that benefits most from a conditioner containing catatonic polymers.

14   What should you look out for on the client's skin during consultation?

15   Describe the rotary massage movement.

16   What is one effect of the friction massage movement?

17   What is the importance of aftercare?

18   Why are manufacturer's instructions important?

19   Which one of the following is the most important reason why the cold water should be turned on first when rinsing the hair during shampooing?

   a. To prevent waste and reduce costs by using less hot water
   b. To rinse the basin clean before commencing the shampooing service
   c. To make sure the cold water is running really cold
   d. To prevent scalding by mixing the hot water into the cold water

20   Why is it important to keep the shower spray heads clear, especially in hard water areas?

6 Cutting facial hair using basic techniques

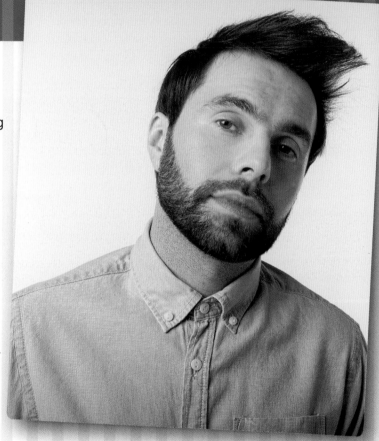

QUALIFICATION SIGNPOSTING

This chapter will help your studies of the following qualifications:

❖ Level 2 NVQ Diploma in Barbering.
❖ Level 3 NVQ Diploma in Barbering.
❖ City & Guilds Level 2 VRQ Certificate in Barbering Techniques.
❖ City & Guilds Level 2 VRQ Award, Certificate and Diploma in Barbering.
❖ City & Guilds Level 2 VRQ Diploma in Women's and Men's Hairdressing.
❖ City & Guilds Level 3 VRQ Diploma in Barbering.
❖ ITEC Level 2 and 3 VRQ Awards, Certificates and Diplomas in Barbering and Men's Hairdressing.
❖ VTCT Level 2 and 3 VRQ Certificates and Diplomas in Barbering.
❖ VTCT Level 2 and 3 VRQ Diploma in Barbering Studies.

For further information on the qualifications covered by this chapter see the qualification mapping grid at the front of the book.

LEARNING OBJECTIVES

In this chapter you will learn:

◆ The importance of cutting and styling facial hair in the barber's shop.

◆ The traditional and current facial hair shapes.

◆ The consultation requirements prior to cutting facial hair.

- About the tools and equipment used when cutting facial hair.

- How to prepare for cutting facial hair.

- The cutting techniques used for cutting facial hair.

- Facial haircutting procedures for beards, moustaches, sideburns and eyebrows.

- How to finish facial hair cutting.

- The aftercare advice necessary after facial hair cutting.

- The specific health and safety requirements for cutting facial hair.

INTRODUCTION

The beard and moustache have played an important role in men's fashions throughout the ages. At one time most men wore a beard, a moustache or long sideburns, but the popularity of the clean-shaven appearance increased following the introduction of safety razors and electric shavers. Today there is again a marked increase in the popularity of beards and moustaches, especially with young men, who now often wear short styles such as a goatee beard. Since 2003 the month of November each year has seen significantly more men around the world wearing moustaches. Starting in Melbourne, Australia November has increasingly been referred to as 'Movember' as during this month men around the world are challenged by the charity the 'Movember Foundation' to grow a moustache and raise funds and awareness for prostrate and testicular cancer and men's mental health. This introduces men new to wearing facial hair to the look of wearing a moustache. Some of these men will go on to try different facial hair shapes during the year. So, make sure your skills and barber's shop are ready to meet the needs of these new facial hair clients! For more information on the Movember Foundation visit their web page http://uk.movember.com/

This chapter looks at the basic techniques used for cutting facial hair to maintain existing shapes and covers:

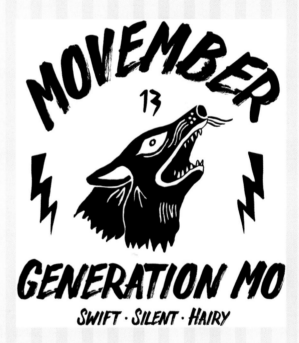

- Cutting and styling facial hair – including traditional and current shapes.

- Consultation prior to cutting facial hair.

- Tools and equipment.

- Preparation for cutting facial hair.

- Cutting techniques.

- Facial haircutting procedures.

- Finishing and aftercare advice.

- Health and safety.

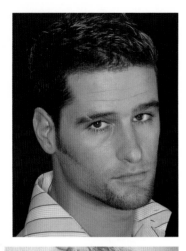

Cutting and styling facial hair

The purpose of cutting facial hair is both to shorten the hair and to style it into shape. This is achieved with scissors or clippers, which are usually used with a comb to perform cutting techniques described as 'scissors-over-comb' or 'clippers-over-comb'.

Sometimes clippers are used with a comb attachment such that the hair is cut at a predetermined length. This attachment is relatively easy to use, and has become popular with many men for keeping their beards and moustaches in shape between barber's shop visits.

Traditional and current beard and moustache shapes

Over the years many beard, moustache and sideburn shapes have been developed – sometimes eyebrows have also been shaped, although most often this work has just been to reduce their length and baulk. Some shapes can be described as traditional, as men first started wearing them many hundreds of years ago. Some of these traditional shapes may also be described as being current shapes, because men today are still wearing the shape or because the shape is currently fashionable. Yet other shapes are new, as they have only just been developed for the look that men like today: these too can be described as current shapes.

The barber must be familiar with many different traditional and current shapes, and able to visualize the right shape for each client and advise them accordingly. Here are some basic beard and moustache shapes for you to consider.

In the past beards, moustaches and sideburns would often be dressed into different styles using various dressings, **pomades** or wax. These made the hair very stiff and enabled the wearer to create intricate styles, such as the traditional handlebar moustache. Dressing creams, pomades, waxes and gels are sometimes used to style facial hair today, but usually only to smooth stray hairs or to create definition or texture on longer beards.

> ### KEY DEFINITION
>
> Pomade: A substance or ointment used to groom and fix the hair in place. Originally oil or wax based and shiny in appearance but now may be water based for easier removal.

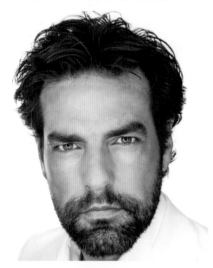

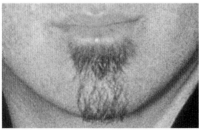

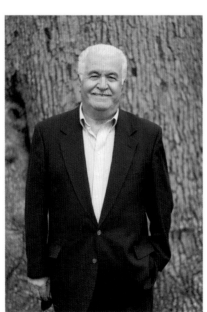

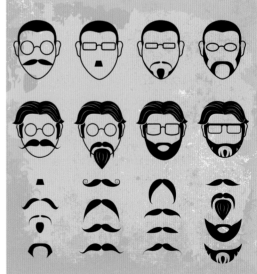

Examples of facial hair shapes

Consultation prior to cutting facial hair

When cutting to maintain the beard, moustache or sideburn shape it is important to consider the client's face shape and hairstyle. You should think of these as being integrated parts of one style, or one total look and trim the facial hair – be it beard or moustache, sideburn or eyebrow shape to suit.

Men are often very particular about their beard, so before you start work carefully consider each of the following factors.

◆ What does the client want?

◆ Why does he have a beard or moustache or long sideburns?

◆ Look for signs of broken skin, abnormalities on the skin, or any unusual facial features or beard growth patterns – are there any contraindications?

◆ What is the facial hair type – type S1, W2, C3 or K4?

◆ What are the facial hair characteristics –

◆ Is the beard hair fine, medium or coarse?

◆ Is the beard growth dense or sparse?

◆ Does the density of beard growth vary around the face?

◆ Pay attention to the client's face shape.

◆ Pay attention to the length and shape of his hairstyle.

HEALTH & SAFETY

Before you start cutting, you must carry out a thorough consultation. Be sure to identify any **adverse conditions** of the hair or skin that may be present. It is particularly important to establish whether you have reason to suspect any infection or infestation, as this would prevent you from cutting the facial hair.

Hair growth patterns

Hair growth patterns are the way in which individual hairs or a section of the beard may grow in a particular direction. Hair growth patterns must be identified because they determine both the shape that can be created and the techniques that you should use. Some clients have very strong hair growth patterns in their beard, such as hair whorls: these should be cut by following the direction of hair growth around the whorl.

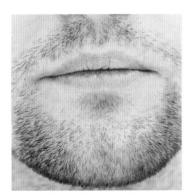

Hair growth patterns

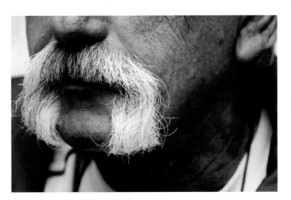

Short horseshoe moustache

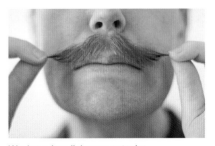

Waxing a handlebar moustache

See **CHAPTER 4** pages 60–62 for full details of hair types and classifications.

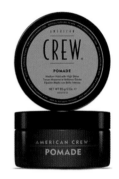

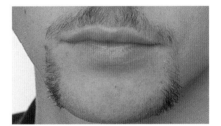

Thin Mexican moustache

It may help you to read **CHAPTER 4**, 'Client care for men' for more detailed information on consultation before reading this section.

KEY DEFINITION

Adverse conditions: Conditions on the client's face or facial hair that may affect what services can be provided or change how the service should be provided.

TIP ✓

It is usually far better to go *with* the direction of beard growth than to go against it, especially when cutting strong growth patterns.

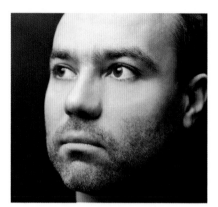

Dense facial hair growth

TIP ✓

Especially with new clients, it is important when cutting existing beard shapes to look for variations in the density of growth: the hair may have been left long in some areas to disguise very sparse growth or to cover a scar. Cutting the hair too short in these areas would expose the skin, and might well annoy or embarrass the client.

Different face shapes require different beard and moustache shapes. These are explained in more detail in CHAPTER 14, 'Designing facial hair shapes'.

Texture

The texture of hair in a beard, sideburn or eyebrow can be fine, medium or coarse. Young men usually have fine facial hair, but as men get older their facial hair often becomes much coarser. Fine hair and hair types S1 and W2a and b are usually easier to cut, but some fuller styles will be more difficult to create. Coarse hair, particularly hair types W2c, C3 and K4 are often more difficult to cut, and is liable to fly in all directions during cutting – extra care must be taken to protect the client's and your own eyes. Coarser hair lends itself to many different beard shapes, but you must also consider the density of growth.

Density

Hair density is the amount of hair that grows in a given area of skin. Some men have a very dense beard growth, which is sometimes known as a *blue beard* because the density of growth gives the skin a blue tinge which remains even after shaving. Indeed, this could be the main reason why the client has grown a beard.

The density of beard growth often varies around the face. Some men have dense growth around their chin, cheeks and top lip, but sparse growth between the bottom lip and chin. Others have dense growth only on their top lip. Yet others have dense growth everywhere except on the top lip. And in others the density of growth may be very sparse, preventing the client from growing certain beard or moustache shapes.

Face shape and facial features

It is important to identify the client's face shape and consider his facial features so that you can avoid damage to the skin and so that you can maintain the most suitable shape. You must make careful note of the following:

◆ The size and position of the mouth.

◆ The width of the top lip.

◆ The shape of the nose.

◆ The shape of the jaw and chin.

◆ Any unusual features, such as moles, dimples or scarring.

Features on a face

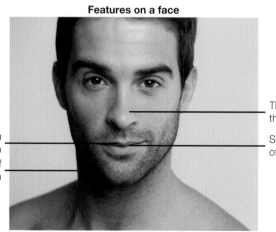

The shape of the nose

Size and position of the mouth

The width of the top lip

The shape of the jaw and chin

HEALTH & SAFETY

Take extra care when cutting very coarse or dense beards. The hair is liable to fly in all directions while it is being cut. If necessary, make sure the client's eyes are well protected with clean cotton wool pads or tissues, and keep your own face well away from the work. If you find the hair is very strong and springy, you may need to wear safety glasses to protect your eyes.

EDWARD HEMMINGS Creative Director at Alan d Hairdressing Education

" A beard, sideburns or moustache, and often all three are important style features for many men. And eyebrows are certainly the norm! Without good skills in cutting all types of facial hair the barber will likely not meet these clients' needs or those of their barbering business. "

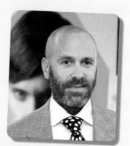

Tools and equipment

Tools

All haircutting tools must be well-balanced, sharp, clean and safe to use. Here are the main tools required for cutting facial hair.

Scissors Scissors are available in different sizes, ranging from 10 cm to 18 cm in length. Most barbers prefer scissors around 15 cm, but you need to find out what feels comfortable given the size of your hand and the job you are doing.

Thinning scissors are used to remove bulk without removing length.

Read the section on haircutting tools in CHAPTER 7, 'Cutting men's hair using basic techniques'; the information and rules explained there also apply to tools for cutting facial hair.

TIP ✓

◆ Use the mirror regularly during cutting to ensure that the shape is centralized and symmetrical.
◆ Pay particular attention to where the beard or sideburns meet the hairstyle, and ensure that they blend together.

Clippers Clippers may be either hand-operated or electric. Hand clippers are not usually used today unless electricity is unavailable, such as during a power cut.

Electric clippers may be powered by either mains electricity or rechargeable batteries. They are the preferred choice today because of their power, accuracy and convenience when compared to hand clippers. They are used to create outlines or when using clippers-over-comb techniques. Detachable comb attachments are also available, which give a wide range of predetermined cutting lengths. These allow for very fast removal of hair and are sometimes used to reduce the length of the beard, which is then finished with scissors and clippers (without the comb attached).

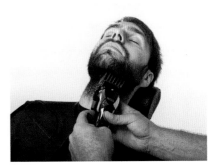

Using clippers with comb attached

Razors Razors are sometimes used to shave part of the face, to emphasize the beard or moustache style. Disposable-blade razors are best because they are more hygienic.

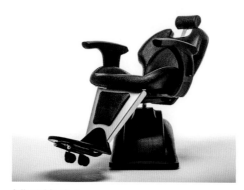

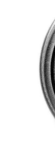

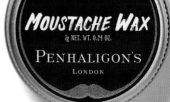

Adjustable chair

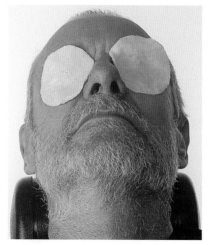

A prepared client – cotton pads should protect the eyes where necessary

Equipment

The client should be seated in an adjustable chair which can be positioned so that the client can recline comfortably. The chair should have a headrest and the height of the chair should be adjustable so that you do not have to bend uncomfortably.

Preparation for cutting facial hair

1   Carry out your consultation with the client. Look for signs of broken skin, abnormalities on the skin, and unusual beard growth patterns.

2   Determine the client's wishes and confirm what is to be done.

3   Position the client in a reclining chair so that you can work on the beard. Ensure you provide support for his head.

4   Before you begin work, gather together all the tools and equipment you will need.

5   Gown the client and place a clean towel across their chest, tucked in at the neck.

6   Where necessary, protect the client's eyes with tissue or cotton wool pads that have been moistened with warm water. The moisture helps the pads stay in place and will be soothing for the eyes. Make sure the tissue or pads are not *too* wet, however: they should be nearly dry.

7   Carefully comb the beard, disentangling the hair as necessary. Look out for areas of sparse growth, scarring or other unusual features you may not have seen earlier.

Scissors-over-comb technique

Cutting techniques

The following cutting techniques are commonly used when cutting facial hair to shape.

Scissors-over-comb Scissors-over-comb cutting is performed by first lifting a section of hair, and then cutting straight across. When cutting beards and moustaches you should take small sections of hair: these are usually lifted with the comb as the hair is quite short. Some barbers, especially when working on longer hair, use the tips of their scissors to lift the sections of hair: the hair is then picked up on the comb and positioned ready for cutting.

Scissors-over-comb is often used to create graduated effects by adjusting the angle and length of each section. Be sure to use the fine teeth of the comb and the tips of the scissors when working around the lips.

Accompanying video available for scissors-over-comb. Please scan this QR code.

Clippers-over-comb Clippers-over-comb or trimmer-over-comb cutting is often used instead of scissors-over-comb techniques, especially on longer, coarser and denser beards. Generally, the same effects possible with scissors can be achieved using clippers. Smaller clippers or trimmers are easier to use on moustaches and when working around the lips, as the blades are smaller and more accurate.

Freehand cutting Freehand cutting is the cutting of hair without first taking the hair into a section or holding the hair in place with the comb or hand. It is often used to remove individual hairs or small amounts of hair when finishing a style, and is usually performed with the tips of the scissors. When cutting beards and moustaches it is used to smooth the outline shape and remove stray hairs.

Razoring Razoring is sometimes used to create clean outlines and emphasize a shape. It is performed with a razor, which may be either an open razor or a safety razor. Disposable-blade razors are best because they are more hygienic. Electric razors are also sometimes used.

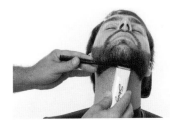

Trimmer-over-comb technique

Accompanying video available for trimmer-over-comb. Please scan this QR code.

Cutting procedures

THE SHORT BEARD

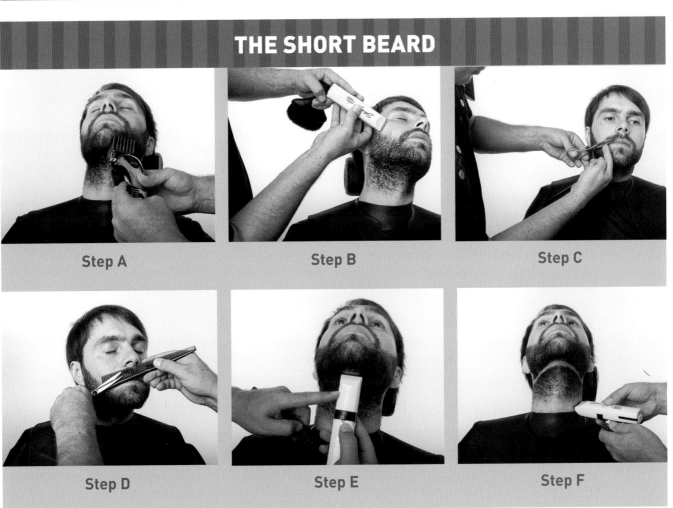

Step A

Step B

Step C

Step D

Step E

Step F

(continued)

THE SHORT BEARD (*Continued*)

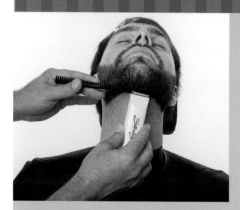 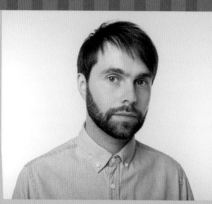 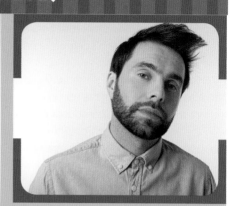

Step G   **Step H**

1. Protect the client's clothes and eyes and if necessary protect their eyes with dampened cotton wool pads. Comb the beard carefully, disentangling the hair where required.

2. Start at one side of your client and begin cutting the beard hair, using the scissors- or clippers-over-comb technique or, as here using a clipper attachment. Again, make sure you blend the beard and head hair to suit the overall look (a).

3. Keep working down the side of the face, cutting the hair to the length determined by the beard shape. Do not cut the moustache at this stage. If the beard shape is to be longer towards the chin you should gradually increase the length as you work down the beard.

4. Repeat this on the other side. Keep looking in the mirror to make sure that the beard is symmetrical.

5. Move to the centre of the beard and cut the hair, using scissors- or clippers-over-comb techniques or the clipper attachment. Blend the two sides into the final shape. If you wish to create a pointed beard, angle your comb towards the point of the chin; otherwise blend the two sides together to create an even, continuous effect.

6. Cut the other outlines on the cheeks, chin or above the moustache, as required. Refer to the mirror to keep the outlines symmetrical (b).

7. Move to one side of the moustache. Carefully outline the moustache along the top lip to create the required shape, using the tips of your scissors or the trimmers (c).

8. Repeat this on the other side of the moustache.

9. Using your comb, lift small sections of the moustache hair and cut this to the required length using scissors or clippers (d). The clipper attachment is not really suitable here.

10. Blend the moustache into the beard, as required by the overall shape.

11. Lift the client's chin and carefully cut the neck outline to the correct height (e). The best height is usually about 2 cm below the jawline, but always consider your client's wishes.

12. The neck outline may be graduated to create a natural effect, or cut into a clean line for a more defined look. The centre of the outline (below the chin) should be cut slightly higher than at the sides to compensate for the skin in the centre moving further up as the head goes back. The difference should be about 1 cm. This will appear level when the head is returned to its normal position (f). Remove hair outside of this line.

13. If necessary, shave the areas outside the outlines (see Chapter 12).

14. Graduate the outlines to blend them with the skin, where required (g).

15. Finish the shape by combing the hair into place (h).

HEALTH & SAFETY

◆ Always protect the client's eyes from hairs, which may fly up during cutting, especially on very coarse beards. Keep your own face away from your work; wear safety glasses for protection.

◆ To ensure the client's comfort, remove excess hair cuttings from his face and neck at frequent intervals.

Accompanying video available for cutting the neck outline. Please scan QR code.

TIP ✓

The procedure for cutting a short beard into shape is basically the same as for cutting a long beard, but many barbers use a clipper attachment to first cut the beard to a predetermined length, and then finish with scissors and comb.

TIP ✓

◆ When determining the correct height for the neck outline you should consider the overall shape and length of the beard. If the outline is too low it will be visible below the chin when viewed from the front: this can appear untidy. If it is too high, however, the outline will be visible across the side of the face.

◆ Outlines can be achieved by cutting the hair either with close-cutting clippers or with an electric razor. The outline hair may also be removed completely by shaving with a razor, which should be used following the shaving procedure described in Chapter 12, Shaving services.

It may help you to read CHAPTER 12, 'Shaving services' for more information on shaving around outlines of the facial hair shape.

THE LONG BEARD

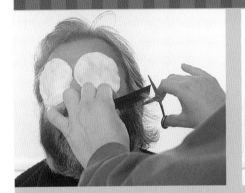
Step A

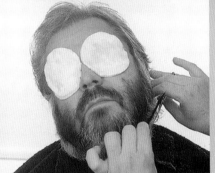
Step B

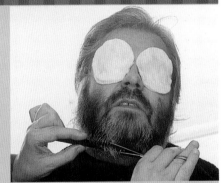
Step C

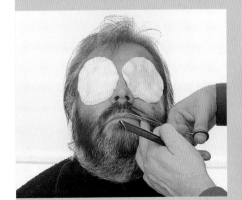
Step D

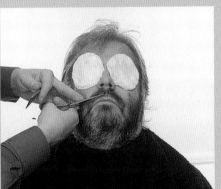
Step E

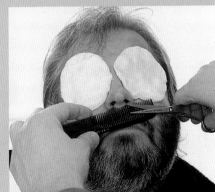
Step F

(continued)

THE LONG BEARD (Continued)

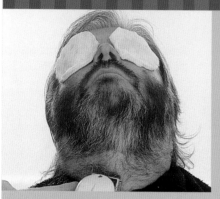

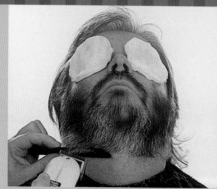

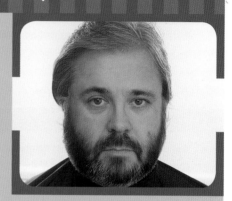

Step G   **Step H**   **Step I**

1. Protect the client's clothes and if necessary protect their eyes with dampened cotton wool pads. Comb the beard carefully, disentangling the hair where required.

2. Start at one side of your client (it does not matter which), and begin cutting the beard hair using the scissors- or clippers-over-comb technique (a). Start in the area where the sideburns join the head hair. Make sure you blend the beard and head hair to suit the overall look.

3. Keep working down the side of the face (b), cutting the hair to the length determined by the beard shape. Do not cut the moustache at this stage. If the beard is to be longer towards the chin you should gradually increase the length as you work down the beard.

4. Repeat this on the other side. As the shape develops, keep looking in the mirror to make sure that the beard is symmetrical.

5. Move to the centre of the beard and cut the hair using scissors- or clippers-over-comb technique, as before (c). Take small sections, blending the two sides into the final shape. If you wish to create a pointed beard, angle your comb towards the point of the chin; otherwise blend the two sides together to create an even, continuous effect.

6. Move to one side of the moustache. Carefully outline the moustache along the top lip to create the required shape, using the tips of your scissors or the clippers (d). Use the fingers of your other hand to guide and support the scissors or clippers whilst cutting.

7. Repeat this on the other side of the moustache (e).

8. Using your comb, lift small sections of the moustache hair and cut this to the required length. Use the tips of your scissors and small, careful movements (f).

9. Blend the moustache into the beard, as required by the overall shape.

10. Lift the client's chin and carefully cut the neck outline to the correct height (g).

11. Cut the other outlines on the cheeks, chin or above the moustache, as required. Refer to the mirror to keep the outlines symmetrical.

12. Shave the areas outside the outlines if necessary (see Chapter 12).

13. Graduate the outlines to blend them with the skin, where required (h).

14. Finish the shape by combing the hair into place (i).

TIP ✓

Cut the centre of the outline below the chin around 1 cm higher than at the sides to compensate for the skin moving up whilst the head is held back.

ACTIVITY: CASE STUDY – ANDREW

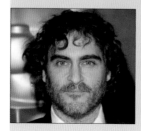

Andrew is a 30-year-old new client in your barber's shop. He requests that you reshape his contemporary beard look. During the consultation you notice he has a harelip. Describe the action that should be taken regarding Andrew's request?

TIP ✓

Commercial service times for cutting facial hair
You must allow sufficient time for the facial hair cutting service to be completed correctly but within the maximum time allowed by your barber's shop. Remember that your work must not appear to be rushed and your client's needs must be met, but you must work within commercial times.

A CONTEMPORARY FACIAL HAIR LOOK–GOATEE BEARD

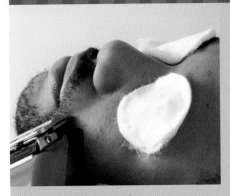

Step A

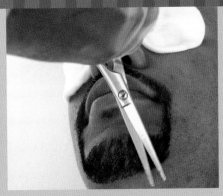

Step B

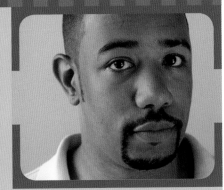

Step C

1. Prepare the client, protect the eyes if necessary and detangle the facial hair.
2. Start at one side of your client and begin cutting the beard to the correct length. Scissors or clippers-over-comb or a clipper comb attachment can be used as preferred.
3. Keep working down the side of the face, cutting the hair to the length determined by the beard shape.
4. Repeat this on the other side. Keep looking in the mirror to make sure that the beard is symmetrical.
5. Blend the two sides into the final shape.
6. Cut the outlines on the cheeks, chin and above the moustache, as required. Refer to the mirror to keep the outlines symmetrical (a).
7. Graduate the outlines to blend them with the skin, where required. Use freehand cutting to remove any stray hairs and ensure an even finish (b).
8. Finish the shape by combing the hair into place (c).

ACTIVITY: CASE STUDY – BOB

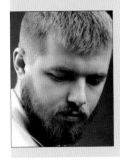

Bob is a regular client in your barber's shop. He requests that you reshape his long beard – it has been 3 months since his last beard trim due to his working away and he hasn't even shaved. Bob wants the neckline redefined and the hair outside removed, although not shaved. During the consultation you notice he has a strong hair whorl directly under the centre of his chin. What action should be taken regarding Bob's request?

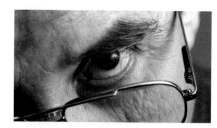

Eyebrow shaping

The client's eyebrows may need cutting and shaping as part of the haircut or facial hair cutting service. Younger men don't often need eyebrow work but as men get older the eyebrows can become very long and coarse and your client may want them trimmed.

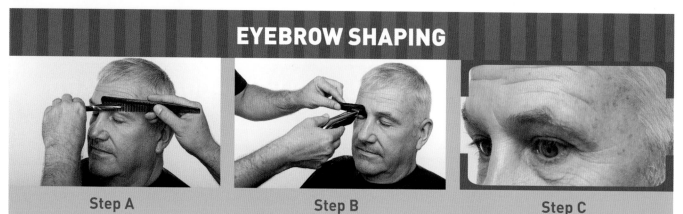

EYEBROW SHAPING

| Step A | Step B | Step C |

Make sure you can offer this service, here is a method used:

1. Prepare the client and detangle the hair.
2. Start at one side of your client and begin cutting the hair using scissors-over-comb (a). Remember to brush away hair cuttings from the client's face to maintain their comfort.
3. Repeat the cutting process on the other side. Clippers-over-comb can also be used, although cordless trimmers are easier to use around the eyes than corded clippers (b). Keep looking in the mirror to make sure that the eyebrows are even and symmetrical.
4. If required eyebrows can be outlined by carefully moving the trimmers along the top outline, similar to outlining a beard. Remember to refer to the mirror so that the outlines are symmetrical. Make sure not to cut into the main eyebrow shape as the effect would appear unnatural (c).
5. Finish the eyebrow shape by combing the hair into place.

Finishing and aftercare advice

Threading Some barbers' shops now offer threading services that can be used as an alternative to trimmers when shaping the eyebrow outline. See CHAPTER 1, 'Barbering – from its origins to the present day' for more information.

After cutting a styling aid may be applied to help smooth the hair, particularly on longer beard and moustache shapes. Use the mirror regularly to check the balance and symmetry of the shape as you dress it.

Comb the client's head hair into style, if required, and allow the client to see your work.

Remember to advise your client on how to maintain their look at home. Here are some ways you can help them achieve good results:

◆ Products to use – suggest which products will help them maintain and improve their facial skin and hair. Remember to stress that facial hair benefits from the use of shampoo and conditioner rather than soap, particularly long beard shapes. This is a good opportunity to highlight the benefits of these and any finishing products you have used and to recommend they buy these from your barber's shop.

◆ How to use products – show the client how the products should be used to achieve the best effects (you can highlight this to them as you style and finish their hair). Help them find and understand the manufacturer's instructions.

◆ How to maintain and style their facial hair look – show the client where to shave outside the outline shape. Discuss good grooming techniques – regular combing, cleaning, exfoliating and moisturising. Answer any questions the client may have.

◆ When the next barber's shop appointment should be made – remember that facial hair will usually soon become untidy and the next cut required within 4 weeks. Encourage the client to book before leaving if your barber's shop has an appointments system.

Health and safety

Read CHAPTER 13, 'Face massage services' for further information on good skincare routines.

Everyone in the barber's shop has a duty to work safely and keep their environment safe. It is particularly important to consider health and safety when cutting facial hair because of the risks associated with using electricity and the risk of cutting the skin.

Here are some important health and safety factors that you must consider when providing haircutting services:

Avoid infection

It may help you to read CHAPTER 2, 'Health and safety in the barber's shop' for general information on working safely in the barber's shop.

◆ If the client has any cuts or abrasions on his face, or you suspect that an infection or infestation is present, you must not carry out the work.

◆ Pay special attention to hygiene when cutting facial hair, because of the risk of cross-infection through open cuts.

◆ Use only clean tools and equipment.

Protect the eyes

◆ You must make sure that the client's eyes are protected from hairs during cutting. Asking the client to close their eyes is the minimum requirement but you must use tissues or cotton wool pads if the hair cuttings are likely to fly up over the face. Keep your own face away from your work too; if necessary, wear safety glasses.

Work safely with razors

◆ Open and safety razors have very sharp blades and must always be handled and used with great care.

◆ When it is not being used or when it is being carried, always close the handle to protect the blade of an open razor.

◆ Never place razors or other cutting tools in your pockets.

◆ Always sterilize a fixed-blade razor before each use.

◆ When using a detachable-blade open razor, always use a new blade for each new client.

◆ Used razor blades, called sharps, must be disposed of correctly in accordance with your barber's shop policy. Soiled disposable materials should be placed in sealed plastic bags for removal.

Work safely with electricity

◆ Always handle and use electrical equipment with care, and in accordance with the manufacturers' instructions.

◆ Never place or use electric clippers or other electrical equipment near water.

◆ Do not go near electrical equipment that is lying in water – first switch off the power at the mains.

◆ Before commencing work, visually check that electrical equipment is safe to use. Check that the cable has not frayed or been pulled, and that the plug is not loose.

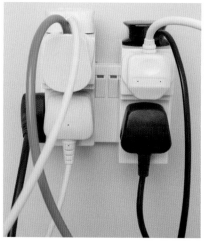

When using and storing electrical equipment, pay attention to the position of cables.

Never overload sockets. Do not plug too many items of electrical equipment into the same socket.

Follow the manufacturer's instructions for the care of your clippers. To avoid damage, be sure to clean and lubricate the blades regularly.

Electrical equipment must be regularly tested, and given a certificate of testing confirming that it is safe for use. The barber's shop owner will ensure that this is carried out, as required.

Be prepared for accidents

Make sure that you know the whereabouts of your barber's shop's first-aid kit.

Keep yourself up-to-date with your barber's shop's first-aid and accident procedures.

Don't overload electrical outlets!

IMAGE GALLERY

Visit the online image gallery on this book's accompanying website to see other inspirational men's beard and moustache shapes.

BRINGING IT ALL TOGETHER

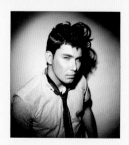

Summary

1   Facial hair is cut to shorten the hair and to style it into shape. This is achieved with scissors or clippers, which are usually used with a comb to perform cutting techniques described as 'scissors-over-comb' or 'clippers-over-comb', or with a clipper attachment.

◆ In the past beards, moustaches and sideburns would often be dressed into different styles using various dressings, pomades or wax.

◆ Wearing a beard or moustache is increasingly popular. The 'Movember' charity has particularly encouraged men to grow a moustache during November each year.

2   The client's beard, moustache or sideburn shape, face shape and hairstyle should be thought of as being integrated parts of one style.

◆ The facial hair type and characteristics affect how the hair is cut:

    i. Hair types W2c, C3 and K4 are often more difficult to cut.

    ii. Young men usually have fine facial hair, but as men get older their facial hair often becomes much coarser.

    iii. Coarse hair is often more difficult to cut, and is liable to fly in all directions during cutting – extra care must be taken to protect the client's and your own eyes.

    iv. The density of beard growth often varies around the face.

3 Use the mirror regularly during cutting to ensure that the shape is centralized and symmetrical.

4 Prepare the hair by combing out any tangles using a comb with widely spaced teeth.

5 Clippers-over-comb cutting is often used instead of scissors-over-comb techniques, especially on longer, coarser and denser beards.

6 When determining the correct height for the neck outline you should consider the overall shape and length of the beard. If the outline is too low it will be visible below the chin when viewed from the front: this can appear untidy.

7 Cut the centre of the outline below the chin around 1 cm higher than at the sides to compensate for the skin moving up whilst the head is held back.

8 Remember to stress that facial hair benefits from the use of shampoo and conditioner rather than soap, particularly long beard shapes.

9 Never place razors or other cutting tools in your pockets.

◆ Before commencing work, visually check that electrical equipment is safe to use – check that the cable has not frayed or been pulled, and that the plug is not loose.

10 Always handle and use electrical equipment with care, and in accordance with the manufacturers' instructions.

Activities

1 Visit a library or use the Internet to research the different types of traditional beard shapes that have been popular in different eras over the past 2000 years. Compare these to shapes worn today and note the key differences.

2 Find out the range of expected service times for cutting facial hair in your barber's shop. What are the minimum and maximum times allowed? What maximum times are specified by your qualification?

Check your knowledge

1 Describe the differences between traditional and current beard and moustache shapes.

2 Describe a hair whorl.

3 Which of the following facial hair types is usually the easiest to cut?

    a. S1b

    b. K4a

    c. W2c

    d. C3a

4 Describe how hair density affects the choice of facial hair shape.

5 List five facial features that must be considered before cutting facial hair.

6 Describe the beard and moustache shapes most suited to a client with a long face.

7 State when razors would be used in cutting beards and moustaches.

8 List two reasons for using freehand techniques when cutting beards and moustaches into shape.

9 Describe the special safety precautions that must be taken into account when cutting facial hair that are not normally required when cutting hair.

10 Describe how to check that electrical equipment is safe before use.

11 Where should razors never be placed?

12 Which of the following statements is correct?

    a. The outline under the chin should be cut straight across so that it appears level.

    b. The outline under the chin should be cut higher in the middle so that it appears level.

7 Cutting men's hair using basic techniques

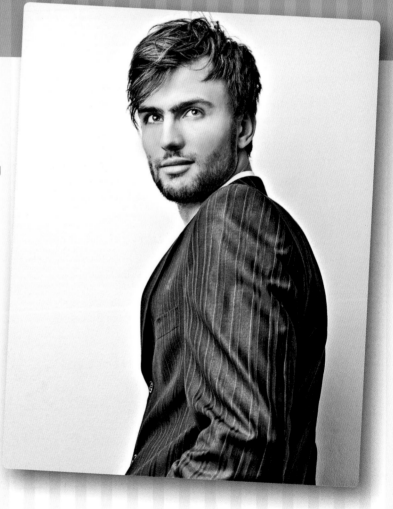

QUALIFICATION SIGNPOSTING

This chapter will help your studies of the following qualifications:

❖ Level 2 NVQ Awards and Diploma in Barbering.

❖ City & Guilds VRQ Level 2 Award, Certificate and Diploma in Barbering.

❖ ITEC Level 2 VRQ Award, Certificate and Diplomas in Barbering and Men's Hairdressing.

❖ VTCT Level 2 VRQ Certificates and Diplomas in Barbering and Barbering Studies.

For further information on the qualifications covered by this chapter see the qualification mapping grid at the front of the book.

LEARNING OBJECTIVES

In this chapter you will learn:

◆ About cutting and styling men's hair – including barbering principles for outlines, sideburns and neckline shapes.

◆ The consultation requirements prior to cutting men's hair.

◆ About the tools and equipment used.

◆ How to prepare for cutting men's hair.

◆ About the cutting techniques – including wet and dry cutting.

◆ The cutting procedures.

◆ About finishing the haircut.

◆ About aftercare for cutting hair.

◆ The health and safety requirements for cutting hair.

INTRODUCTION

Competent haircutting is the foundation of all good hairdressing, and cutting skills are amongst the most important that any hairdresser has. These skills are particularly important to the barber because most clients visiting the barber's shop want their hair cut. Indeed, some barbers perform few, if any, other services.

This chapter looks at the basic techniques the barber uses for cutting men's hair. It covers the following topics:

❖ Cutting and styling men's hair – including barbering principles for outlines, sideburns and neckline shapes

❖ Consultation prior to cutting men's hair.

❖ Tools and equipment.

❖ Preparation for cutting men's hair.

❖ Cutting techniques – including wet and dry cutting.

❖ Cutting procedures.

❖ Finishing.

❖ Aftercare.

❖ Health and safety.

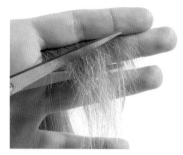

Split ends

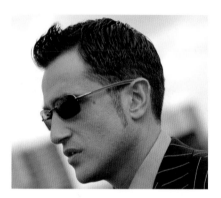

Cutting and styling men's hair

The main purpose of cutting hair is to style the hair into shape. Both the hair length and the hair thickness can be removed, either to create a completely new look or just to **trim** the client's current look back into shape. Cutting also removes any split ends (*fragilitas crinium*) that may be present, thereby improving the condition and appearance of the hair.

Men's haircutting is achieved with scissors and clippers, although razors are also sometimes used as required to shave the outlines, thin the hair or produce textured effects. Club cutting with scissors-over-comb and clippers-over-comb techniques is most often required.

Sometimes the clippers are used with a comb attachment that positions the blades to cut the hair at a predetermined length. These are particularly useful for creating short looks on longer hair, as the long hair can be removed quickly and easily to produce a rough shape ready for finishing.

The haircut

The haircut has an important role in all hairdressing because it is the basis on which all other hairstyling takes place. It determines how the hair can be later dressed and styled, and how easy that styling will be. A good haircut design should make the client look and feel good and will be easy to manage. Indeed, remember that most men want a style that is 'easy to maintain'.

Barbering Principles There are many similarities between cutting men's hair and women's hair. Often the same cutting techniques can be used and sometimes men and women wear the same looks, but there are usually subtle differences in the shapes that are required and in the methods that are used to achieve them. **Barbering principles** have evolved over time as being particularly suitable for dealing with the **characteristics** that typically affect men's hair and for creating the most suitable men's hairstyles and beard and moustache shapes. Facial hair, dense hair growth on the neck and male-pattern alopecia (baldness), which usually occur in men only, must be especially considered.

There are also distinct differences between masculine and feminine shapes. Masculine shapes are usually more square and angular and are suited to most men, while feminine

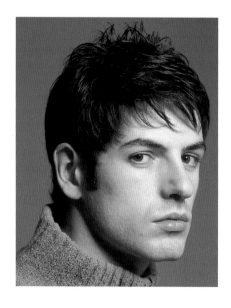

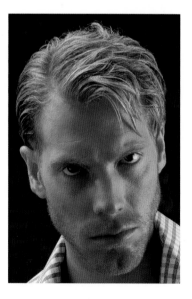

shapes tend to be fuller and more rounded. Taller, less full or leaner shapes are also more flattering on most men, so minimal thickness at the back and sides is often required.

Remember that these are just basic principles, however: they should be adapted to take account of factors such as the client's wishes, his face shape and his hair growth patterns. The client consultation will help you determine which of these shapes is best suited to the particular client.

Most men, and many women too, wear short layered looks. These are popular because they require minimal blow-styling and dressing, and so are easy for clients to maintain. Many of these haircuts are so short that the styling details are quite subtle: precise cutting movements and accurate cutting angles are required. Often only very small amounts of hair are removed at a time until the desired effect is achieved – great care is needed, as the hair is too short to hide any mistakes. Most short layered looks are graduated at the back and sides. The outlines of these haircuts are often emphasized, and these require careful attention.

Cutting outlines

Many men have dense hair growth outside the natural hairline, particularly on the face and in the nape areas, whereas most women have soft, natural hairlines with few hairs growing outside. On women the outline usually requires little further definition, but on most men the haircut must be outlined or it appears untidy and unfinished.

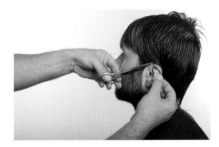

Cutting outlines around the ears

In the past, outlines were cut with scissors and by shaving. The shaving was performed with an open razor and was used to remove all unwanted hair from outside the haircut outline. This produced a smooth, close finish that helped to extend the life of the haircut as the hair took longer to grow back. Today, outlines are usually shaped with the points of the scissors and with electric clippers, which can cut the hair nearly as close as when shaved. Shaving is still used sometimes, when a particularly close finish is required. Many barbers use both scissors and clippers throughout the outlining of a haircut. The choice of tool and technique is determined both by the needs of the haircut and by the barber's personal preference.

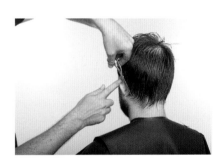

Cutting the outline into the nape

Here are some important points to remember about outlining men's haircuts:

◆ On most men the haircut must be outlined or it will appear untidy and unfinished.

◆ Follow the natural hairline wherever possible, particularly when outlining short haircuts. Avoid making unnecessary cuts into the natural hairline, especially around the ears and at the sides of the nape. (Such cuts would appear harsh and unnatural, and the haircut would soon appear untidy when the hair started to grow back.)

◆ Many outlines, particularly on shorter styles, appear more natural if they are gently tapered in the nape and at the bottom of the sideburns.

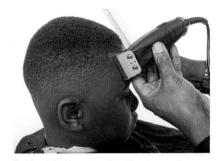

Cutting into the natural outline to create definition

◆ Some African-Caribbean men have outlines created at the front to add definition to their style.

DON'T BE TEMPTED   X

In basic work the key barbering principles should be followed closely. In advanced work the principles are more flexible, but even then they are still considered and followed unless the look specifically requires a different approach. Don't be tempted to break them without good reason or the lack of barbering knowledge will be obvious to all in the resulting haircut!

TIP   ✓

Remember: barbering principles are especially important when cutting outlines!

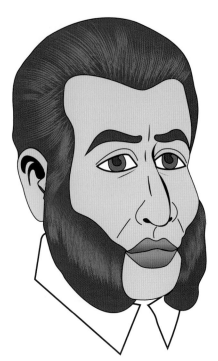

Mutton chops sideburns

Cutting sideburns

At one time most men wore a beard, a moustache or long sideburns. The sideburns were often grown so long that they reached the bottom of the jawbone, and long distinctive sideburn shapes such as mutton chops became a prominent feature in men's fashion for many years. The introduction of the safety razor in about 1905 helped to establish the popularity of the clean-shaven appearance, and men started wearing their sideburns much shorter.

Today, sideburns are important in most men's haircuts, particularly on shorter styles because the sideburns are more visible. Many young men are now wearing longer sideburns, often shaped into points or other more elaborate designs. Most men, however, want sideburn shapes that are less prominent, with the emphasis on creating a natural, balanced look. The face shape and the hairstyle should be used to determine the correct choice of sideburn shape for each client.

Here are some important points to remember about cutting sideburns:

◆ Most men's haircuts are improved by having sideburns. When cut to the correct length sideburns help to balance the haircut and create an attractive, masculine frame to the face.

◆ Avoid cutting the length of the sideburns higher than the top of the ear and into the hairline, as this creates a particularly harsh and unnatural effect. Men sometimes do this inadvertently when shaving, so offer advice on how to avoid this (see the tip below and Chapter 12, 'Shaving services').

◆ A drop of about 2 cm from the top of the ear is often acceptable, but remember to take into account other factors.

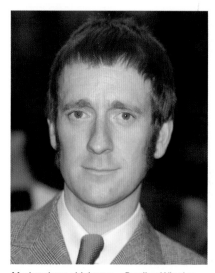

Modern long sideburns – Bradley Wiggins

It may help you to read CHAPTER 6, 'Cutting facial hair using basic techniques' for more detailed information on cutting facial hair.

TIP ✓

To ensure that the sideburns are cut level, place the thumb of each hand high on each sideburn. Whilst looking in the mirror, slide one thumb down until the desired length is reached. Slide the other thumb down until both thumbs are level. Memorize the position of the thumbs – you can note a position on each ear as a point of reference. Now cut each sideburn to the correct length.

Consider sharing this tip with your clients, many of whom may have difficulty keeping their sideburns level when shaving.

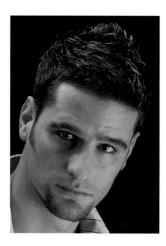
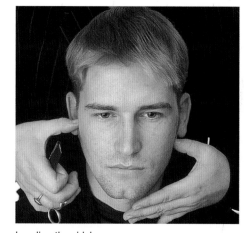

Leveling the sideburns

◆ Always ensure that the sideburns are cut level. Do not use the ears to determine the level of the sideburns, as they themselves are seldom level.

◆ Pay particular attention to where the haircut meets the sideburns and ensure that they blend together. You should think of these as being integrated parts of one style. Do not cut straight across the sideburns when outlining the haircut – this would produce a line across the sideburn through which the skin could be seen. The sideburns should be outlined by following down their natural hairline, adjacent to the ear.

> **TIP** ✓
>
> Remember: it is especially important to follow barbering principles when cutting necklines on shorter layered looks!

Neckline shapes

The outline of the haircut in the nape is called the neckline shape. The neckline is particularly important in men's hairdressing: the neckline is often visible and the natural neck hairline is usually less well defined as hair often grows densely on the neck.

Over the years three basic neckline shapes have been developed to produce the looks that men like whilst ensuring that the haircut does not become untidy too quickly when the neck hair grows back. The three shapes are:

◆ *Squared neckline shapes* These are sometimes known as a square cut.

◆ *Tapered neckline shapes* These are sometimes known as a taper cut or fade cut.

◆ *Rounded neckline shapes* These are sometimes known as a Boston neckline.

Cutting a squared neckline

Squared neckline shapes Squared neckline shapes have clean distinct outlines that form a square shape. They can be achieved with scissors or electric clippers, which are often inverted and used to cut the neckline straight across. The neckline should be cut into a square corner where it meets the outline at the sides of the nape.

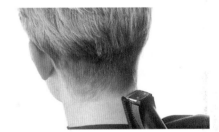

Cutting a squared neckline

These outlines must be cut to follow the natural hairline, or a true square-cut shape will not be produced. Do not make any cuts into these outlines, as they would appear harsh and unnatural and the removed hair would soon grow back to make the haircut appear untidy. If required, the square-cut neckline may be gently tapered to produce a softer, more natural finish.

Tapered neckline shapes Tapered neckline shapes have soft, graduated outlines that follow the natural hairline in the nape. They are far less severe than a squared neckline. The hair may be graduated through most of the back and sides of the head, or it may just be applied to the last few centimetres of hair at the bottom of the nape. Tapered necklines are usually achieved with scissors-over-comb and clippers-over-comb cutting techniques, though clipper attachments can also be used. In some looks the taper is faded so that no outline is visible at all, such as the skin fade that is popular with some African-Caribbean men.

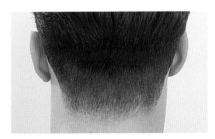

A tapered neckline

As with squared necklines, it is important that the outlines at the sides of the nape are cut to follow the natural hairline. Indeed, the whole neckline shape should still appear squared, but without any distinct outlines.

Rounded neckline shapes Rounded neckline shapes are similar to squared neckline shapes. They too have distinct outlines and appear square-shaped, but the

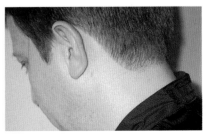

Rounded neckline

TIP ✓

Cut the *sides* of the nape outlines before cutting *across* the neckline. This will help you to judge the proportions of the head and neck more clearly, and so determine the correct height at which to cut the neckline.

When cutting necklines, remember to take into account any hair growth patterns in the nape such as nape whorls, and ensure that these do not distort the required shape.

It may help you to read CHAPTER 4, 'Client care for men' for more detailed information on consultation before reading this section.

corners of the neckline are then gently rounded. Rounded necklines can be achieved with scissors or electric clippers. Avoid making the shape too round, as rounded shapes are more feminine and are not usually suited to most men; also, any hair removed by such round shapes will soon grow back and make the haircut appear untidy. If required, rounded neckline shapes may be gently tapered to produce a softer, more natural finish.

Consultation prior to cutting men's hair

A successful haircut will always begin with a thorough consultation. The correct haircut design for each client relies on careful consideration of many different factors, which can only be identified through a consultation. Always make time to discuss the client's requirements and expectations with them, whether they are a new or a regular client.

HEALTH & SAFETY

A thorough consultation will ensure that you identify any adverse conditions of the hair or skin that may be present. It is particularly important to establish whether a suspected infection or infestation is present: these are contraindications that would prevent you from carrying out the haircut.

EBRU ALKAYA Senior Educator and part of International Creative Team at Alan d Hairdressing Education

❝ Great haircutting skills are fundamental to your success as a barber – it really is what being a barber is all about! Get these basic cuts right and you will have the foundation for a fantastic barbering career. ❞

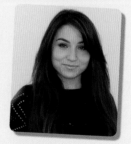

See CHAPTER 4 pages 60–62 for full details on hair types and classifications

Here are some of the critical factors you must consider when cutting men's hair.

◆ Identify the client's requirements, then give them advice on suitable styles. Agree the final effect to be achieved.

◆ Look for signs of broken skin or any abnormalities on the skin or hair.

◆ Look for signs of any unusual hair growth patterns, and identify the natural fall of the hair.

◆ What is the hair type – type S1, W2, C3 or K4 (sometimes called VC4)?

◆ What are the hair characteristics

    ◆ Is the hair fine, medium or coarse?

    ◆ Is the growth dense or sparse?

    ◆ Does the density of growth vary around the head – does the client have male pattern alopecia?

◆ Is the client wearing an added hairpiece?

◆ Does the client have a beard or a moustache?

◆ Determine the features of the client's head, face and body. Is the client wearing spectacles or a hearing aid?

◆ Take into account the approximate age of the client.

◆ Consider the client's lifestyle.

Hair growth patterns

Hair growth patterns are the way in which individual hairs or a section of the hair may grow in a particular direction. Hair growth patterns must be identified because they determine both the looks that can be created and the techniques that you should use. Some clients have very strong hair growth patterns: these need careful attention to produce the best effects, and sometimes just to prevent the hair from sticking straight up!

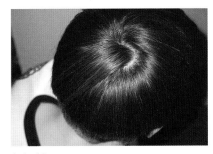

A double crown

Here are some unusual hair growth patterns and the most suitable ways of cutting them.

Double crown With a double crown the hair is usually best left longer. If cut too short, the hair will stick up and will never lie flat.

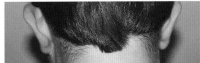

Nape whorls

Nape whorl A nape whorl may be found at either side of the nape, and sometimes at *both* sides. It can make the hair difficult to cut into a straight neckline – often the hair naturally forms a V-shape. Tapered neckline shapes may be more suitable, but sometimes the hair is best left long so that the weight of the hair overcomes the nape whorl movement.

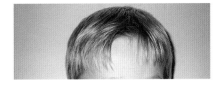

A cowlick

Cowlick The cowlick is found on the hairline at the front of the head. It makes cutting a straight fringe difficult, particularly on fine hair, because the hair often forms a natural parting. It is usually better to cut the hair following this shape. Sometimes a fringe can be achieved by leaving the layers longer so that they weigh down the hair.

Widow's peak The widow's peak growth pattern appears at the front hairline. The hair grows upward and forward, forming a strong peak. It is usually better to cut the hair into styles that are dressed back from the face, as any fringe would be likely to separate and stick up. Short cropped styles or a parting may also be suitable, and sometimes a fringe is possible if the layers are left long.

Texture

The texture of hair can be fine, medium or coarse. Fine hair can be easy to cut, but some fuller styles will be more difficult to create and 'steps' are often more easily produced. Coarse hair can be more difficult to cut and is liable to fly in all directions during cutting, particularly on very short styles, so extra care must be taken to protect the client's and

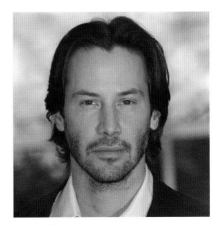

A widow's peak

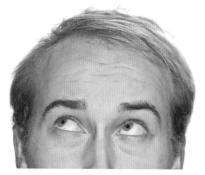
Male-pattern alopecia

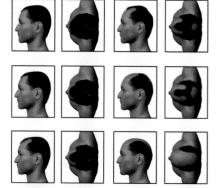
Male-pattern alopecia – for many clients this is a particularly anxious time

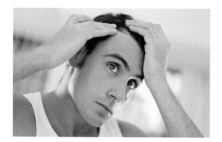
Reduction in hair density during onset of male-pattern alopecia

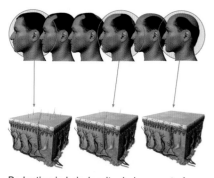
Typical stages of male-pattern alopecia

your own eyes. It is important when cutting very coarse hair to use sharp cutting tools and to take small cutting sections.

Type

Hair type may be tight curly, curly, wavy or straight. Each hair type must be considered because the different types will behave differently when cut, so particular cutting techniques are more suited to some types than others. Here are some examples.

◆ *Tight curly hair – Type K (VC) 4* – Tight curly hair is often very difficult to cut with scissors-over-comb techniques, so scissors- or clippers-over-fingers and freehand cutting techniques are mostly used. Razor-cutting is not usually suitable.

◆ *Curly hair – Type C3* – Curly hair will coil back after being stretched during cutting, so remember not to cut it too short! Scissors- or clippers-over-comb techniques may be more difficult to use efficiently and accurately on curly hair, so cutting over the fingers is usually best.

◆ *Wavy hair – Type W2* – Any of the cutting techniques can be used with wavy hair, but the position of the waves requires careful attention. Careful cutting is needed to ensure that the resulting wave movement suits the required look. Cutting the crests of the waves too short can make the hair stick up: dressing the hair into shape would then be difficult.

◆ *Straight hair – Type S1* – Straight hair – and especially fine straight hair – requires small, accurate sections to be used or marks and 'steps' may become visible. Straight hair may be cut with any of the cutting techniques, but razor-cutting on fine hair is usually not required.

Density

Hair density is the amount of hair that grows in a given area of the scalp. It determines the choice of hairstyle that can be created and affects the techniques that are used.

Baldness Many people experience a noticeable reduction in the density of their hair as they get older. Common baldness is the most frequent cause of this hair loss. It can affect both men and women, but it is much more common in men. Indeed, about 50 per cent of men experience some hair loss by the age of 50, so many men must accept the likelihood of going bald, especially if their fathers have lost their hair.

Most baldness in men is caused by male-pattern alopecia. This is a hereditary condition in which some hair follicles stop producing **terminal hairs** and revert to producing vellus-type hairs that cannot be seen.

It is thought to result from the influence of the male hormone called androgen. The affected follicles usually follow a distinct pattern, the Hamilton pattern, which is seen in men throughout the world.

The exact causes of male-pattern alopecia are still not fully understood, but over the years many different cures have been tried, usually with little success. Some men try to disguise the advanced stages of baldness by creating an unusually low parting in their remaining hair – sometimes unsympathetically referred to as a 'comb-over': make sure you do not use this term. The parted hair section is then grown long and combed up and over the bald area. This strategy is not particularly successful, as the section of hair may be many centimetres in length and is easily blown about when outdoors. Large amounts of sprays and dressings may be used to hold the hair in place, but the effect this creates is often unnatural and may simply cause the long strands of hair to be blown up together, exposing the scalp beneath and leading to considerable embarrassment.

> ### TIP ✓
>
> Before cutting the hair, especially with new clients, always look for signs of male-pattern alopecia or of alopecia areata: the hair may have been left long in some areas to cover the baldness. Cutting the hair too short in these areas would expose the skin, which would not go unnoticed!

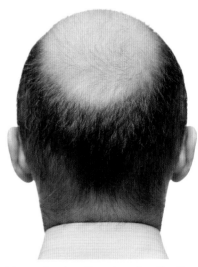

Advanced male-pattern alopecia – Hamilton pattern

On most bald men, short layered looks and leaner haircut shapes are usually more flattering. These looks are more natural and more manageable, although men are often anxious about 'going short' on the first occasion, especially if they usually have long hair.

The impact of baldness on men should not be underestimated. During the consultation, handle this subject with great care. Always respect the client's wishes, especially with men who wish to retain the style with a low parting or who wear added hairpieces.

> ### KEY DEFINITION
>
> Terminal hair: The longer hair that occurs on the head, arms, legs, eyebrows and pubic areas, and on the face and chest in men.

> ### TIP ✓
>
> If your client prefers to have the combed-over effect the ends of the hair in the long hair section combed across the top of the head must be tapered and thinned to ensure that they blend in with the hair at the other side of the head. This is achieved with scissor tapering techniques applied to small sub-sections of the hair at a time. Use a slithering, backwards-and-forwards movement.
>
> Take great care not to cut the hair too short, or it will no longer reach the hair on the other side and the scalp will become visible. Never just cut this section of hair straight across: if you did, a harsh line would be clearly visible.

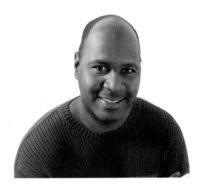

Advanced Hamilton pattern male-pattern alopecia

Added hairpieces Some bald men wear added hairpieces because they prefer the look that these create. Cutting a new hairpiece into shape is a specialist service that should be attempted only by those competent in this type of work. Further studies will be necessary if you are interested in acquiring these skills.

Some barbers specialize in providing such services and establish long and profitable relationships with their clients, but often the manufacturer or supplier of the hairpiece carries out this work. However, any barber will benefit by being able to *recognize* that an established hairpiece is worn and by knowing how to cut the client's natural hair to suit.

Here are some important things to remember about working with hairpieces.

♦ *Full hairpieces* Men who wear full hairpieces usually remove the hairpiece before visiting the barber's shop. They often have their natural hair cut short because it is not visible when the hairpiece is worn.

♦ *Smaller hairpieces and toupees* Some barbers leave smaller hairpieces and toupees in place while they cut the client's natural hair. The hairpiece hair is sectioned at the bottom and held out of the way with cutting clips to gain access to the natural hair beneath. (Do not use brightly coloured butterfly clips – these would

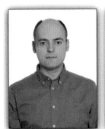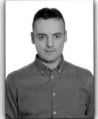

The contrast and appeal of wearing a toupee?

certainly embarrass the client.) This method of cutting is sometimes preferable because it allows the barber to determine the correct length at which the natural hair should be cut and so blend the hairpiece in more effectively. Scissors-over-comb cutting techniques are used, and great care must be taken as any cuts to the hairpiece will not grow back!

◆ *Removing hairpieces* Hairpieces are usually held in place by special double-sided sticky tape. They should be removed by the client themself, to avoid causing any discomfort.

> **TIP** ✓
>
> If the client has a beard or moustache you must think of these as being integrated parts of one style. Choose a haircut shape to suit the total look.

> **TIP** ✓
>
> If the client wears spectacles or an external hearing aid, ask them to remove them while you cut their hair, but remember to take them into account during cutting. Some spectacles may cause the hair to stick out if it is not cut correctly. Hearing aids often clip over the back of the ear, and the client may wish you to leave the hair longer to disguise this.

Features

The features of the client's head, face and body must all be noted to ensure that you choose the most suitable haircut shape. Every haircut should be designed to suit the head and face shape. Your decisions about the hair length, thickness and balance must all relate to the features of these underlying structures.

Careful consideration must be given to each of the following:

◆ The shape of the face – round, square, oblong, long, short or whatever.

◆ The size and position of the ears.

◆ The size and shape of the nose.

◆ The shape of the jaw and chin.

◆ Any unusual features, such as a high front hairline.

◆ The way the head and body are held.

◆ The length and width of the neck.

Different head and face shapes require different haircut shapes. Here are some examples.

◆ *A round face* Choose a haircut shape that is dressed higher at the front and top. The sides should be less full, or leaner. Avoid full, round shapes, as they would make the face appear more round.

◆ *A large head and face* A large, full haircut shape may be more suitable, as a small shape can appear lost and out of proportion, but the shape of the face must also be considered.

◆ *A small head and face* The smaller face is more suited to less full, leaner haircut shapes: the face would appear swamped by large, full and fussy styles.

◆ *A large nose* Fuller shapes with side partings usually help to diminish a large nose. Avoid centre partings and dressing the hair straight back off the forehead.

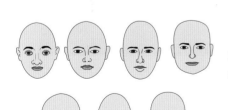

Face and head shapes

> **TIP** ✓
>
> Use the mirror regularly during cutting to ensure that the developing shape is balanced.

◆ **A tall person** Taller shapes accentuate the person's height, so flatter shapes are better.

◆ **A short person** Flatter shapes will make short people appear shorter, so taller shapes are usually best.

◆ **A long face** Choose a shape that is fuller at the sides and shorter on the top. This will help to make the face appear less long.

◆ **A square face** Taller shapes are often more suitable. They should be short and less full at the sides, but longer and higher towards the top.

◆ **An oval face** An oval face shape is considered to be the ideal because most hair-cut shapes will suit it. Remember to take into account the client's other features, however, such as the position of his eyes and ears.

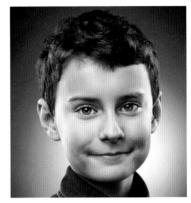

Simple haircuts usually work best for younger clients

Age

The client's age must be considered because people of different ages usually require different hairstyles.

◆ **Children** – mostly require simple hairstyles that need little or no dressing and styling, so shorter styles are often best. But remember: it is the client's wishes that count, and with children this means the parents' wishes too!

◆ **Teenagers** – wear many different styles. Some of these are common to older age groups, but many young men want highly personalized styles. This age group is often prepared to carry out daily grooming, blow-styling and dressing to achieve their chosen look. Distinctive and sometimes quite extreme looks are required, which may be either short or long.

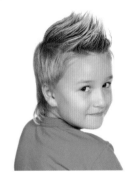

Some children (and parents) prefer a more personalised look

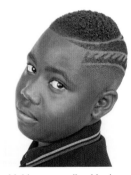

Sometimes a highly personalised look

TIP ✓

Remember to follow your salon's policy for providing services to young children. Ensure that a parent or guardian has confirmed the requested service, especially where radical styling or a change is requested it is better to take the time to check before completing the work than it is to explain an unwanted new look to an unhappy parent.

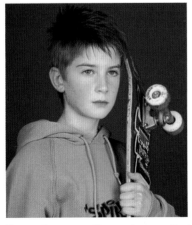

Younger teenagers often want personalized looks, but make sure the parent or guardian agrees before agreeing to radical work!

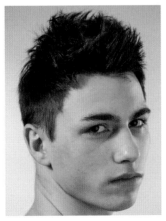

Looks for older teenagers are usually personalized

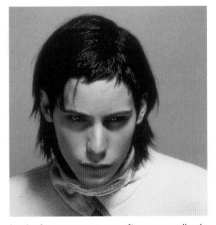

Looks for young men are often personalized

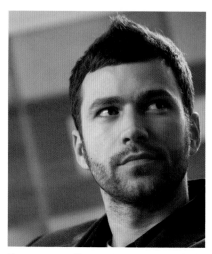

Younger men often want contemporary looks

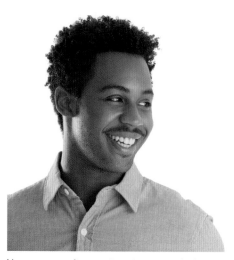

Younger men often want contemporary looks

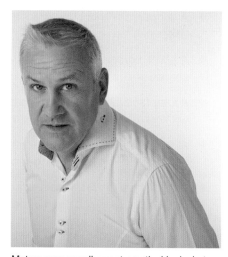

Mature men usually want practical looks but these too can be fashionable!

◆ *Young men* – usually require fashionable but practical styles which are easy to manage and are in keeping with their chosen style of clothing. Preferred styles are often similar to those worn by teenagers, but usually less extreme.

◆ *Mature men* – usually require practical styles that are easy to maintain. Shorter shapes are most popular, but remember clients differ and younger looks might be preferred.

Lifestyle

The client's lifestyle also affects the choice of haircut design. Busy men may not have the time to look after fussy styles; long hair may not be suitable for those who take part in a lot of sport, as drying the hair can take too long. Particular jobs sometimes require particular hair-cuts – for example, short haircuts are required for those in the army, fire service or police.

Tools and equipment

Tools

All haircutting tools must be well-balanced, sharp, clean and safe to use. Here are the main tools required for cutting men's hair.

Scissors Scissors are available in different sizes, ranging from 10 cm to 18 cm. Barbers usually prefer scissors around 15 cm in length, but it depends on what feels comfortable in the size of your hand and for the job you are doing.

Haircutting scissors should be held with the thumb through one handle and the third finger through the other. Only the blade that is operated by the thumb should move when the scissors are being used. This method will produce the most accurate results and it provides the most control and stability, which is vital when cutting around delicate areas such as the ears.

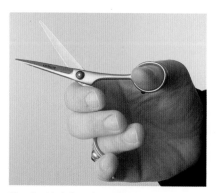

Standard hairdressing scissors

TIP ✔

Do not let other barbers use your scissors. They become accustomed to your grip and can become blunt more quickly if used by others.

TIP

Develop your skills by using the scissors before you start cutting any hair. A good exercise is to open and close the scissors several times whilst moving up along a flat vertical surface such as a broom handle. Concentrate on making the thumb blade move whilst keeping the other blade still. Make the movements slowly at first – increase the speed only when you become more proficient.

Good-quality hairdressing scissors can be quite expensive, but they will last you for many years if you look after them. Only ever use them for cutting hair, or they will quickly become blunt. Keep them clean, and always remove loose hairs, grease and any dirt before disinfecting or sterilizing them. Never use dirty scissors because of the risk of passing infection from one client to another.

Clean and lubricate the scissors regularly, and especially before using them on each new client. Many different disinfectants, alcohol wipes and disinfectant sprays are available for this purpose.

Thinning scissors are used to remove bulk without removing length. The blades are serrated so that when the blades are closed only some of the hairs are cut. One or both of the blades may be serrated, and scissors are available with different numbers and sizes of serrations. The size and number of the serrations determine how many hairs are cut when the blades are closed.

Clippers Clippers may be either hand-operated or electric. Hand clippers are operated by squeezing the handles together. They are seldom used today unless there is no access to electricity, such as during a power cut.

Electric clippers or trimmers may be powered by either mains electricity or rechargeable batteries, and are operated by an electric motor or a magnetic coil.

Electric clippers are the preferred choice today because of their power, accuracy and convenience in comparison with hand clippers. They are available in three different designs:

◆ **Detachable-blade electric clippers** These have a wide range of blade sizes available and tend to be operated by powerful electric motors, making them suitable for all types of work. The blades are easily changed, as the new selected blade is simply pushed on to the clipper head when required. The blades are quite delicate though and must be handled carefully to avoid dropping them. Detachable-blade clippers are easy to clean. The blades and a blade storage box can usually be purchased separately if not provided with the clippers. Some detachable blade clippers now also include adjustment to produce a variable taper effect.

> **TIP** ✓
>
> Make sure that you change detachable blades over a working surface to avoid them dropping to the floor and being damaged.

◆ **Adjustable-blade electric clippers** Adjustable-blade clippers are very versatile, as the blades can be set across a wide range of cutting depths, although the range does not usually cut quite as close as the closest cutting detachable blade. Adjustable-blade clippers, sometimes called variable taper clippers are preferred by many barbers, as they are self-contained and the barber does not need to carry additional blades. This makes them easy to transport and very suitable for freelance work. They are usually operated by a magnetic coil, which means they are quieter and therefore less frightening for smaller children. The blades can be easily dismantled for cleaning. Some adjustable-blade electric clippers now have predetermined depth settings to make it easier to select a specific cutting depth, helping the barber work consistently.

> **TIP** ✓
>
> Ensure scissors are always kept sharp by using professional sharpening services.

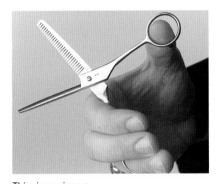

Thinning scissors

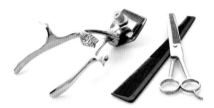

Hand operated clippers, thinning scissors and taper comb

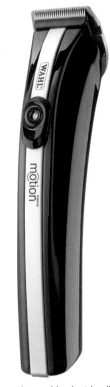

Premium rechargeable electric clippers with detachable and adjustable blades

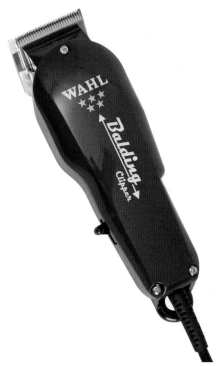
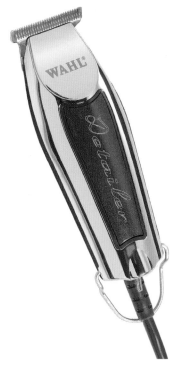

Fixed balding blade corded electric clippers   Non-detachable blade electric trimmers

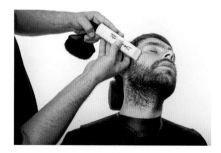

TIP ✓

A wide range of accessories is available for all types of clippers and trimmers, including:

◆ Detachable comb attachments with different cutting lengths: Number 1 = 3 mm, 2 = 6 mm, 3 = 10 mm and 4 = 13 mm.

◆ Storage units.

◆ Charging units (where relevant).

◆ Cleaning equipment and products.

◆ Lubricants.

◆ ***Non-detachable-blade electric clippers/trimmers*** Non-detachable-blade electric clippers or trimmers, as they are often called, are mostly used for outlining haircuts and facial hair shapes, especially around the lips, and for cleaning hair from the nape. Indeed, they are sometimes used to remove hair from the nape area in women's hairdressing. They are usually smaller than detachable-blade and adjustable-blade clippers and so are easier to use in confined areas, such as under the nose. Closer cutting blades are usually fitted and units are normally operated by less powerful electric motors or magnetic coils. The blades can usually be dismantled for cleaning.

Clippers are equipped with a range of different blade sizes for different purposes. The number 000 blade is good for removing hair from outside the outlines, whilst the number 1 blade is best for clipper-cutting the hair to remove bulk.

Here are the most common approximate sizes available; remember that slight variations are sometimes used by different manufacturers.

TIP ✓

Some clippers are now fitted with ceramic blades that should never need sharpening.

	Blade sizes	Cutting length of blade
Detachable blades	0000	A very close cut (similar to shaving – sometimes called balding blades)
The blades are available in a wide range of sizes	000	0.3 mm (a close cut)
	00	0.4 mm
	0	0.8 mm
	0A	1.2 mm
	1	3.3 mm
	1A	4.0 mm
	11/2	4.8 mm
	2	6.4 mm
	3	7.9 mm
Adjustable blade	From 000 to 1	As above
Moving a small lever alters the cutting length of the blade (Hand-operated clippers often have adjustable blades.)		
Non-adjustable blade	A fixed setting between 000 and 1. A cutting length of 1.8 mm is often popular	As above

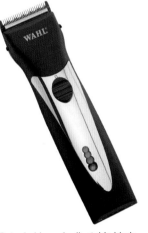

Texturizing and razoring blades Recently detachable texturizing blades and razoring blades have become available for some clippers. The cutting edge of texturizing blades resembles castellated scissors. They have preset gaps in the guard so that more hair is removed in just these areas in order to produce different textured effects within the haircut. Razoring blades too can produce textured effects but these mainly give results similar to traditional razoring.

Detachable and adjustable blade
rechargeable/mains clippers

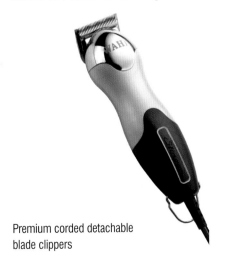

Premium corded detachable
blade clippers

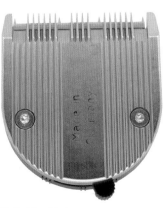

Texturizing blade

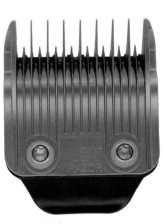

Razoring blade

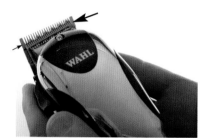

Incorrectly set blade – the cutting blade is not level with the stationary blade

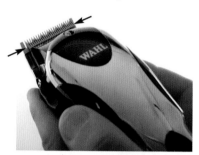

Correctly set blade – the blades are level

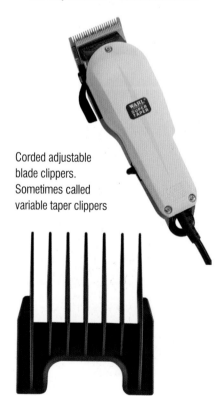

Corded adjustable blade clippers. Sometimes called variable taper clippers

TIP ✓

Choosing a clipper/trimmer

Buying clippers and trimmers is a significant investment for the busy barber. They can cost hundreds of pounds and will be used in most, if not all haircuts and facial hair work in the barber's shop. They must be powerful and precise enough to do the work required, without losing their cutting edge, power or overheating and must be tough enough to shrug off the bumps and knocks likely in a busy barber's shop. Here are some important features you should look for:

Corded clippers/trimmers

- Powerful heavy duty motor.
- Variable speed control to power through dense work but maintain precision cutting in finer detailed work.
- Long and robust quality electrical cable.

Rechargeable clippers/trimmers

- Clear charge status indicators.
- Long running time and short recharge cycle for rechargeable clippers/trimmers.
- Simple charging operation and battery care – charging station and NiMH battery with no memory effect.

Common features

- Lightweight and ergonomic design to prevent fatigue and ensure fine detail control.
- Quality finish and choice of look to match your barber's shop décor.
- Simple to dismantle, clean and maintain.
- Supplied with cleaning equipment and lubricant.
- Range of quality quick release cutting attachments is supplied/available.
- Clear instructions for use.
- Long and effective warranty.

Detachable comb attachments are also available for electric clippers, which give a wide range of predetermined cutting lengths. These allow for very fast removal of hair and are sometimes used to reduce the length of the hair and produce a rough shape, which is then finished with scissors and clippers (without the comb attached). The combs are available in sizes ranging from a number 8, which will leave the hair about 25 mm long, to a number 1, which will leave the hair only about 1–3 mm long after cutting. The most popular sizes are the number 3, which leaves the hair about 10 mm long, and the number 4, which leaves the hair about 13 mm long.

Razors Razors are used in men's haircutting to shave outlines, to thin and style the hair, or to produce textured effects. Disposable-blade razors are preferable because they are more hygienic. For cutting hair these are sometimes called hair shapers. Detailed information on razors is provided in Chapter 12, 'Shaving services'.

Combs Combs are available in various different sizes for different purposes. Cutting combs are usually thin and pliable, with fine teeth at one side and coarse teeth at the other. The coarse teeth should be used for most combing and sectioning, while the fine teeth are good for detailed work and close cutting. The barber comb, sometimes called a 'taper comb' is specifically designed for this purpose. It is very thin and pliable and the side with the fine teeth narrows to a point. This makes the comb easier to use when producing fine tapered finishes, especially in confined areas, such as around the ears.

A cutting comb should fit comfortably in the hand and be easy to move into all the positions required during cutting.

Neck brush A neck brush is required to remove excess hair cuttings and to maintain the client's comfort throughout the service.

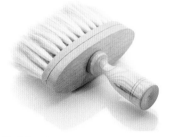

A standard cutting comb and a barber's 'taper' comb

Equipment

The client should be seated in an adjustable chair, which can be positioned at the correct height so that the hair can be worked on efficiently.

Preparation for cutting hair

1   Carry out your consultation with the client.

2   Determine the client's wishes and confirm what is to be done. Use photographs or pictures to help clarify the required shape.

3   Before you begin work, gather together all the tools and equipment you will require.

4   Gown the client, placing a clean tissue or neckstrip between the client's neck and the gown. A cutting collar may then be placed on top of the gown. Some barbers use a clean towel instead of a cutting collar, particularly if the hair is wet. This should be placed across the client's back and be tucked in at the neck.

5   Position the client in a chair so that the hair can be worked on efficiently.

6   Carefully comb the hair, disentangling it if required. Look out for areas of sparse growth, scarring or other unusual features you may not have seen earlier.

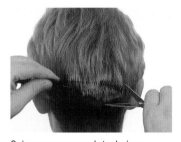

Neck brush

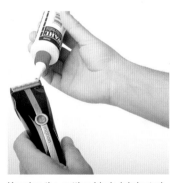

Barber's chair

Basic cutting techniques

The techniques used for cutting men's hair are generally the same as those used in women's hairdressing. The barber understands, however, that differences exist in the way the techniques are used and in the effects they achieve.

The following cutting techniques are commonly used when cutting men's hair.

Club cutting

In club cutting, the sections of the hair are cut straight across to produce blunt ends which are all cut at the same length. Small sections are required, particularly on coarse, dense hair, or the hair ends will not be level. This technique may be used on wet or dry hair.

Here are the main methods of club cutting used in men's hairdressing.

Scissors-over-comb The scissors-over-comb technique is performed by lifting a section of hair and then cutting it straight across. When cutting short hairs in the nape you should take extra-small sections of hair, which are usually lifted with the comb.

Keeping the cutting blade lubricated

Scissors-over-comb technique

TIP ✓

Make sure that your scissors are fully closed before using the tips to lift sections of hair when doing scissors-over-comb or the open blade will snag the hair and cut it short near the roots.

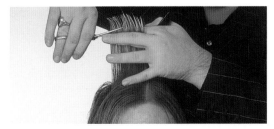

Clubbing over the fingers

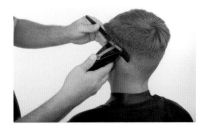

Clipper-over-comb

Some barbers use the tips of their scissors to lift the longer sections of hair, which are then picked up on the comb and positioned ready for cutting. Ensure that you use the coarse teeth of the comb and the main part of the scissors when cutting the interior of the hair cut, and the fine teeth and the tips of the scissors when working around the ears and nape.

Scissors-over-comb is mostly used on shorter styles, particularly to create graduation in the nape and at the sides.

Clubbing over the fingers

Clubbing over the fingers is very similar to the scissors-over-comb technique – indeed, it might be called 'scissors-over-fingers'. It is performed by lifting a section of the hair, which is then combed out and transferred to the fingers. The fingers slide up the section of hair to the correct position for cutting, and the hair is then cut straight across. The hair may be held at different angles, and different sizes of sections may be used, to create the amount of graduation required.

Clubbing over the fingers is mostly used on longer styles and to cut the top of many short styles.

Clippers-over-comb

Clippers-over-comb can be used instead of scissors-over-comb and clubbing-over-the-fingers techniques, especially on long, coarse and dense hair, and particularly if it is being taken much shorter. Many of the same effects possible with scissors can also be achieved using clippers. Clippers are best used on dry hair.

Freehand cutting

Freehand cutting is the cutting of hair without first taking the hair into a section or holding the hair in place with the comb or hand. It is often used to remove individual hairs or small amounts of hair when finishing a style, or for producing textured effects. It is usually performed with the tips of the scissors.

Freehand cutting can be particularly useful when cutting tight curly or curly hair, and is often used on beards and moustaches to smooth the outline shape and remove stray hairs. Tapered effects can also be achieved freehand by using sliding and slicing movements.

Accompanying video available for scissors-over-comb. Please scan this QR code.

Accompanying video available for clubbing over the fingers. Please scan this QR code.

Accompanying video available for clippers-over-comb. Please scan this QR code.

Accompanying video available for freehand cutting. Please scan this QR code.

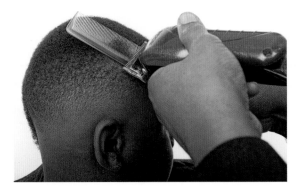

Clipper-over-comb

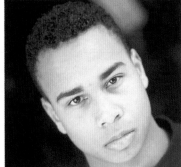

Tight curly hair – type K4a hair

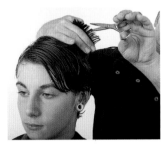

Scissor thinning or point cutting

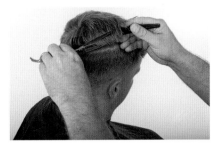

Cutting with thinning scissors

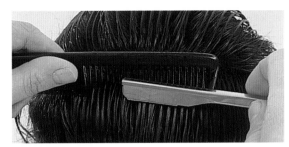

Thinning with a razor

Thinning

Thinning techniques are used to remove bulk and thickness without affecting the overall length. Thinning is achieved by cutting just *some* of the hairs in a section of hair, while leaving others uncut so that the length of the overall section remains unchanged. The hair should be cut only in the middle third of the section: if it is cut too close to the roots, the resulting short hairs will stick straight out.

Here are the most common methods used for thinning men's hair.

Scissor thinning   Scissor thinning is achieved using a similar action to that used in scissor tapering, but here the open scissor blades are moved along the hair section in one long movement. The hair may also be cut with the points of the scissors, known as point cutting or pointing – this technique should be used in the middle of the hair section. Sometimes it is used to thin the ends of the hair and to create softer lines.

Cutting with thinning scissors   Thinning scissors have serrated blades: when closed, they cut only some of the hairs. They should be used in the middle third of the section or towards the ends.

Thinning with a razor   Thinning with a razor is carried out only on wet hair. It is achieved by placing the razor on the hair at an angle of about 30–40° and then cutting the hair by gentle slicing movements. Gentle actions are required or the hair will be cut straight through!

> **TIP** ✓
>
> Take great care when cutting with a razor. Do not razor-cut the hair too near to the hairline or roots.

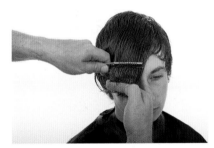

Shaping and thinning with a razor

> **HEALTH & SAFETY**
>
> Razors have very sharp blades and must always be treated with care and respect. Keep the handle closed or cover the blade when not in use, and especially when carrying or passing a razor. Never place a razor in your pockets, and always keep razors out of the reach of children.

Skin fading

Skin fading is the term used to describe very close short graduation with clippers that leaves no visible outline at the back and sides – the hair simply appears to *fade* into the skin. The cut increases from a 0000 sized detachable blade or 000 adjustable blade setting in the nape and around the ears up to a length of several centimetres on the top.

Partings and fringes

Partings   Many men's hairstyles have partings. These can be used in many different ways and to create many different effects. For example, partings may be used to draw attention away from unwanted prominent facial features, such as a large nose or large ears. Centre partings and side partings are often used to divide large hair masses and produce more pleasing and symmetrical shapes, which are also more manageable.

Accompanying video available for thinning with a razor. Please scan this QR code.

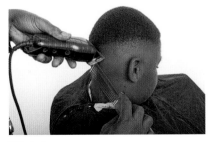

Skin fading

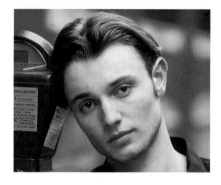

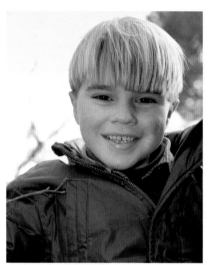

Many men have natural partings. To identify these, comb the wet hair straight back, then push it forward with the palm of the hand: where the hair parts naturally is the natural parting. Such partings should be used, where possible, as the resulting style will be easier to manage. The natural hair growth patterns and the hair fall must all be identified and considered to determine where, if at all, a parting is required.

Fringes The front of the hair may be dressed into a fringe. Men do not often wear full fringes, but many children do. A fringe shape may be short, long, squared, rounded, blunt-cut or tapered.

The client's head and face shape will determine which fringe shape is best. The fringe should not be too heavy or it will appear unnatural, and fringes can even look like artificial hair! Layering is often used to reduce the thickness, and the ends are sometimes tapered to produce a softer line. Hair growth patterns such as a cowlick or widow's peak must be considered as they may make a full fringe impractical. Remember that it is usually better to go *with* the natural hair fall rather than *against* it.

> **TIP** ✓
>
> Remember that hair stretches by up to half its own length when wet. Keep this in mind when you are cutting stretched hair, so that it is not too short when it dries.

Wet and dry cutting

Traditionally, most men visited the barber's shop to have their hair cut dry. A dry cut produced good results and was completed more quickly than a wet cut. Today, many men have their hair washed and then cut wet, but dry cutting is still common.

> **TIP** ✓
>
> If you wish to carry out dry cutting, it is best to wash and dry the hair first. Be sure to explain this to the client first and take their wishes into account.

If the client's hair is greasy and dirty then it must be washed before you can cut it. Wet hair is also required for blow-styling and some cutting techniques, such as razor-cutting, which should always be carried out on wet hair to avoid causing damage to the hair and discomfort to the client. Other cutting techniques are less suitable for use on wet hair, such as some scissor-tapering and clippers-over-comb movements. In general, *scissors* can be used on wet or dry hair, razors must only be used on wet hair, and *thinning scissors* and *clippers* are best used on dry hair.

Layering

The purpose of layering is to produce a series of connected, unbroken layers, with no perceptible lines or 'steps' in-between. Most men wear layered haircuts: these often produce a more masculine shape and are easier to manage.

Here are the two main layered effects that are mostly required in men's hairdressing.

Uniform layering Uniform layering is the process of cutting the sections of the hair to the same length. It can be achieved by holding each section at 90° to the head, and then cutting the hair straight across at the same angle.

Uniform layering is used mostly in longer styles, and to cut the hair on the top of the head in some shorter styles. It is particularly suitable for creating shapes on curly hair.

Graduated layering Graduated layering is the process of producing a difference in length between the layers at the top and the layers at the bottom of a section of hair. This can be achieved by elevating the sections of the hair at different angles and then

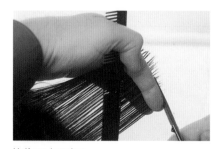

Uniform layering

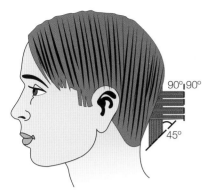

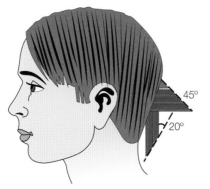

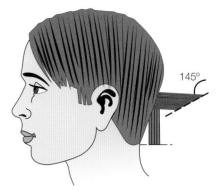

Producing a 45 degree angle of graduation   Producing a 20 degree angle of graduation   Producing a level length

cutting them straight through, or by holding the sections at 90° to the head and then cutting through the section at a different angle. Lifting the sections *higher* and then cutting them will produce a *greater* amount of graduation; holding them *lower* and then cutting will produce *less*.

The gradient between the top and bottom of the hair sections when positioned back on the head is called the angle of graduation.

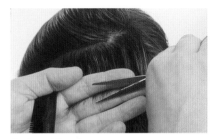

Graduated layering

- ◆ If you hold a section of hair at 90° (a right angle) to the back of the head, and cut it at 90° to the section, you will produce a 45° angle of graduation.

- ◆ If you hold a section of hair at 90° and cut it at 45° you will produce a steeper graduation.

- ◆ If you hold a section of hair at 90° and cut it at 145° you will produce a level length, in which all of the ends of the hair fall level, without graduation.

Many men's haircuts are graduated at the back and sides to produce taller, leaner, more masculine shapes.

Cutting guidelines

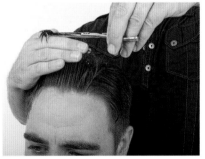

Cutting along the guideline

The cutting guideline is the line that is created by the ends of the hair when a section of hair is held out from the head. Establishing correct guidelines is very important when cutting the hair: if this is not done, the results will be uneven and inaccurate, and will not be likely to meet the client's requirements.

Some cutting guidelines are called the baseline or perimeter line. These are used to determine the outer and inner perimeters of the haircut. These lines are important because they usually provide the basis for the other guidelines to follow.

To produce precise, accurate results, the guidelines should be carefully followed throughout the cutting process. Make sure that a guideline from a previously cut section of hair is clearly visible before cutting the new section of hair. Both the hair length and the line of the cut in the previous section should be used to guide where the next cut is to be made.

When preparing guidelines, many different factors must be considered – the position of the ears, the nose and the eyes, the shape of the head and the position of the hairlines, and so on. During the cutting process the head is often divided into large sections, rows or panels, to ensure that the guidelines are easily seen and to make the hair more manageable. Each of these sections or panels is then sub-divided into sections of hair

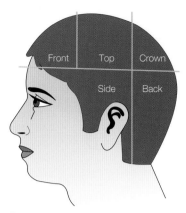

Guide sections

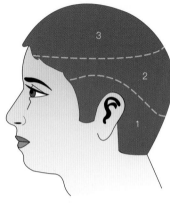

Guide areas

for cutting. The cutting guideline established in one section is transferred from section to section, and panel to panel, so that the resulting haircut is connected throughout to produce an even result.

In men's hairdressing, particularly on shorter styles, the head is often divided into three main areas, which reflect the different shapes that are required and the techniques that are used.

◆ Area 1 includes the hairline, the ear outline and the occipital bone. This is where most of the graduation and tapering is carried out. Usually scissors- or clippers-over-comb techniques are required.

◆ Area 2 is between the occipital bone and the bottom of the crown area. On shorter styles this is where the graduation and taper are blended into the hair in the top section. Thickness is often reduced here to create the taller, less full, more masculine shapes that most men prefer. Usually scissors- or clippers-over-comb and over-fingers techniques are required.

◆ Area 3 covers the rest of the top of the head, starting from the crown area. The blending of area 2 continues, and the lengths of the top and front are determined. Scissors- or clippers-over-comb cutting techniques can be used, but more often scissors- or clippers-over-fingers techniques are required.

Cutting procedures

In cutting men's hair, several different cutting procedures may be followed. Each individual barber will decide where to start and which cutting techniques to use, mainly according to personal preference.

Many different cutting techniques can achieve similar effects. They can also be combined and adapted as necessary, to achieve the required results. The best procedure is one that allows the barber to work accurately and efficiently throughout the whole haircut.

The following examples show how some common men's looks can be achieved using basic techniques.

Short layered looks

SHORT GRADUATION WITH A TAPERED NECKLINE AND RAZOR-THINNING – TYPE S1 HAIR

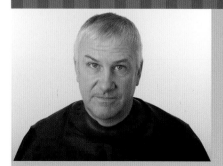

Step A

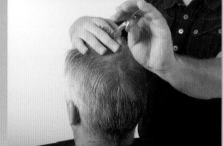

Step B

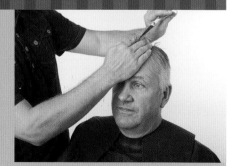

Step C

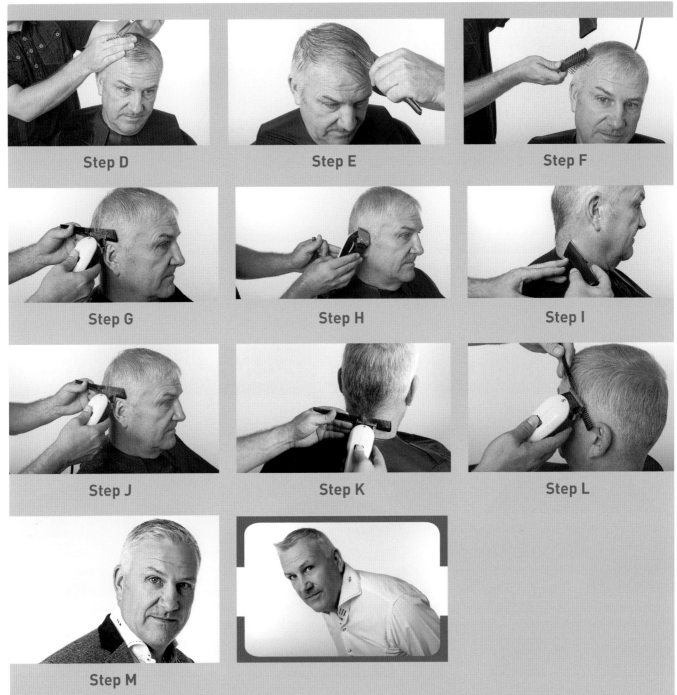

Step D

Step E

Step F

Step G

Step H

Step I

Step J

Step K

Step L

Step M

1. Protect the client's clothes.

2. Comb the hair carefully, disentangling it where required (a).

3. Start in the centre panel at the crown and point cut the top to the correct length. Point cutting will prevent the top forming a solid effect (b).

4. Transfer this guideline to the front (c).

5. Work across the top connecting each guideline until completed (d)

6. Point razor the top to reduce baulk and break up the solid effect (e).

7. Rough dry the hair ready for the scissors-over-comb or clippers-over-comb work (f).

8. If using the clippers, choose the comb attachment for the length of cut you require. (The best size of comb for this look is either a number 3 or a number 4.) Ensure that the comb is securely attached to the clippers. Scissors- or clippers-over-comb techniques may be used instead, if preferred. Start cutting the hair to the required length (g).

(continued)

SHORT GRADUATION WITH A TAPERED NECKLINE AND RAZOR-THINNING – TYPE S1 HAIR (*Continued*)

9. If your client has sideburns, cut the first side to the required length. Carefully outline the sideburn and the hair around the ears down to the nape (h).

10. As you create the outlines, *make sure you do not cut into the natural hairline, particularly at the sides of the nape (i)*.

11. Continue cutting to the guideline from the previous section and the adjacent panel as you work around the head. If the panels are not connected, long hairs will be left between them (j).

12. As you complete the back, position the client's head so that it is bent forward slightly. The neckline must now be tapered to create a natural effect: do not cut it straight across. Use scissors-over-comb or clippers-over-comb techniques. The bottom edge of the comb should be held against the skin, then angled so that the hair will be cut shorter at the bottom and left longer at the top (k).

13. Continue working around the head, cutting the hair to the length determined by the chosen haircut shape and blending into the top. As the shape develops, keep looking in the mirror to make sure your work is symmetrical. Consult with your client at regular intervals to confirm that the developing shape is correct, making adjustments if required (l). Remember to make sure that the sideburns are cut level (see the tip on p. 112).

14. Finish the shape by combing, styling and dressing the hair into place (m).

SHORT GRADUATION, FADED NECKLINE – TYPE K4 HAIR

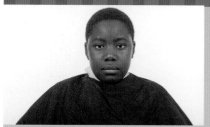

Step A

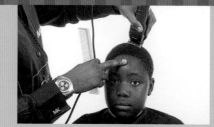

Step B

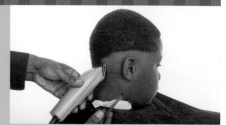

Step C

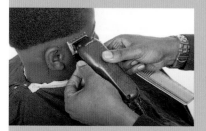

Step D

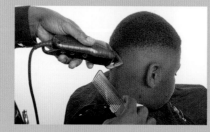

Step E

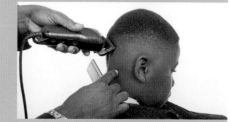

Step F

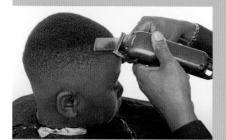

Step G

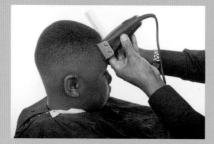

Step H

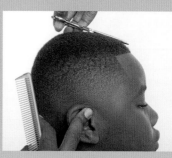

Step I

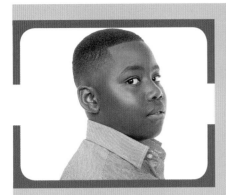

Step J

Uniform length top with faded neckline (using a detachable comb clipper attachment).

1. Protect the client's clothes.
2. Comb the hair carefully, disentangling where required (a).
3. Using a number 1 comb attachment, cut the hair length to length (b).
4. Remove hair using balding blade clippers up to the start of the fade (c).
5. Begin graduating the weight line at the start of the fade using adjustable blade clippers without a comb attachment.

Adjust the blade to decrease the cutting depth – this will gradually remove more hair and the faded effect will appear (d). As the shape develops keep looking in the mirror to make sure that it is symmetrical (e). Consult with your client at regular intervals to confirm that the developing shape is correct, making adjustments if required

6. A number 1 attachment can be used to blend into the top hair (f).
7. Clippers-over-comb is used to finish blending into the top (g).
8. Outline the cut (h).
9. Finish the cut with precise freehand cutting (i).
10. Shave the areas outside the haircut outlines, if required (see Chapter 12, Shaving services).
11. Finish the look by combing, styling and dressing the hair into place (j).

TIP ✓

Before cutting the hair, make sure that you can clearly see the cutting guideline created by the previous section. If the hair is too thick for you to see the guideline through it, you may need to take a thinner section.

UNIFORM LAYERED TOP, GRADUATED WITH A SQUARED OR ROUNDED NECKLINE – TYPE W2 HAIR

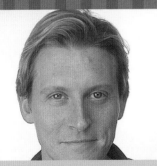

Step A

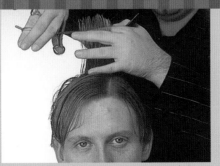

Step B

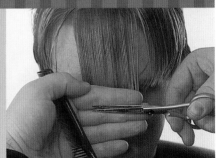

Step C

(continued)

UNIFORM LAYERED TOP, GRADUATED WITH A SQUARED OR ROUNDED NECKLINE – TYPE W2 HAIR (*Continued*)

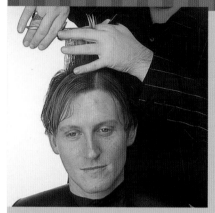

Step D

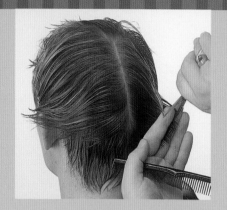

Step E

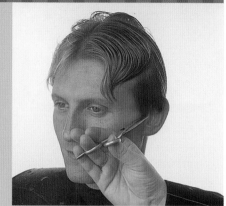

Step F

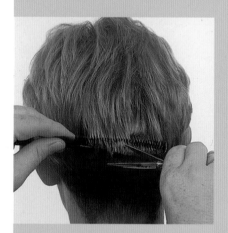

Step G

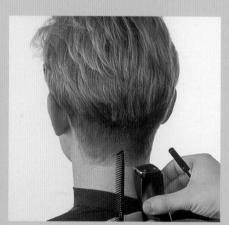

Step H

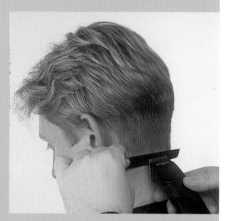

Step I

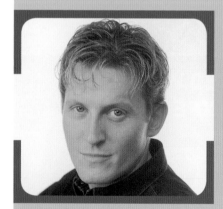

Step J

1. Protect the client's clothes.

Comb the hair carefully, disentangling it where required (a).

2. With the hair wet, section the hair in two by making a parting from ear to ear across the top of the head. Take a section *parallel* to this parting at the crown and hold it at 90° to the head. Cut this section straight across to the correct length using the scissors-over-fingers technique (b).

3. Take a section going down the centre panel towards the front hairline. Hold it at 90° to the head, then cut it to the guideline from the first section. Continue down this panel to extend this guideline through the top.

4. Take the front section forwards and hold it at 90°, then cut it to the required length for the front area. Remember: wet hair stretches, so do not cut it too short (c).

5. Return to the crown area. Take a small section, parallel to the first parting, and hold it at 90° to the head. Cut it to length, following the guideline from the first section. Continue working forward down the centre panel, always cutting to the guideline from the previous section (d).

6. Move to an adjacent panel of hair and repeat the process, making sure that the panels are connected. Keep working around the top of the head, cutting the hair to the length determined by the chosen haircut shape.

7. Transfer the guideline down onto the side of the head by taking a vertical section. Continue cutting the sections through the sides to the required length. The hair length may be graduated to remove weight around the ears, if required, by angling the cut across the section.

8. As the shape develops, keep looking in the mirror to make sure that the shape is symmetrical. Consult with your client at regular intervals to confirm that the developing shape is correct, making adjustments if required.

9. Take a vertical section down the central panel at the back of the head. Hold it at 90° to the head and cut it to the length determined by the guideline (e).

10. Take a further section below this one. The hair length may now be graduated to remove weight in the nape by angling the cut across the section, as required.

11. Move to the adjacent panel of hair and repeat the process, as before. Make sure the panels are connected, or long hairs will be left between adjacent panels.

12. When the back is complete, move to one side of the head. If there are sideburns, note the required length and cut them to shape. Carefully outline the sideburn and the hair around the ears, then move down the sides of the nape with the tips of your scissors. Use the fingers of your other hand to guide and support the scissors or clippers whilst cutting (f).

13. Repeat this on the other side of the head. Ensure that the sideburns are level (see the tip on p. 112).

14. Dry the hair into style.

15. Return to the centre panel of hair at the back of the head and finish the nape area, the neckline and the side outlines, using scissors- or clippers-over-comb techniques (g).

16. Position the client's head so that it is bent forward slightly. Carefully cut the neckline straight across to the correct height. Use the proportions of the head and neck, the length of the hair and the position of the ears to determine the length that is most suitable (h).

17. The neckline may be gently tapered to create a softer effect or the corners may be rounded, if required (i).

18. Shave the areas outside the haircut outlines, if necessary (see Chapter 12, Shaving services).

19. Finish the shape by combing, styling and dressing the hair into place (j).

The procedure described is for a squared neckline. For a rounded neckline, follow this sequence and after the squared shape has been created, simply round off the corners of the neckline.

TIP

Make sure you do not cut into the natural hairline, particularly at the sides of the nape.

TIP

When cutting a squared neckline, the centre of the neckline should be cut slightly higher than at the sides to compensate for the skin in the centre of the neck moving further up as the head goes forward. The difference should be about 5 mm. This will appear level when the head is returned to its normal position.

TIP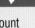

Remember to take into account that wet hair stretches, so do not cut it too short!

UNIFORM LAYER AFRO, TAPERED ROUNDED NECKLINE USING FREEHAND CLIPPER AND SCISSORS WORK – TYPE K4A HAIR

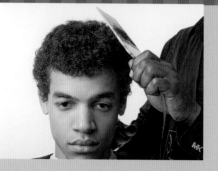

Step A

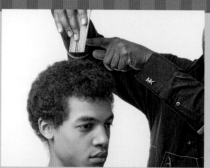

Step B

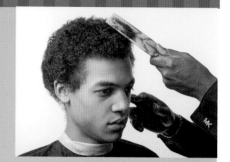

Step C

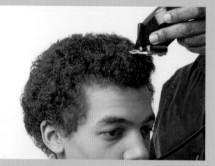

Step D

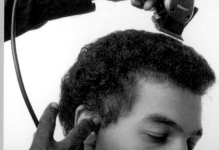

Step E

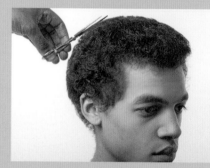

Step F

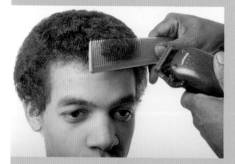

Step G

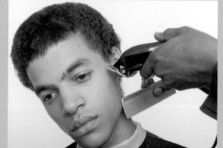

Step H

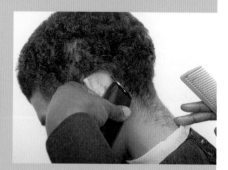

Step I

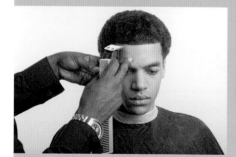

Step J

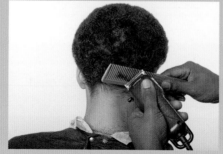

Step K

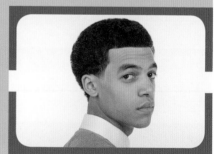

Step L

1. Protect the client's clothes. Comb the hair carefully, disentangling where required with a wide tooth comb (a).

2. Remember that very curly hair will be much longer than it appears as the curls make the hair shrink back. This can be seen by the volume and depth of the hair on the top (b). Freehand clipper and scissor work is used to ensure an even cut.

3. A little hairspray is applied before combing out to help separate and define the hair (c).

4. Using a freehand clipper cut the hair to the required basic length. Keep combing through with a wide tooth comb to ensure an even cut (d).

5. Keep working around the head. As the shape develops keep looking in the mirror to make sure that it is symmetrical. Consult with your client at regular intervals to confirm that the developing shape is correct, making adjustments if required (e).

6. Use freehand scissors to make precise cuts (f).

7. The front, sides and back are shaped, graduated and tapered using clippers-over-comb (g) and (h).

8. Outline around the ears and down to the nape (i).

9. Outline the front (j).

10. Taper the back. The shape should remain square and then just round off the corners (k).

11. Shave the areas outside the haircut outlines, if required (see Chapter 12, Shaving services).

12. Finish the look by combing, styling and dressing the hair into place (l).

SHORT GRADUATION, TAPERED NECKLINE, FREEHAND CUTTING AND SCISSOR THINNING – TYPE C3 HAIR

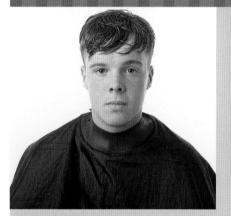
Step A

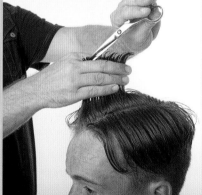
Step B

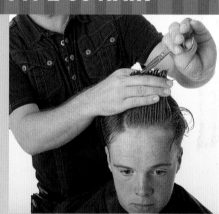
Step C

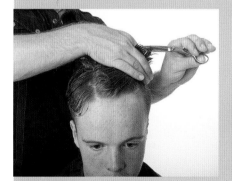
Step D

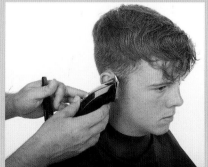
Step E

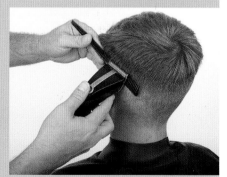
Step F

(continued)

SHORT GRADUATION, TAPERED NECKLINE, FREEHAND CUTTING AND SCISSOR THINNING – TYPE C3 HAIR (*Continued*)

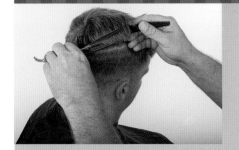
Step G

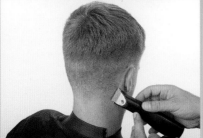
Step H

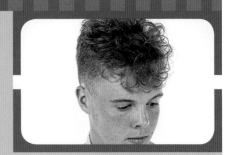
Step I

A tapered neckline (without a detachable comb clipper attachment).

1. Protect the client's clothes. Comb the hair carefully, disentangling where required (a).

2. Take a section of hair at the front using the clubbing-over-fingers technique. Point cut into the ends of the hair section until the hair is at the required length. This will reduce the length and thin the hair to make it a less solid shape. Club cut the sections if you want to retain this solid shape (b).

3. Move across the head taking small sections following the cutting guideline and ensure that each panel of hair is connected, as before (c).

4. Work down into the sides (d).

5. Roughly dry the hair.

6. Outline around the ear and sideburn, cut the sideburn to the correct length (e).

7. Taper the outlines and neckline using clippers-over-comb.

8. Move to one side, or in the centre panel of hair at the back of the head, and cutting the hair using scissors- or clippers-over-comb techniques to the length of cut you require. Blend the shorter lengths into the top (f).

9. Make sure you follow the cutting guideline from the previous sections and adjacent panels as you work. As the shape develops keep looking in the mirror to make sure that it is symmetrical.

10. Reduce the weight where the top blends into the side with thinning scissors (g).

11. Sharpen the outline with close cutting trimmers. *Make sure you do not cut into the natural hairline when creating the outlines, particularly at the sides of the nape* (h).

12. Shave the areas outside the haircut outlines, if required (see Chapter 12, Shaving services) or remove any visible hair using balding blade clippers.

13. Finish the shape by combing, styling and dressing the hair into place (i).

GRADUATED LAYERS – TYPE W2 HAIR

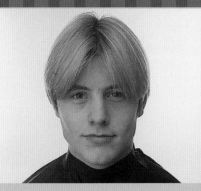
Step A

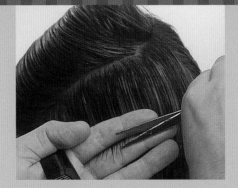
Step B

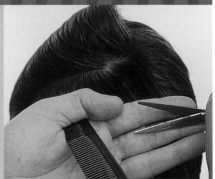
Step C

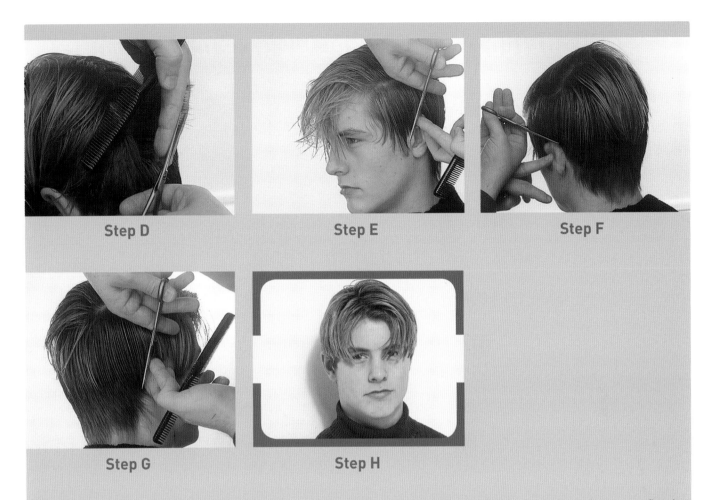

Step D   **Step E**   **Step F**

Step G   **Step H**

In men's hairdressing, graduated layers are often required on the back and sides of the haircut to produce taller, leaner shapes that are more flattering to most men.

1. Protect the client's clothes (a).

2. Comb the hair carefully, disentangling it where required.

3. With the hair wet, make a parting about 2 cm above the hairline, going from the front to the sides, around the ears and down into the nape.

4. Comb the hair at the front of the ear down from this parting to its natural position. Lift it by the width of two fingers to create the required amount of graduation. Cut the hair to the required length (b).

5. Take another section adjacent to the first, and cut it as before (c).

6. At the back of the ear, comb the hair forwards towards the ear, lift it the width of two fingers, and cut it to the guideline from the previous section.

7. Continue cutting the hair along this first section until you reach the nape.

8. Make the second parting above and parallel to the first. Start at the front and comb the hair to its natural fall, then lift it to the same position as before. Cut this section to the guideline created by the first section beneath.

9. Continue down the second parting, taking each section to exactly the same position where you held the hair from the first parting. Ensure that the hair is lifted by the same amount each time, or the graduation will not be consistent.

10. Make further partings, continuing up the head. Pull each section of hair to the same position and cut it to the same guideline.

11. Move to the other side and repeat the process. Ensure that the hair is pulled to the position equivalent to that on the previous side.

12. As the shape develops, keep looking in the mirror to make sure that the shape is symmetrical. Consult with your client at regular intervals to confirm that the developing shape is correct, making adjustments if required.

13. When both sides are complete, cross-check the back area to ensure that the shape is balanced and that the cut is accurate. This may be carried out with either scissors-over-fingers or scissors-over-comb techniques (d).

(continued)

GRADUATED LAYERS – TYPE W2 HAIR (*Continued*)

14. When the back is complete, move to one side of the head. If there are sideburns, note the required length and cut this sideburn to shape. Carefully outline the sideburn and the hair around the ears (e, f).

15. Move down the sides of the nape with the tips of your scissors. Use the fingers of your other hand to guide and support the scissors or clippers whilst cutting (g).

16. Repeat this on the other side of the head. Ensure that the sideburns are level. *Make sure you do not cut into the natural hairline, particularly at the sides of the nape.*

17. Dry the hair into style.

18. Return to the centre panel of hair at the back of the head and finish the nape area, the neckline and the side outlines, using scissors- or clippers-over-comb techniques. The neckline should be squared, tapered or rounded, as required.

19. Shave the areas outside the haircut outlines, if necessary (see Chapter 12, Shaving services).

20. Finish the shape by combing, styling and dressing the hair into place (h).

TIP

When determining the correct height for the neckline you should consider the length of the neck, the position of the ears, the head shape and the length of the hair. If the neckline is too low on a short neck it will make the neck appear shorter; whilst if it is too short on a long neck it will make the neck appear longer. The best height is usually about 3–4 cm below an imaginary line between the bottom of the ears, but always consider your client's wishes before cutting.

The sculpture cut, 'number 1' or full skin fade – type K4b hair

Different variations of the sculpture cut are popular with many men, but most often with young men. The name is derived from the closeness of the cut: it closely follows the features of the head, so the hair appears to be sculpted. It is also sometimes called a 'number 1' after the size of the clipper comb attachment regularly used to achieve the cut. Longer versions of this type of cut have been called 'number 3' or 'number 4', again after the size of comb attachment used.

Traditionally this type of cut was called a crew cut (the length usually being equivalent to that produced with a number 4 comb attachment). However, the crew cut was often achieved with just scissors-over-comb technique, and it required great skill to ensure the same length of cut throughout.

The sculpture cut produces a very masculine shape. It can be quite severe, though variations in length may be used to produce effects to suit the individual client's requirements. The looks created are very easy to manage as no blow-styling or dressing is required. Some men who are partly bald enjoy these looks because the shortness of the hair reduces the effect and impact of the bald areas.

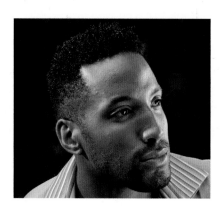

The sculpture cut is particularly suitable for very tight curly hair, where the hair is often taken very close. Indeed, the clippers are sometimes used at the back and sides with no comb attachment, and a skin fade is produced. Adjustable-blade clippers are usually set to their longest setting (equal to a size 1 blade), and the detachable clippers are used with a clipper blade of size 1 or above. Lines and shapes can be channelled (sometimes known as tramlining when used to create simple lines) into the hair on these styles to create elaborate designs.

THE SCULPTURE CUT, 'NUMBER 1' OR SKIN FADE

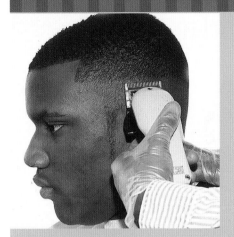

Step A

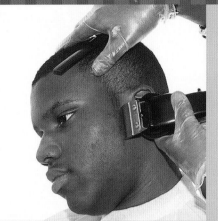

Step B

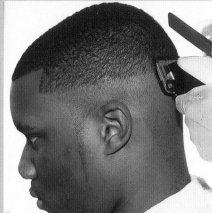

Step C

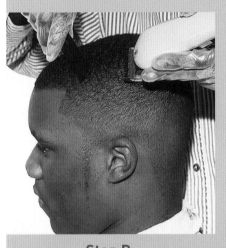

Step D

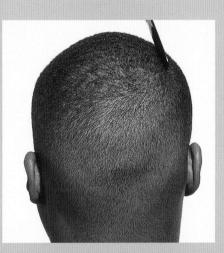

Step E

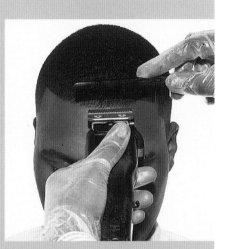

Step F

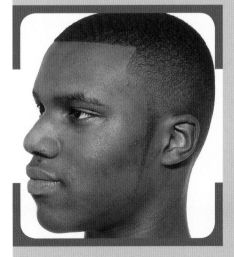

Step G

(continued)

THE SCULPTURE CUT, 'NUMBER 1' OR SKIN FADE (*Continued*)

1. Protect the client's clothes. Comb the hair carefully, disentangling it where required. This barber is wearing gloves to cover recent minor cuts on his hands.

2. Start in the centre panel of hair at the back of the head. Begin cutting the hair using the clippers set to the longest setting or with a size 1 blade. Alternatively, a comb attachment can be used for a less severe effect. The best-sized comb for this look is either a number 1 or a number 2. Before you start, make sure that any comb attachment is securely attached to the clippers.

3. Place the clippers flat against the neck, just below the neckline. Using a *smooth, continuous movement*, push the clippers slowly up the head, keeping them flat against the scalp until you reach the area where you want the taper to begin: in this case the occipital bone. In a smooth *rocking* movement, *pivot* the clippers away from the head to produce the shape and length of hair that you want. Unless the top panels are to be cut this short as well, do not go higher than the occipital bone without pivoting away from the head (a).

4. Move to an adjacent panel of hair, and repeat the process as before. Make sure the panels are connected, or long hairs will be left between them.

5. Keep working around the head, cutting the hair to the length determined by the chosen haircut shape.

6. As the shape develops, keep looking in the mirror to make sure that the shape is even and symmetrical. Consult with your client at regular intervals to confirm that the developing shape is correct, making adjustments if required.

7. Move to one side of the head. If there are sideburns, note the required length for any sideburns and cut this sideburn to shape. Carefully outline the sideburn and the hair around the ears (b).

8. Remove any comb attachment, move down the sides of the nape with the clippers. Use the fingers of your other hand to guide and support the clippers whilst cutting. Repeat this on the other side of the head.

9. Position the client's head so that it is bent forward slightly. Carefully cut the neckline to the correct height. Use the proportions of the head and neck, the length of the hair and the position of the ears to determine the length that is most suitable.

10. The neckline must be tapered to create either a natural effect, or a skin fade effect where the hair appears to fade away. Do not cut it straight across. Use clippers-over-comb technique and set the clippers to cut at the shortest setting, or use a size 000 blade. On longer hair, the bottom edge of the comb should be held against the skin and the clippers moved up or across the comb: the comb must be angled so that the hair will be cut shorter at the bottom and left longer towards the top. On very short hair the clippers are held directly against the scalp. Pivoting the clippers away in a smooth rocking movement blends and fades the neckline.

11. Return to the centre panel of hair at the back of the head. Using a number 1 comb attachment, or a size suitable for the length of hair required, begin to blend the hair where the top of the taper meets the hair on the crown of the head (c).

12. Move across the head, working on small sections and ensuring that each panel is connected to the previous one, blending the two areas together to create an even, continuous effect with no lines.

13. Move across the head, following the direction of hair growth. As you cut, ensure that successive panels of hair are connected (d).

14. Blend together the top panels and the side and back panels where they meet, to create an even, continuous effect (e). You may need to remove the comb attachment to do this.

15. The front hairline may be shaped with the clippers, if required, but avoid making deep cuts into the natural hairline unless the client wishes this effect (f).

16. Comb all the hair through, checking for any long hairs. Remove them with scissors- or clippers-over-comb or freehand cutting techniques. If possible, rinse the hair first to remove the loose hairs and help make any longer hairs more visible.

17. Shave the areas outside the haircut outlines, if necessary (see Chapter 12, Shaving services).

18. Finish the shape by combing the hair into place (g).

TIP

Always comb the hair after each movement with the clippers, to remove loose hairs and ensure that you can see clearly.

Remove excess hair cuttings from the client's face and neck at regular intervals, to ensure that he is comfortable.

ACTIVITY: CASE STUDY – MATTHEW

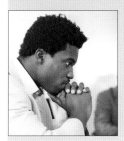

Matthew is a 25-year-old new client in your barber's shop. He requests that you restyle his hair into a modern look. He starts a new job as a fire officer next week. Describe the action that should be taken regarding Matthew's request?

Longer layered looks

Uniform layers (including razor-thinning) – type W2 hair In men's hairdressing uniform layering is not often used throughout the whole haircut, because the shape produced is too round, though it can be used to create some suitable shapes on curly hair. Uniform layering is most often used through the top of the head, with graduated layering being used at the back and sides to produce a taller, leaner and more masculine shape.

UNIFORM LAYERS (INCLUDING RAZOR-THINNING) – TYPE W2 HAIR

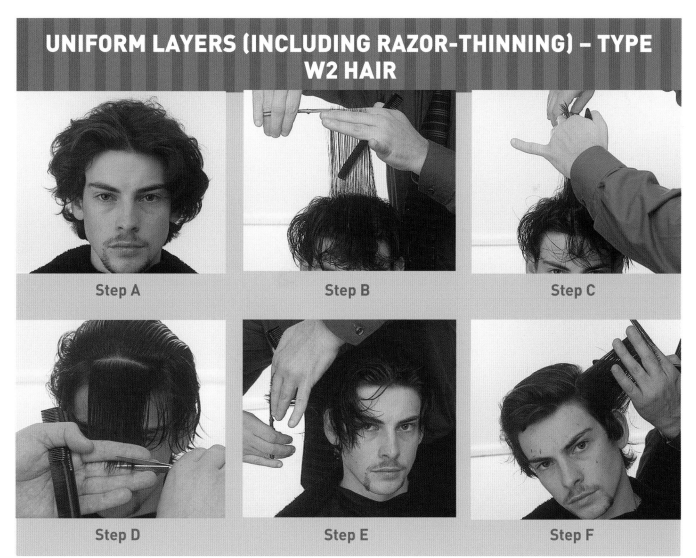

Step A   Step B   Step C

Step D   Step E   Step F

(continued)

UNIFORM LAYERS (INCLUDING RAZOR-THINNING) – TYPE W2 HAIR (*Continued*)

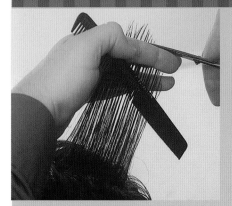

Step G

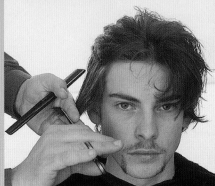

Step H

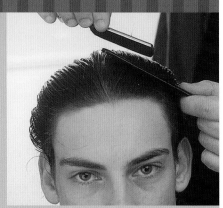

Step I

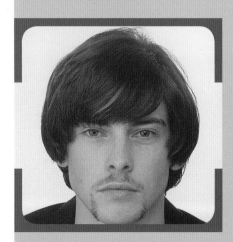

Step J

Protect the client's clothes. Comb the hair carefully, disentangling it where required (a).

1. With the hair wet, section the hair in two by making a parting from ear to ear across the top of the head. Take a section parallel to this parting at the crown, and hold it at 90° to the head. Cut it to length using the scissors-over-fingers technique. Make sure you cut the section straight across at 90° to the head (b).

2. Take a section going down the centre panel towards the front hairline. Hold this at 90° to the head and cut it to the same length. Continue down this panel, but do not cut the front section at this stage (c).

3. Take the front section forwards and hold it at 90° to the head. Cut it to the required length for the front (d). Remember that wet hair stretches, so do not cut it too short.

4. Return to the crown area and take a small section, again parallel to the first parting, and hold it at 90° to the head. Cut it to length following the guideline from the first section. Continue working forward down the centre panel, always cutting to the guideline from the previous section. Move to the adjacent panel of hair and repeat the process. Make sure that the panels are connected. Keep working around the top of the head, cutting the hair to the length determined by the chosen haircut shape.

5. Transfer the guideline down onto the side of the head by taking a vertical section (e).

6. Continue cutting these sections to the required length. The hair length may be graduated to remove weight around the ears, by angling the cut across the section as required (f).

7. As the shape develops, keep looking in the mirror to make sure that the shape is symmetrical. Consult with your client at regular intervals to confirm that the developing shape is correct, making adjustments if required.

8. Transfer the guideline from the front of the first parting at the crown area through into the back of the head (g).

9. Take a vertical section down the central panel at the back of the head. Hold it at 90° and cut it to the length determined by the guideline. Take a further section below this one. The hair length may now be graduated to remove weight in the nape, by angling the cut across the section as required. Move to the adjacent panel of hair, and repeat the process as before. Make sure the panels are connected or long hairs will be left between them.

10. When the back is complete, move to one side of the head (h).

11. If there are sideburns, note the required length and cut this sideburn to shape. Carefully outline the sideburn and the hair around the ears, then move down the sides of the nape with the tips of your scissors. Use the fingers of your other hand to guide and support the scissors or clippers whilst cutting.

12. Cut the neckline to the shape required by the look.

13. The top layers are then cut with a razor to reduce the thickness and to create more texture and movement. The hair must be wet. Comb the hair straight back and start in the centre panel at the front, about 3 cm back from the hairline. Do not start too near the hairline or the resulting short hairs will stick straight up! The hair is then cut, using gentle slicing movements with the razor. The razor and comb should move down the section together as the required amount of hair is removed (i). Take great care, as the razor can easily cut the hair straight through.

14. Finish the shape by combing, styling and dressing the hair into place (j).

ACTIVITY: CASE STUDY – JUSTIN

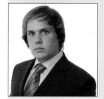

Justin is a 30-year-old new client in your barber's shop. He requests that you restyle his hair into a more modern look that will suit his new job in sales. During the consultation you notice he has a double crown. Describe the action that should be taken regarding Justin's request?

TIP ✓

Outlines can be achieved by cutting the hair with either close-cutting clippers or an electric razor. The outline hair may also be removed completely by shaving with a razor, which should be used following the shaving procedure described in Chapter 12, 'Shaving services'.

Square layers – type C3a hair Square layers are good for creating movement and texture through the interior of a mid-length haircut. On men they are particularly suitable for longer haircuts because they produce a shape that is more square and angular, and thus more masculine. They also help make longer hair more manageable.

SQUARE LAYERS – TYPE C3A HAIR

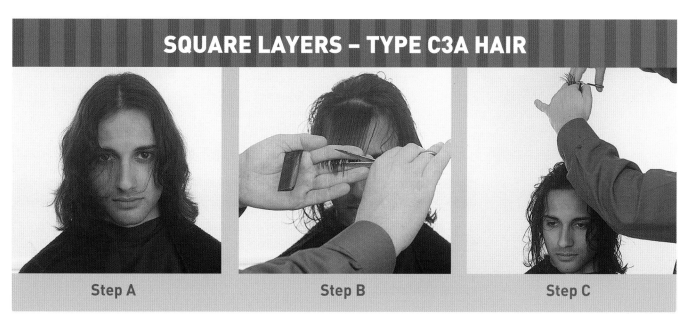

Step A   Step B   Step C

(continued)

SQUARE LAYERS – TYPE C3A HAIR (*Continued*)

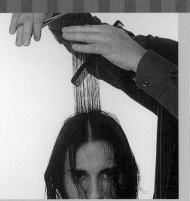

Step D

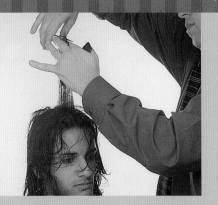

Step E

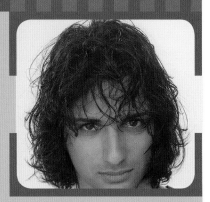

Step F

1. Protect the client's clothes. Comb the hair carefully, disentangling it where required (a).

2. With the hair wet, make a centre parting from the forehead to the nape.

3. Create two sections in the nape, running slightly diagonally from the centre parting outwards to the bottom of the ears. Starting in the middle of these two sections, comb the hair down and cut it to the required length with the scissors-over-fingers technique. Continue cutting straight across these sections to produce a square line.

4. Take two more diagonal sections, about 2 cm higher and running parallel to the first. Cut the hair to the guideline, sometimes called a baseline, which was created in the nape. Continue the baseline around onto the sides.

5. Continue working up the head, taking 2 cm sections, until all of the hair at the back has been cut to this baseline.

6. Move to the front of the head and take a diagonal section about 2 cm wide on the side from the centre parting to the top of the ears. Cut this section up from the baseline created at the bottom of the sides. Continue cutting up along the section to the required length for the hair at the front. Do not cut the front too short or the layers through the head will be too short (b).

7. Repeat this on the other side. Check that the sides are level.

8. Create a section going down the centre panel from the front hairline to the nape. Take the section at the front and hold the hair straight up at 90° to the head. Cut this to the guideline that will now be visible coming up from the sides. This will create a new guideline on the top that determines the length of the square layers throughout the interior of the haircut (c).

9. Continue cutting this guideline across the central panel to the crown area.

10. Take a next section of the central panel from below the crown area and comb it straight up to the same position as the last section on the top of the head. Cut this section to the guideline on the top to produce a square layer and retain the length at the back (d).

11. Repeat this down the rest of the central panel, making sure that the hair is all combed straight up to the same position and cut to the top guideline.

12. Move to the adjacent panel of hair at the back and repeat the process, making sure that the panels are connected.

13. Keep working around the crown, imagine that the crown is the hub of a wheel, and the panels of hair are each of the spokes. Follow this process until the hair at the back is connected with the hair at the sides (e).

14. If there are sideburns, note the required length and cut them to shape. Ensure that they are level. Remove any unwanted hair from outside the outline, shaving these areas if necessary (see Chapter 12, Shaving services).

15. Finish the shape by combing, styling and dressing the hair into place (f).

> **TIP**
>
> Make sure you cut each section on the top straight across at 90° to the head or a uniform layered effect will not be achieved.

ACTIVITY: CASE STUDY – GEORGE

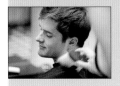

George is a 40-year-old new client in your barber's shop. He requests that you restyle his hair into a modern look. During the consultation you notice he has a strong whorl in the neckline. Describe the action that should be taken regarding George's request?

Finishing

When possible the hair should be rinsed after cutting to remove any loose hair on very short styles as the short hairs can be difficult to remove.

Styling products may then be applied, and the hair dried and dressed in accordance with the requirements of the desired look. Use the mirror regularly to check the balance and symmetry of the shape as you dress it.

Show the client the finished result and apply final finishing products if required. Provide advice and tips on aftercare styling and products, as appropriate.

Aftercare advice

Remember to advise your client on how to maintain their look at home. Here are some ways you can help them achieve good results:

◆ Products to use – suggest which products will help them maintain and improve their hair and scalp and hairstyle. This is a good opportunity to highlight the benefits of any shampoo, conditioning and finishing products you have used and to recommend the client buy these from your barber's shop.

◆ How to use products – show the client how the products should be used to achieve the best effects (you can highlight this to them as you style and finish their hair). Help them find and understand the manufacturer's instructions.

◆ How to maintain and style their look – show the client where to shave outside the sideburn outline shape. Discuss good grooming techniques – regular combing, cleaning and drying tips. Answer any questions the client may have.

◆ When the next barber's shop appointment should be made – remember that shorter hair will usually soon become untidy. The next cut is often required within 4 weeks. Encourage the client to book before leaving if your barber's shop has an appointments system.

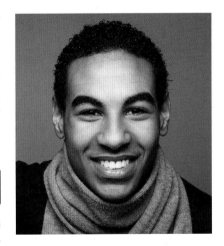

Health and safety

It is important to consider health and safety when cutting hair because of the risks associated with using electricity and the risk of cutting the skin. Here are some important health and safety factors that you must consider when providing haircutting services:

Avoid infection

◆ If the client has any cuts or abrasions on his head, or you suspect that an infection or infestation is present, you must not carry out the haircut.

◆ Pay special attention to hygiene when cutting hair, because of the risk of cross-infection through open cuts.

◆ Use only clean tools and equipment. Use alcoholic wipes and sprays to keep clippers clean and disinfected between clients.

It may help you to read CHAPTER 2, 'Health and safety in the barber's shop' for general information on working safely in the barber's shop.

Work safely with razors

◆ Open and safety razors have very sharp blades and must always be handled and used with great care.

◆ When it is not being used or when it is being carried, always close the handle to protect the blade of an open razor.

◆ Never place razors or other cutting tools in your pockets.

◆ Always sterilize a fixed-blade razor before *each* use.

◆ When using a detachable-blade open razor, always use a new blade for *each* new client.

◆ Used razor blades, called sharps, must be disposed of correctly in accordance with your salon policy. Soiled disposable materials should be placed in sealed plastic bags for removal.

Work safely with electricity

◆ Always handle and use electrical equipment with care, and in accordance with the manufacturers' instructions.

◆ Never place or use electric clippers or other electrical equipment near water.

◆ Do not go near electrical equipment that is lying in water – first switch off the power at the mains.

◆ Before commencing work, visually check that electrical equipment is safe to use. Check that the cable has not frayed or been pulled, and that the plug is not loose.

◆ When using and storing electrical equipment, pay attention to the position of cables.

◆ Never overload sockets. Do not plug too many items of electrical equipment into the same socket.

◆ Follow the manufacturers' instructions for the care of your scissors and clippers. To avoid damage, be sure to clean and lubricate the blades regularly.

◆ Electrical equipment must be regularly tested, and given a certificate of testing confirming that it is safe for use. The salon owner will ensure that this is carried out, as required.

Be prepared for accidents

◆ Make sure that you know the whereabouts of your salon's first-aid kit.

◆ Keep yourself up-to-date with your salon's first-aid and accident procedures.

◆ If the client's skin is cut while you are cutting his hair, stay calm and explain what has happened. Follow your salon's first-aid and accident procedures. *Here is an example of what you should do. Give the client a clean dressing and ask them to apply it against the cut until the bleeding stops. A new dressing or plaster may then be applied by the client if needed.* **Do not touch the cut yourself.** *If the cut is more serious, advise the client to seek medical attention as soon as possible. If any gowns or towels have been soiled, seal them in a plastic bag and launder them at a high temperature as soon as possible. Remember to wear gloves when handling contaminated items!*

◆ If you cut your *own* skin while you are cutting a client's hair, stay calm and explain what has happened. Follow your salon's first-aid and accident procedures. *Here is an example of what you should do. Excuse yourself from the client and rinse the cut under cold running water to remove any hairs. Apply a clean dressing against the cut, until the bleeding stops. A new dressing or plaster may then be applied. If the cut is more serious, seek medical attention as soon as possible. If any gowns or towels have been soiled, seal them in a plastic bag and launder them at a high temperature as soon as possible. Gloves should then be worn to protect the cut and dressing.*

IMAGE GALLERY

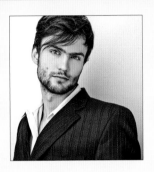

Visit the online image gallery on this book's accompanying website to see other basic haircut looks.

BRINGING IT ALL TOGETHER

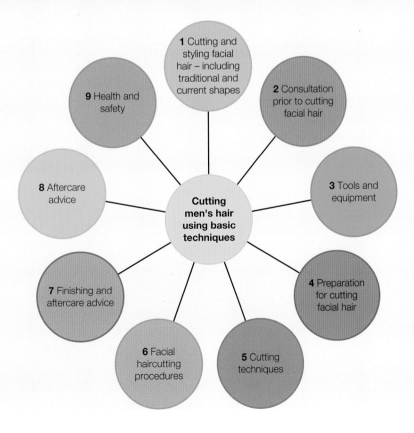

Cutting men's hair using basic techniques

1 Cutting and styling facial hair – including traditional and current shapes

2 Consultation prior to cutting facial hair

3 Tools and equipment

4 Preparation for cutting facial hair

5 Cutting techniques

6 Facial haircutting procedures

7 Finishing and aftercare advice

8 Aftercare advice

9 Health and safety

Summary

1   The main purpose of cutting hair is to style the hair into shape. Both the hair length and the hair thickness can be removed, either to create a completely new look or just to trim the client's current look back into shape.

   There are also distinct differences between masculine and feminine shapes. Masculine shapes are usually more square and angular and are suited to most men, while feminine shapes tend to be fuller and more rounded. Taller, less full, or leaner shapes are also more flattering on most men, so minimal thickness at the back and sides is often required. Barbering principles define how men's hair should be cut and styled.

   Follow the natural hairline wherever possible, particularly when outlining short haircuts. Avoid making unnecessary cuts into the natural hairline, especially around the ears and at the sides of the nape. (Such cuts would appear harsh and unnatural, and the haircut would soon appear untidy when the hair started to grow back.)

   Avoid cutting the length of the sideburns higher than the top of the ear and into the hairline, as this creates a particularly harsh and unnatural effect.
   The outline of the haircut in the nape is called the neckline shape. The neckline is important in men's hairdressing: the natural neck hairline is usually less well defined as hair often grows densely on the neck. There are three main shapes: tapered, squared and rounded.

2   Hair growth patterns must be identified because they determine both the looks that can be created and the techniques that you should use.
   On most bald men, short layered looks and leaner haircut shapes are usually more flattering.

3   All haircutting tools must be well-balanced, sharp, clean and safe to use. Adjustable-blade clippers are very versatile, as the blades can be set across a wide range of cutting depths. A cutting comb should fit comfortably in the hand and be easy to move into all the positions required during cutting.

4   When preparing clients always carefully comb the hair, disentangling it if required. Look out for areas of sparse growth, scarring or other unusual features you may not have seen earlier.

5   In club cutting the sections of the hair are cut straight across to produce blunt ends which are all cut at the same length. The scissors-over-comb technique is performed by lifting a section of hair and then cutting it straight across. When cutting short hairs in the nape you should take extra-small sections of hair, which are usually lifted with the comb.

   Clippers-over-comb can be used instead of scissors-over-comb and clubbing-over-the-fingers techniques, especially on long, coarse and dense hair, and particularly if it is being taken much shorter. Freehand cutting can be particularly useful when cutting tight curly or curly hair, and is often used on beards and moustaches to smooth the outline shape and remove stray hairs. In general, *scissors* can be used on wet or dry hair, razors must only be used on wet hair and *thinning scissors* and *clippers* are best used on dry hair.

   Uniform layering is the process of cutting the sections of the hair to the same length.

6   Many different cutting techniques can achieve similar effects. They can also be combined and adapted as necessary, to achieve the required results. The best procedure is one that allows the barber to work accurately and efficiently throughout the whole haircut.

7   Show the client the finished result and apply final finishing products if required.

8   Provide the client with advice and tips on after-care styling and products, as appropriate. Suggest which products will help them maintain and improve their hair and scalp and hairstyle. This is a good opportunity to highlight the benefits of any shampoo, conditioning and finishing products you have used and to recommend the client buy these from your barber's shop.

9   Pay special attention to hygiene when cutting hair, because of the risk of cross-infection through open cuts.

Activities

1   Research the options available for sharpening and reconditioning scissors. Produce a report setting out the features and benefits of each option and

present this to your manager. With the manager's permission, recommend the best options to your colleagues.

2   Visit local wholesalers and use the Internet to search manufacturers' sites to research the types of electric clippers and trimmers and blades and attachments that are available. Produce a chart showing the features and benefits of each item, especially noting things like ease of use, maintenance requirements, life expectancy and any unique features. You can then use the information to help you and your colleagues choose the equipment that is most suitable for your requirements.

Check your knowledge

1   Describe why outlines are important in men's haircutting.

2   Describe the three main neckline shapes in men's hairdressing.

3   Outline the best way of dealing with a double crown.

4   Describe the condition thought to be the cause of male-pattern alopecia.

5   Describe the looks usually most suitable for men with male-pattern alopecia.

6   Describe how added hairpieces are secured to the head.

7   Describe the look least suited to a client with a round face.

8   The cutting length of a size 1 clipper blade is:

   a. 1.2 mm
   b. 3.3 mm
   c. 4.0 mm
   d. 4.8 mm

9   Why must clipper blades be checked before use and especially after being dismantled?

10   Describe how to identify a client's natural parting.

11   State which cutting technique(s) should be carried out on dry hair and not carried out on wet hair.

12   Describe the angle of graduation produced if you hold a section of hair at 90° to the head and club cut it at 90°.

13   State why it is important to establish and follow the correct cutting guideline.

14   Which of the following statements is correct?

   a. Sideburns should be cut level by using the same position on each ear as a guide.
   b. Sideburns should be cut level by memorizing their position whilst looking in the mirror.

15   Describe the action that should be taken if, about to cut a client's hair, you suspect an infestation is present on their head.

16   Describe the action you should take if you were to cut yourself whilst cutting a client's hair.

8 Drying and finishing men's hair

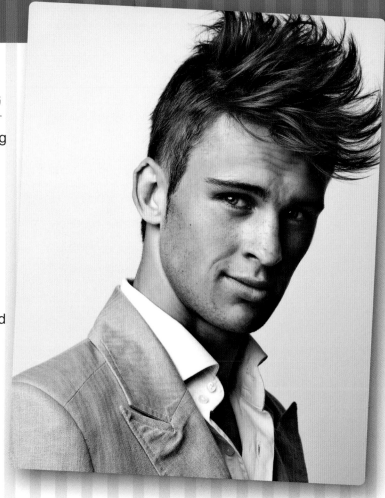

QUALIFICATION SIGNPOSTING

This chapter will help your studies of the following qualifications:

❖ Level 1 NVQ Diploma in Barbering.
❖ Level 2 NVQ Diploma in Barbering.
❖ City & Guilds Level 2 Certificate in Barbering Techniques.
❖ City & Guilds Level 2 Award, Certificate and Diploma in Barbering.
❖ City & Guilds Level 2 Diploma in Women's and Men's Hairdressing.
❖ City & Guilds Level 3 Diploma in Barbering.
❖ ITEC Level 1 VRQ Certificate in Barbering.
❖ ITEC Level 2 VRQ Awards, Certificates and Diplomas in Barbering and Men's Hairdressing.
❖ VTCT Level 2 VRQ Certificates and Diplomas in Barbering.
❖ VTCT Level 2 VRQ Diploma in Barbering Studies.

For further information on the qualifications covered by this chapter see the qualification mapping grid at the front of the book.

LEARNING OBJECTIVES

In this chapter you will learn:

◆ About the theory of blow-drying.

◆ The requirements of consultation for blow-drying.

◆ How to prepare for blow-drying.

◆ About the styling products, tools and equipment used.

◆ The blow-drying techniques – including blow-waving, finger drying, scrunch drying and natural drying.

◆ The finishing techniques and aftercare advice needed.

◆ How to maintain health and safety.

INTRODUCTION

Blow-drying is not just about drying the hair. It is the art of styling wet hair with brushes, combs or fingers whilst blow-drying it with a hand held hairdryer. Today, many men enjoy having their hair shampooed and 'blow-styled', so the barber must understand how the hair is to be professionally dried and finished.

The techniques used for blow-drying and styling men's hair are very similar to those used in women's hairdressing. Some might have said there is no difference, but the barber understands that differences exist in the way that the techniques are used, and in the different effects that they achieve.

This chapter examines how blow-drying and styling techniques are used in men's hairdressing. It covers the following:

❖ The theory of blow-drying.

❖ Consultation for blow-drying.

❖ Preparation for blow-drying.

❖ Styling products, tools and equipment.

❖ Blow-drying techniques – including blow-waving, finger drying, scrunch drying and natural drying.

❖ Finishing techniques and aftercare advice.

❖ Health and safety.

KEY DEFINITION

Hygroscopic: A substance that attracts and absorbs moisture.

See CHAPTER 4, 'Client care for men' for more information on hair structure.

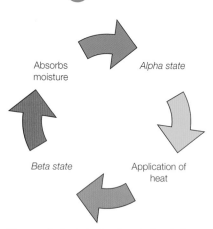

Absorbs moisture

Alpha state

Beta state

Application of heat

Changes in the hair structure during drying

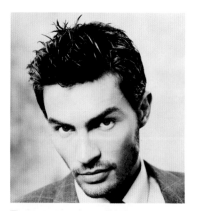

The correct product will help support textured effects

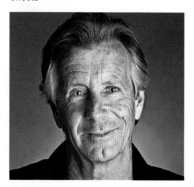

The correct amount of volume will control the hair and maintain a natural effect

The theory of blow-drying

Blow-drying works by stretching and temporarily changing the hair structure.

Wet hair is very elastic and can stretch by up to 50 per cent of its original length. It is stretchy because the weaker hydrogen bonds and salt links, which form part of the hair cortex are temporarily broken. The application of heat then softens the hair and causes it to stretch and mould to the new shape created by the brush, comb or fingers. The hair structure is then changed from its original state, called the *alpha state* (not stretched) to the *beta state* (stretched).

The new shape is only temporary because hair is **hygroscopic**: it absorbs moisture. Eventually moisture from the atmosphere will enter the hair and the polypeptide chains will recoil to return the hair its natural alpha state. Washing the hair in hot water will return the hair to its natural state immediately.

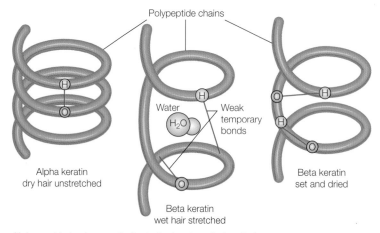

Polypeptide chains

Alpha keratin dry hair unstretched

Water H_2O

Weak temporary bonds

Beta keratin wet hair stretched

Beta keratin set and dried

Alpha and beta changes in the hair structure during drying

Consultation prior to blow-drying

Blow-drying is usually carried out immediately following a shampoo or a shampoo and haircut, where it is used to produce the final look that the haircut has created. Consultation for blow-drying is likely to have been included in the consultation *before* the haircut, but you must still make sure that time is always set aside to discuss the client's requirements with them.

> **TIP**
>
> Most men do not want too much volume in the finished blow-dried style. Usually you should avoid creating root lift in the back and sides. Use a partial blow-waving technique to create definition and reduced volume.

Here are some of the factors that must be considered when blow-drying men's hair.

◆ Identify the client's requirements. Give him advice on suitable styles and agree the final effect to be achieved.

◆ Look for signs of any unusual hair growth patterns.

◆ Identify the natural fall of the hair.

◆ Determine whether the hair is coarse or fine.

Many men prefer not to have too much volume created in the finished blow-dried style. You should pay particular attention to this during the consultation and ensure that you choose suitable brushes and techniques for creating the amount of volume required.

It may help you to read CHAPTER 4, 'Client care for men' for more information on consultation.

ERIK LANDER Education Director, Habia

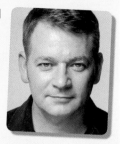

" A great haircut is only half the story; good drying, styling and finishing skills are all important to bring out the potential of the cut. And remember, this is a great opportunity to provide good aftercare advice to help your client manage their look at home – winning you a happy, loyal client and an opportunity to sell retail. "

Preparation for blow-drying

Following the consultation and before you begin work; gather together all the products, tools and equipment you will require. You must also prepare the client and their hair.

Preparing the client

Remove any wet towels and make sure your client is comfortable. If the hair has just been cut, ensure that all the hair cuttings are removed.

Preparing the hair

1   Shampoo and towel-dry the hair.

2   Comb out any tangles using a comb with widely spaced teeth.

3   Apply a suitable blow-styling aid, if the hair or the style requires it. Tell your client why you advise using the styling aid and make sure your client agrees before you apply it!

Products, tools and equipment

Styling and finishing products

There has been a large increase in the range of styling and finishing products available that have been produced specifically for men. These products are designed to work well on different hair types and to support a wide range of style effects. They perform particularly well on short styles, which are worn by many men.

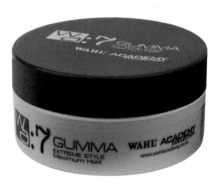

Hair wax

Men's products often contain little or no perfume and are available in packaging specifically designed to be attractive to men. These products work just as well on women's hair and can support many women's styles. Similarly, general styling products can be used equally well on men's hair, although these are less likely to sell as retail products to the male market.

Styling products are often versatile and many can be applied to the hair either before or after blow-drying, but some products are designed for use specifically before or after

TIP ✓

Read all manufacturers' instructions carefully to ensure that you can get the best performance from their products.

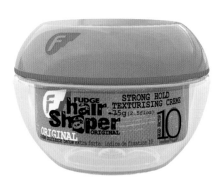

blow-drying. Products that are applied *before* are designed to protect the hair and help the styling process by providing added support to the style. Products that are applied *after* blow-drying impart shine and help to achieve and retain the finished style.

Some products bond to the internal structure of the hair and help the hair to retain moisture, as well as to retain the style. Yet others are designed to help the process of moulding and shaping the hair. A good knowledge of products and their use will help you to choose the most suitable products for creating different styles and effects.

> ## TIP ✓
>
> Manufacturers are constantly developing new styling products. Keep your product knowledge up-to-date by visiting the wholesalers, reading industry magazines and talking to manufacturers' representatives. Trying different products within the barber's shop and on your own hair will help you identify their strengths and limitations and maximize their potential in your work.

Whatever they are intended to do, most styling products will contain one or more of the following.

- *Plasticizers* These coat the hair, help mould it to shape, and then support the finished hairstyle.

- *Moisturisers* These retain the hair's natural moisture while resisting the absorption of further moisture from the atmosphere, as this moisture would make the hair structure revert to its alpha state, causing the style to drop.

- *Protectors* These protect the hair from the heat of the dryer and the adverse effects of the environment, particularly from the effects of ultraviolet rays from the sun.

Two types of products are especially common in men's hairdressing today.

- *Blow-styling aids* These are used to help mould the hair into shape. They support the finished hairstyle and protect the hair from the heat of the drying process, whilst also adding volume. They are available in a variety of strengths, ranging from 'firm hold' to 'ultra hold', and they are usually available as lotions, sprays, mousses and gels.

- *Dressing and finishing aids* These are used to retain the finished style. Some aids can also increase the shine, and improve the apparent condition of the hair. They are often used to give definition and texture to selected sections of hair, particularly on short styles, and are commonly available as mousses, gels, creams, oils and waxes.

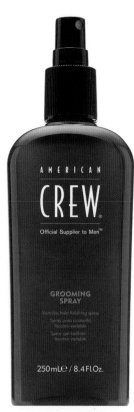

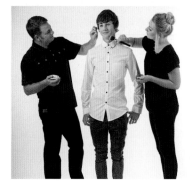

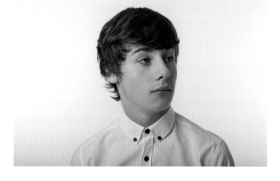

Tools

Brushes Brushes are available in many different shapes and sizes. Next to the hairdryer they are probably the most important item you will need.

Each brush is designed for a particular purpose, although often, with experience, it is possible to achieve similar effects with different brushes. Some brushes are designed to help you dry the hair quickly and are good for general shaping. Others are good for creating volume or for creating waves.

Here are some brushes commonly used in men's hairdressing:

◆ *Half-round plastic brushes* are good for creating smooth finishes and for general shaping (a). They can be used to build volume into the style during drying and can also be used to produce larger waves during blow-waving.

◆ *Half-round, flat or straight bristle brushes* can be either wood or plastic but in both cases they have short stiff bristles that grip the hair well (b, c). Bristle brushes are many barbers' preferred choice for blow-drying and especially blow-waving, as they can be used to produce large or small waves or partial waves where definition is required without a full wave being visible. They are often used to define partings and to control areas of hair without building too much volume into the style. They are equally good for straightening and smoothing the hair.

◆ *Vent brushes* (d) have vents which allow the air to flow through easily and so aid quick drying. They are very easy to use and are often used by barbers after styling with half-round brushes, to break up the style, smooth and straighten or to create a textured effect.

◆ *Circular brushes* are available in many different sizes. Small-diameter brushes are better for short to medium-length hair and produce a curled effect. Larger-diameter brushes work well on medium to long hair and produce a softer curl. Circular brushes are used more often for creating women's hairstyles than men's, but some may be used for blow-waving or for dealing with longer hair (e).

Combs Combs required include wide-toothed combs for disentangling the hair after it has been shampooed, and cutting combs or straight combs for sectioning longer hair

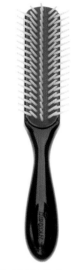

(a) Half-round plastic brush

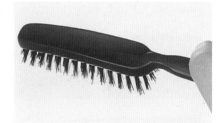

(b) Plastic bristle brush

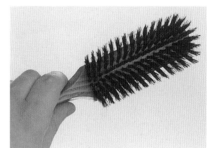

(c) Wooden bristle brush

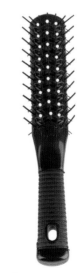

(d) Vent brush

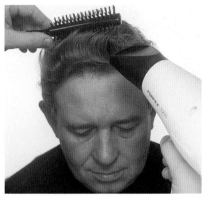

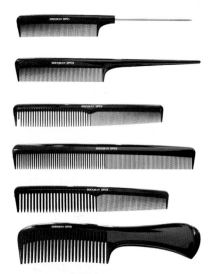

(e) Circular brush being used in blow-waving

before blow-drying. Cutting combs may also be used for creating waves during blow-waving but they must be heat-resistant.

Metal combs too are available, and may be used during blow-waving. They should be used with great care, as the metal can become quite hot from the heat of the dryer, but it is this heat that helps to fix the hair into the intended new shape. Only professional combs should be used.

Equipment

The most important piece of blow-drying equipment is, of course, the hand held hair-dryer. There are many models to choose from, but essentially the dryer should have adjustable speeds and temperatures, and be light and easy to hold – remember that whilst working you will be holding the dryer out for long periods. A professional-quality dryer should be your preferred choice, as this will have several functions and be adequately constructed to give many years of trouble-free service with minimum maintenance.

The dryer must include a nozzle to concentrate and direct the airflow, which is particularly important for blow-waving, creating definition and for men's hairdressing in general. The dryer should also have a diffuser, which disperses the airflow to dry the hair without moving it out of place. This method of drying produces an effect similar to that of natural drying and is often used in 'scrunch drying' (described below).

Blow-drying techniques

TIP

Commercial service times for blow-drying and finishing
You must work to commercially acceptable times in the barber's shop. This means allowing sufficient time for the service to be completed correctly but within the maximum time allowed. Remember that your client's needs must be met and your work must not appear to be rushed but you must work within commercial times.

TIP ✓

Always use a comb with widely spaced teeth for disentangling the hair, or the hair will pull and may break!

HEALTH & SAFETY

Metal combs retain heat and can burn the scalp so take extra care when using them.

It may help you to read Chapter 4, 'Client care for men' for more information on hair types and characteristics.

Your choice of blow-drying techniques will be based upon a number of important factors, including hair type and hair characteristics. Here are the main factors to consider:

- The hair type: known as Type 1 or S1 (Straight), Type 2 or W2 (Wavy), Type 3 or C3 (Curly) and Type 4 or VC4 (or K4) (Very Curly and sometimes called Kinky).

- The hair texture – fine, medium or coarse.

- The natural hair fall – growth patterns and length.

- The density – quantity of the hair per square centimetre.

- The current haircut – will the cut support the desired look?

- The desired style.

Different types of hair may require different techniques and can produce different effects. Thick, coarse hair is often the easiest to blow-dry, as it can be moulded to produce strong effects; however, it can take longer to dry and if particularly thick can be more difficult to shape. Fine hair often requires the use of styling aids to help thicken the hair and support the finished style.

A variety of different blow-drying techniques may be used to create the different effects required in men's hairdressing. Many of these techniques are also used to dry and style women's hair, but here we will consider their use for creating men's hairstyles.

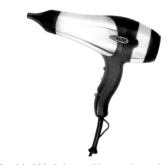

Hand-held hairdryer with nozzel attachment fitted

Blow-drying

Blow-drying is drying the hair with a hand-held hairdryer. It can be used just to dry the hair, but it is usually used to dry the hair into a shape or style.

A traditional blow-drying method

Traditional looks tend to have less volume and they often use blow-waving to define areas such as partings. Here are some examples:

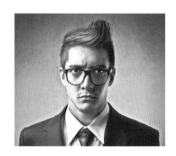

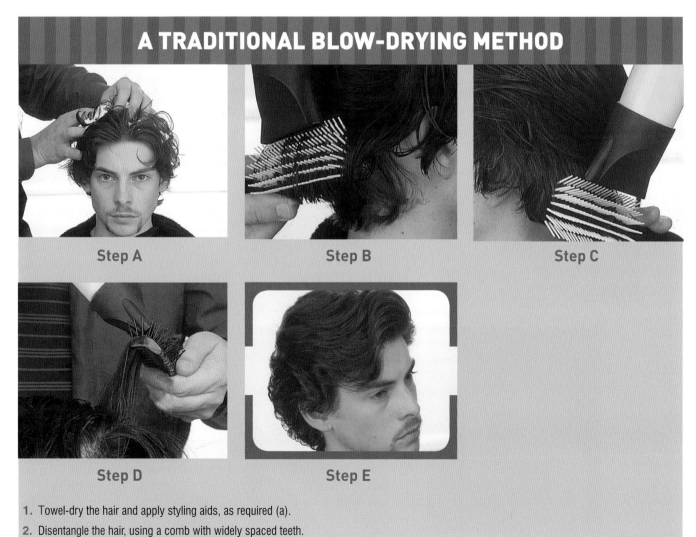

A TRADITIONAL BLOW-DRYING METHOD

Step A

Step B

Step C

Step D

Step E

1. Towel-dry the hair and apply styling aids, as required (a).
2. Disentangle the hair, using a comb with widely spaced teeth.

3. If the hair is particularly long (below shoulder) or one-length, cleanly divide it into small sections, using plain clips if required. If the hair is short, use the brush to divide the area of hair you are going to dry into manageable sections. Take horizontal sections for hair that is to go down, and vertical sections for hair that is to go back.

4. Lift the section of hair with the brush, and direct the heated airflow at the root area first – but not at the scalp, or it will burn. The angle at which you lift the hair will determine the amount of volume that is created (b).

5. Work methodically and ensure that you keep any wet hair away from the hair you are drying, or have already dried. Only use clips to secure the hair when necessary and make sure they are plain. (Remember: try not to use brightly coloured clips as these might embarrass your client!)

6. During drying, always direct the airflow away from the roots and towards the ends of the hair (c). Do not direct the airflow from the ends to the roots, or the cuticles will be blown open and the hair will become dull, rough and easily tangled.

7. Keep moving the brush as you direct the warm air over the section you are drying. Visualize the moulding process that is taking place as you manipulate the dryer, brush and hair (d). Make sure the section is fully dry. If the hair is long, allow it to cool before removing your brush – or use the cold-air button on your dryer if it has one.

8. Finish the style by dressing with combs or brushes. Apply finishing products, if required (e).

TIP ✓

When blow-drying, use the mirror regularly to check the balance of the style as it develops.

TIP ✓

Make sure you use the correct angle of lift to achieve the amount of volume required – remember many men prefer not to have too much volume in the finished style.

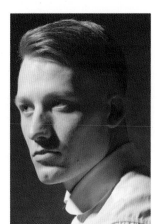

HEALTH & SAFETY

Check that the temperature setting on your dryer is correct prior to starting work. Test that the temperature is suitable by directing the airflow against the back of your hand.

Take care not to burn the hair or scalp by leaving the airflow directed in one place for too long.

Blow-drying contemporary looks

Contemporary looks are created mostly using the same blow-drying and styling techniques but often have more volume, sometimes the cut is disconnected and the blow-styling is used to emphasize the difference. Here are some examples.

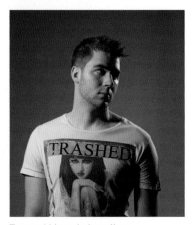

Textured blow-drying effect

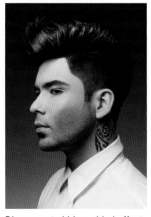

Disconnected blow-dried effect

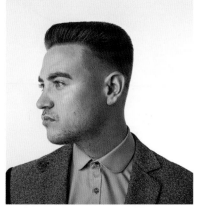

Flattop

ACTIVITY: CASE STUDY – SIMON

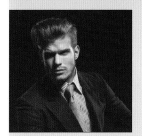

Simon is a new client in your barber's shop. He requests a shampoo cut and blow-dry. Simon wants a disconnected look. What advice should be provided regarding Simon's request?

Blow-waving

At one time blow-waving was very popular in men's hairdressing. Many men would have waves styled into their hair. Some had them going straight back; others had them going forward; yet others used waves in partings or at the sides to control the hair and keep it brushed back. Today, blow-waving is sometimes seen as being old-fashioned as people visualize a head full of tightly formed waves. Indeed, styles full of very visible waves are not currently in vogue, but the barber understands that blow-waving skills are essential to create definition and reduce volume in men's hairdressing.

Blow-waving may only be used on hair that is over about 6 cm in length, as the length of hair must be sufficient to allow the wave to form. It can be used very effectively to control unruly hair, particularly naturally curly or wavy hair. The waves should be created following the natural fall of the hair: this makes it easier to blow-wave and will ensure that the style is retained for as long as possible. It will also be much easier for clients to manage their own hair in this way.

Waves are often used *within* blow-drying to create movement that controls the hair and supports the style, in the same way that the hair may be permed to help support a desired style. The blow-drying is then completed with a vent brush, or Denman brush to break up the hair and leave a casual finish or smooth effect with few or no waves visible.

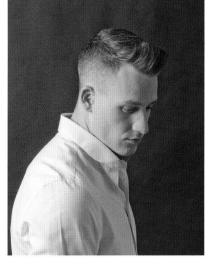

A versatile contemporary look

HEALTH & SAFETY

Take extra care not to burn the scalp when blow-waving, as the nozzle also concentrates the heat!

TIP

Blow-waving is much easier to achieve if you use a nozzle on the dryer.

Always towel-dry the hair before blow-waving, but make sure that the hair is still quite damp or the waves will not form.

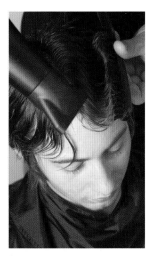

Creating the second wave

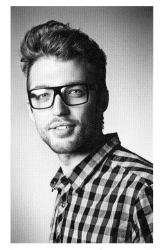

Loose waves create texture and movement in natural looks

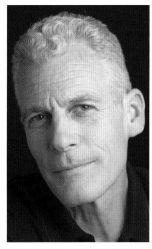

A classic blow waved effect

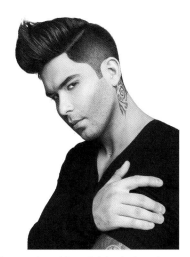

Blow-waving adds underlying body and support even though the waves are not visible

A BLOW-WAVING METHOD

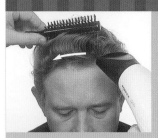

Step A Direct the airflow

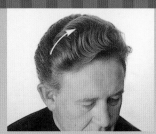

Step B Create the second wave

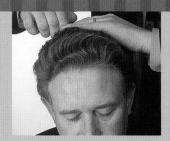

Step C Finish with a comb or brush

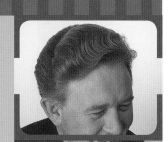

Step D The finished look – remember these waves can be softened by finishing drying across the waves using a vent brush

1. Towel-dry the hair and apply styling aids as required. The hair should be left quite damp.

2. Disentangle the hair, using a comb with widely spaced teeth.

3. Start at the front hairline and follow the hair's natural movements.

4. With a suitable brush or a wide-toothed comb, make a backward movement for about 5 cm and grip the hair. Turn the brush or comb slightly and, whilst gripping the hair, make a slight forward movement that produces the shape of a wave.

5. Direct the warm airflow along the trough created against the brush or comb, moving in the opposite direction to the brush or comb. Use a nozzle attachment on the dryer to concentrate the airflow (a).

6. Keep moving the airflow along the hair until the hair is dry, taking care not to burn the hair or scalp. Leave the hair to cool for a few seconds, or use the cold-air button on your dryer to fix the wave before moving onto the second wave.

7. The second wave is created in a similar way to the first, but in the opposite direction (b).

8. Keep working through the hair, creating waves where required, following the hair's natural fall. Create each wave in the opposite direction to the previous one, until the style is complete.

9. The shorter areas of hair should be dried smoothly to follow the movement of the last wave and to meet the style requirements.

10. Finish the style by dressing with a comb, or use a vent brush for a broken or textured effect (c).

11. Apply finishing products, if required (d).

TIP ✓
Do not keep trying to create waves on dry hair – use a water spray and start again!

TIP ✓
Blow-waving is a skill that takes a lot of practise to develop. Good co-ordination is required in both hands. Practise by blow-waving just three consecutive waves before you try to do more.

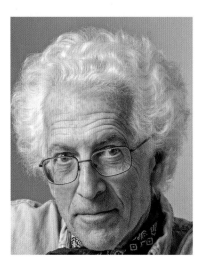

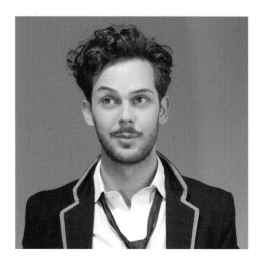

Blow-waving in contemporary styles

Blow-waving may be used to create movement that supports a wide range of styles. Many of these styles incorporate just three wave movements to achieve the required control and support.

The following method illustrates how blow-waving three consecutive wave movements may be used to produce a traditional style with a parting, without creating unwanted volume. This technique may then be applied in creating many different styles and effects.

BLOW-WAVING TO CREATE A TRADITIONAL STYLE

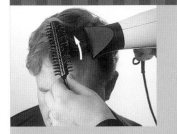

Step A First wave

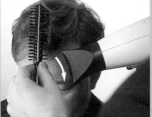

Step B Second wave

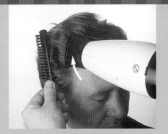

Step C Third wave

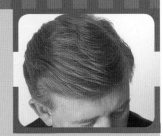

Step D

1. Towel-dry the hair and apply styling aids as required. The hair should be left quite damp.
2. Disentangle the hair, using a comb with widely spaced teeth.
3. To find the natural parting, comb the hair back, then push it forward slightly with the palm of your hand. The hair will fall between the front hairline and the crown: this is the natural parting.
4. Start at the front hairline section of the parting.
5. With a suitable brush or wide-toothed comb, make a backward movement away from the parting for about 5 cm and grip the hair. Turn the brush or comb slightly and, whilst gripping the hair, make a slight forward movement towards the parting, to produce the shape of a wave with the trough going up towards the crown.
6. Direct the warm airflow along the trough created against the brush or comb, moving in the opposite direction to the brush or comb (a).
7. Keep moving the airflow along the hair until it is dry, taking care not to burn the hair or scalp. Do not direct the airflow too deeply into the trough. The intention is to create movement, as opposed to a full wave. Let the hair rest for a few seconds or use your cold-air button to cool the hair and fix the movement before moving onto the second wave movement.
8. The second wave movement is created in a similar way to the first, but in the opposite direction. The movement is really a series of short movements with the dryer to mould the hair around the front hairline. The trough of the wave moves towards the face. Keep working through the hair until you reach the other side (b).
9. Make the third wave movement in the opposite direction, so that the trough of the wave goes back up towards the crown (c). You will notice that this turns the hair to go down or slightly back on the side opposite the parting.
10. The shorter areas of hair should be dried smoothly to meet the style requirements.
11. Finish the style by dressing with a comb, or use a vent brush for a more broken or textured effect. Apply finishing products, if required (d).

Other techniques

Finger drying

In finger drying the hair is styled by pulling, teasing and lifting with the fingers while the airflow from the dryer is used to mould the hair to the shape that has been created. The

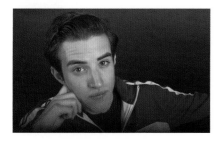

method results in fullness and soft billowing shapes which have little definition and so create a casual finished look.

Scrunch drying

Scrunch drying is a form of finger drying using a diffuser rather than a dryer with or without a nozzle. It produces softer shapes and is used more often in women's hairdressing than men's, primarily because it is usually used on longer hair to produce a casual, ruffled effect that is particularly suitable for women. It may be used on men, but a more masculine result is often required. Scrunch drying is usually carried out with a diffuser attachment on the dryer.

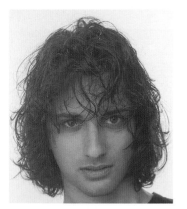

Natural drying

Natural drying is simply leaving the hair to dry naturally. Some men choose natural drying when it suits the hairstyle they are wearing.

In the barber's shop, natural drying is usually assisted by the application of heat from infrared lamps or accelerators or by blow-drying with a diffuser attachment. Essentially, the main characteristic of this method is that the hair is not styled during drying but is left to dry in its natural fall.

A finger dried look

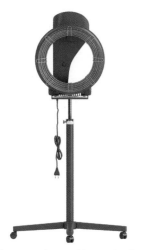

ACTIVITY: CASE STUDY – LEE

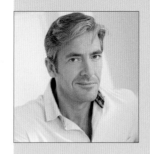

Lee is a 52-year-old regular client in your barber's shop. He requests a shampoo, blow-dry and neck shave as he is attending an important meeting later today. He wants a side parting and normally brushes the sides back. It is a windy day. What action should be taken regarding Lee's request?

Scrunch drying

Finishing techniques and aftercare advice

After drying, the style should be finished by combing or brushing. Some styling aids may be applied at this time to help smooth the hair while it is being dressed. Use of the comb will produce a smooth result, whereas a brush is likely to produce a more broken or textured effect. Use the mirror regularly to check the balance and symmetry of the style as you dress it.

When the desired effect has been achieved, finishing aids such as hairspray or wax may be applied to help retain it.

Remember to advise your client on how to maintain their look at home. Here are some ways you can help them achieve good blow-drying and finishing results:

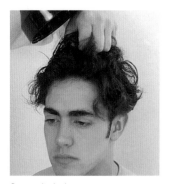

A heat lamp can be used to accelerate natural drying

◆ Products to use – suggest which products will help them achieve the look. This is a good opportunity to highlight the benefits of the products you have used to blow-dry, style and finish their hair and to recommend they buy these from your barber's shop.

◆ How to use products – show the client how the products should be used to achieve the best effects (you can highlight this to them as you style and finish their hair). Help them find and understand the manufacturer's instructions.

◆ How to dry and style their hair – show the client the basics of drying and styling and answer any questions they may have.

Health and safety

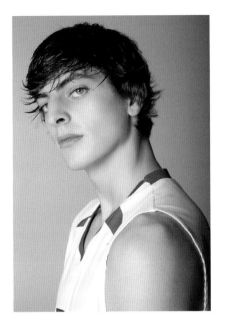

Everyone in the barber's shop has a duty to work safely and keep their environment safe. It is particularly important to consider health and safety in blow-drying, because of the risks associated with using electricity and the risk of burning the skin with the heat from the drying equipment.

Here are some important health and safety factors that you must specifically consider when providing blow-drying services.

Work safely with electricity

◆ Electrical equipment must always be handled and used with care, in accordance with the manufacturers' instructions.

◆ Never use or place a hand-dryer or other electrical equipment near water.

◆ Do not go near electrical equipment that is lying in water – switch off the mains power first.

◆ Before commencing work, visually check that electrical equipment is safe to use – check that the cable has not frayed or been pulled, and that the plug is not loose.

◆ Pay attention to the position of cables when using and storing electrical equipment.

◆ Never overload sockets by plugging too many items of electrical equipment into the same socket.

◆ Electrical equipment must be regularly tested and given a certificate of testing to confirm that it is safe to use. Your barber's shop owner will ensure that this is carried out, as required.

It may help you to read CHAPTER 2, 'Health and safety in the barber's shop' for more information on working safely in the barber's shop.

Avoid accidents

◆ Follow the manufacturer's instructions for the care of your dryer. Ensure that you clean the air filter regularly, to avoid overheating.

◆ Take care not to let the client's or your own hair or clothes get drawn into the air inlet at the back of the dryer.

◆ Always direct the airflow away from the scalp – this avoids burning, and produces a better, smoother blow-dried result.

◆ Use only clean tools and equipment.

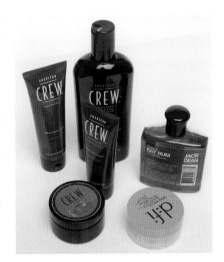

Be prepared for accidents

◆ Make sure that you know the whereabouts of your barber's shop's first-aid kit.

◆ Keep yourself up-to-date with your barber's shop's first-aid and accident procedures.

IMAGE GALLERY

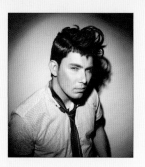

Visit the online image gallery on this book's accompanying website to see other inspirational men's hairstyles.

BRINGING IT ALL TOGETHER

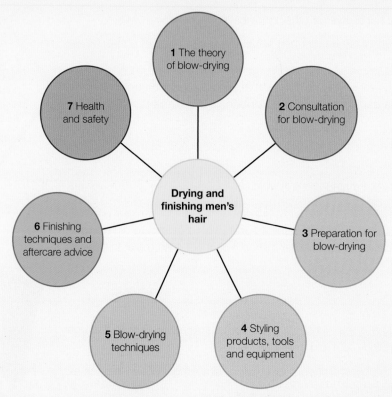

Summary

1 The process of shampooing and conditioning is mostly the same for men and women. Some products do differ, usually in their perfume and packaging.

2 During blow-drying the hair structure temporarily changes from its original natural state, called the *alpha state* (not stretched) to the *beta state* (stretched).

3 Consultation for blow-drying is likely to have been included in the consultation *before* the haircut, but you must still make sure that time is always set aside to discuss the client's requirements with them.

4 Prepare the hair for blow-drying by shampooing, towel-drying and combing out any tangles using a comb with widely spaced teeth.

5   Protectors protect the hair from the heat of the dryer during blow-drying.

◆   Half-round, flat or straight bristle brushes are often used to define partings and to control areas of hair without building too much volume into the style. They are equally good for straightening and smoothing the hair.

6   The angle at which you lift the hair whilst blow-drying will determine the amount of volume that is created.

◆   Many men prefer not to have too much volume in the finished style.

◆   Blow-waving may be used to create movement that supports a wide range of styles.

◆   Finger drying involves styling the hair by pulling, teasing and lifting the hair with the fingers while the airflow from the dryer is used to mould the hair to the shape.

7   Help clients find and understand the manufacturer's instructions for aftercare products that you recommend they buy from your barber's shop.

8   Before commencing work, visually check that electrical equipment is safe to use – check that the cable has not frayed or been pulled, and that the plug is not loose.

Activities

1   Visit local wholesalers and research the styling and finishing products available for men's hairdressing. Organize your findings into product groups, based on what they do. Compare the different alternatives and short-list those that provide the best features for your purposes. Work out how these might be recommended to clients as part of your aftercare advice. Compare this shortlist with the list of products in your barber's shop created earlier in this chapter. You can then recommend additional products to your manager.

2   Practise the blow-waving technique until you can link at least three consecutive waves together in a fluid, unbroken sequence before moving onto waving a full head. Investigate how this technique can assist in creating contemporary looks.

3   Find out the range of expected service times for drying and finishing hair in your barber's shop. What are the minimum and maximum times allowed? What maximum times are specified by your qualification?

Check your knowledge

1   Describe the changes that take place in the hair structure during blow-drying.

2   Describe the effect that a humid atmosphere has on blow-dried hair.

3   Describe the importance of considering volume when blow-drying men's hair.

4   List two things that should be done to prepare the client's hair before blow-drying.

5   State the purpose of plasticizers in a styling product.

6   What type of tool is most suitable for blow-waving?

a. Vent brush
b. Round brush
c. Half-round brush
d. Comb

7   What type of comb should be used for disentangling hair?

8   When should a nozzle be used on a hand held hairdryer?

9   Describe why it is important to consider airflow when blow-drying and blow-waving hair.

10 What should you do if the hair becomes dry before the style has been achieved?

a. Apply hairspray to the hair and continue blow-drying
b. Increase the heat setting and hold the dryer still until the *beta state* is formed
c. Decrease the heat setting and move the dryer more slowly until the *alpha state* is formed
d. Moisten the hair with a water spray and continue blow-drying

11 Describe natural drying.

12 How do you check that hairdryers are safe to use?

13 What action should be taken if a hairdryer was accidentally left on a wet surface?

14 Why is it important to take care with the inlet of a hairdryer?

9 Colouring men's hair

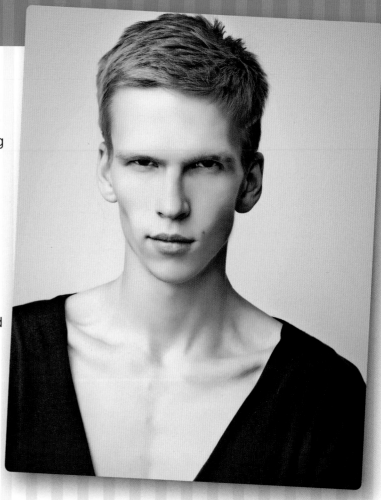

QUALIFICATION SIGNPOSTING

This chapter will help your studies of the following qualifications and units:

- ❖ Level 1 NVQ Certificate in Hairdressing and Barbering.
- ❖ Level 2 NVQ Diploma in Barbering.
- ❖ Level 3 NVQ Diploma in Barbering.
- ❖ City & Guilds Level 2 Award, Certificate and Diploma in Barbering.
- ❖ City & Guilds Level 2 Diploma in Women's and Men's Hairdressing.
- ❖ City & Guilds Level 3 Diploma in Barbering.
- ❖ ITEC Level 2 VRQ Diploma in Barbering.
- ❖ ITEC Level 2 and 3 VRQ Awards, Certificates and Diplomas in Barbering and Men's Hairdressing.
- ❖ VTCT Level 2 and 3 VRQ Diplomas in Barbering.
- ❖ VTCT Level 2 and 3 VRQ Diploma in Barbering Studies.

For further information on the qualifications covered by this chapter see the qualification mapping grid at the front of the book.

LEARNING OBJECTIVES

In this chapter you will learn:

◆ The basic principles of colouring.

◆ The different types of hair colourants.

◆ About lightening hair.

◆ The consultation requirements for colouring men's hair.

◆ About colouring in men's hairdressing.

INTRODUCTION

Traditionally, hair colouring has not often been required as a service in the barber's shop, so few barbers developed or offered colouring services. Some men seeking colouring services would visit 'unisex' or women's hair salons, whilst others relied on retail colourants and coloured their hair themselves, sometimes with alarming colour results! Colouring has featured in fashionable men's looks, such as the 'highlighted' looks that were popular in the 1980–1990s. Partial hair colouring and lightening have been more popular with men: although some men have had full-head colours, usually to mask grey hairs, it has mostly been women who have requested colouring services. Today, it is still the case that fewer men have their hair coloured, but some have recognized that colouring can provide depth, tone and texture to enhance a new haircut or to make an old hairstyle more interesting – for some hair colour is an important style statement! The barber's shop today should have colouring services at their disposal to ensure all their clients' hairdressing needs can be considered during consultation. Surely the contemporary barber

should be prepared to meet these clients' needs rather than see them access retail products for home use or other salons, with the potential that their business will be permanently lost?

This chapter is designed to provide an insight into how hair colouring and lightening, including bleaching, can be used in men's hairdressing. If you are new to colouring and lightening hair and intend to become expert, you will need to undertake more detailed studies of the principles and techniques of colouring, which are mostly the same for both men and women.

Here are some of the topics covered in this chapter:

❖ The basic principles of colouring.

❖ The different types of hair colourants.

❖ Lightening, including bleaching.

❖ Consultation for colouring men's hair.

❖ Colouring in men's hairdressing.

❖ Gallery of images for colouring in men's hairdressing.

Detailed technical information on colouring and lightening for those who wish to become expert can be found in other books within the Cengage Learning series.

The basic principles of colouring

Before reading this section it may be helpful if you read Chapter 5, 'Client care for men'.

Some basic facts about colour

Colour helps us to interpret the world we see around us. Indeed, it is often used to provide information and instructions. Colour makes things appear more interesting and attractive. It can affect our moods; make things appear warm or cold, subdued or vibrant. On hair it can make subtle or dramatic changes to a person's appearance, benefits that have been recognized in hairdressing for many years.

Why we see colour

White light such as normal daylight is actually a mixture of light of many different colours. These become visible only when a prism scatters the light, or when raindrops scatter sunlight to display the different colours in a rainbow. The range of colours that we see, from red to violet, is called the visible spectrum.

The colours that we see are the result of different parts of the light being absorbed and reflected. Consider a red object, for example. When white light falls on this, the red light in the spectrum is reflected, and all of the other colours in the white light are absorbed. The reflected light is what reaches our eyes, so the object looks red.

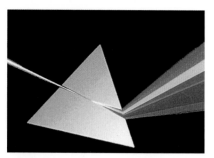
The colour spectrum from visible light

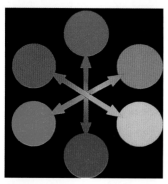
The colour circle

Natural hair colour

TIP	✓

The hair colour we see is reflected light: a portion only of the light falling on the hair. Natural daylight contains the complete spectrum – all the colours of the rainbow. Artificial lights, however, contain only some of them. Fluorescent lights tend to neutralize red and warm colours, while tungsten lights tend to add warmth and reduce ash effects. Natural daylight is the best light for showing the true hair colour.

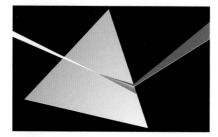
Red light reflecting and others being absorbed

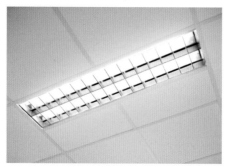
Fluorescent light

Tungsten light

Colour pigments

The natural colour of hair is due to granules of a pigment called melanin. The type of this pigment, and how much there is of it, determines the colour.

Daylight

Melanin is present within the hair cortex. The light falling on the hair passes through the hair cuticle, as this is translucent. The light is then reflected by the melanin. The colour we see is therefore determined by the colour that the melanin reflects.

There are two main types of melanin present in the hair:

◆ Eumelanin is responsible for black and brown hair.

◆ Pheomelanin is responsible for red and blond hair.

Most people have a mixture of the two types of **melanin** in their hair. Their natural hair colour is formed by the quantity of each type of pigment that is present.

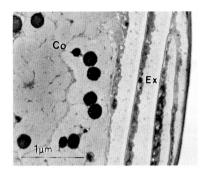

Melanin granules in the cortex of the hair ($1\mu m$ is 1/1000th of 1 mm)

White hair – going grey!

Age and other factors such as stress can affect the production of natural hair pigments. As we get older, our new hairs have reduced levels of pigment – or, in the case of white hair, no pigment at all. Your client may have asked you, 'am I going grey yet?'

Over time, the proportion of hairs on the head with reduced pigment or no pigment increases, and so the overall colour of the hair changes. Grey hair is the result of a large number of white hairs growing amongst the naturally coloured hairs; thus the hair is not actually turning grey – it is becoming white but looks grey mixed with the still coloured hairs. The amount of white hair is often described as a percentage of the whole head. For example, if half of the hairs are white and half are still naturally pigmented, the hair is described as being '50 per cent grey', or 10 per cent if about one in ten hairs are white. Often these white hairs are concentrated at particular parts of the head and as a consequence the percentage of white is different, such as around the temples.

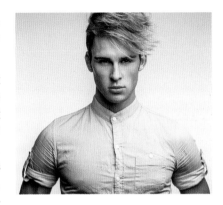

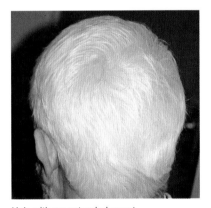

Hair with no natural pigment

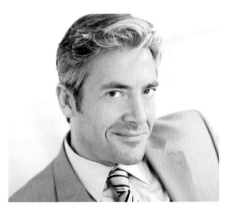

Changes in the level of pigment occur over time

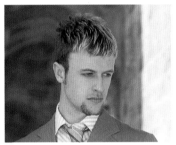

Describing colour

Naturally pigmented hair colours are often simply described as being blond, red, brown or black. Although these descriptions are adequate for general use, they are not precise enough for professional hair colouring. The International Colour Chart (ICC) was developed so that hair colours could be accurately identified and described – both the natural hair colour and the desired or 'target' hair colour.

Each hair colour is described in levels of depth and tone. Depth refers to how light or dark the colour is. This is determined by the intensity of the pigments in the hair. Tone refers to the colour that is seen. This is determined by the combination of different pigments present.

The different shades of colour are numbered, starting with 1 for black through to 10 for lightest blond. Additional numbers are then added to each shade to identify the huge range of tones that are possible.

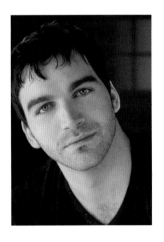

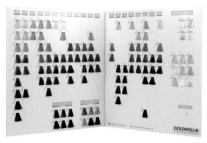
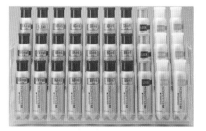

ICC chart

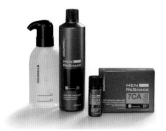

Colouring products

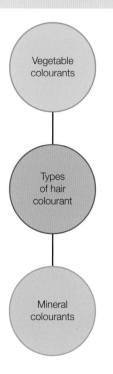

Men's colouring products

> **KEY DEFINITION**
>
> Colourant: A substance added to something else to cause a colour change.

Vegetable colourants

Types of hair colourant

Mineral colourants

The International Colour Chart

Colour	Depth	Colour	Tone
1/0	blue-black	–/0	natural
2/0	black	–/1	special ash
3/0	dark brown	–/2	cool ash
4/0	medium brown	–/3	honey gold
5/0	light brown	–/4	red/gold
6/0	dark blond	–/5	purple
7/0	medium blond	–/6	violet
8/0	light blond	–/7	brunette
9/0	very light blond	–/8	pearl ash
10/0	extra light blond	–/9	soft ash

Hair colourants

Colouring is the general term used to describe the various techniques and processes that are used to change hair colour. It is achieved through a process that adds colour pigments to the hair in the form of natural or synthetic dyes.

The history of hair colouring goes back many thousands of years. People have changed their natural hair colour for many reasons, sometimes to meet the requirements of a religion or society, but most often to express their individuality and create a look that they like.

Colourants used – from early hair colouring to present day

Over the years, various methods and lotions have been used to change the colour of hair. Around 2000 years ago the Egyptians used the powdered leaves of the henna plant to colour hair red. The Romans used a mixture consisting largely of ash, sodium bicarbonate and lime to lighten the hair. Many other natural and artificial ingredients have been used, with varying degrees of success. In the early 1800s, however, hydrogen peroxide was discovered, and more modern methods of colouring were established. Today, most hair **colourants** are derived from either vegetable or mineral extracts.

Vegetable colourants

Vegetable colourants are made from the flowers or stems of different plants, such as henna. For example, camomile, made from the flowers of the camomile plant, is used to brighten light blond hair.

Mineral colourants

Mineral colourants are made from either metallic dyes or aniline derivatives. Metallic dyes are used to coat the surface of the hair, and are sometimes used in hair colour restorers, though they are not often used in the salon.

Special care must be taken to identify whether mineral colourants have been used as metallic dyes are incompatible with hydrogen peroxide, and peroxide forms part of many hairdressing products used in colouring, bleaching and perming. An **incompatibility** test should be carried out when the use of metallic dyes is suspected.

Aniline derivatives

Aniline derivatives are synthetic dyes made from ingredients found in crude oil. They are used in most modern hair colourants and are known as para dyes.

These types of dye can cause a skin reaction, so a skin test is carried out before they are applied.

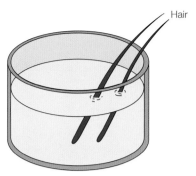

No reaction – hair and selected product are compatible

HEALTH & SAFETY

Follow the manufacturers' instructions for testing carefully. Do not apply products containing para dyes to a client who has had a positive reaction to a skin test. Do not apply products containing hydrogen peroxide to hair that has produced a positive reaction to an incompatibility test.

Make sure that you keep a record of the skin test and its results and a record of your consultation and the client's responses in case of problems.

Ask the client to check their responses and sign to confirm they are correct.

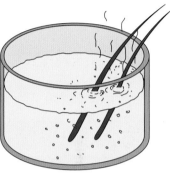

Reaction (between chemicals in product already on hair) – hair and product are incompatible

Groups of hair colourants

In hair colouring the colourant products used are often described simply as 'colouring products' or 'colour products'. These hair colour products are then usually grouped according to how long they remain on the hair. They include temporary, semi-permanent, quasi-permanent and permanent colours.

KEY DEFINITION

Incompatibility: Two or more substances that do not work well when mixed together; they sometimes react badly.

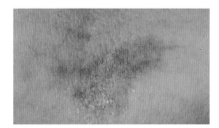

Allergic reaction to skin test

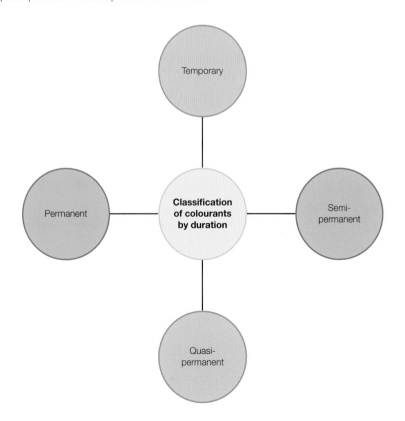

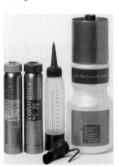

Permanent hair colouring products

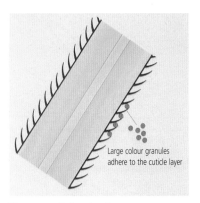

Temporary hair colouring

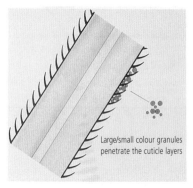

Semi-permanent hair colouring

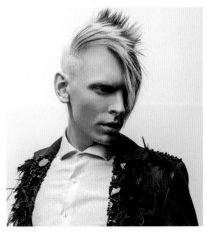

Some clients prefer vibrant colours

Temporary colours

Temporary colours are available as lotions, mousses, and creams, sprays gels, and so on. They contain large colour molecules which coat the hair cuticle. They do not penetrate into the hair cortex or affect the natural hair colour, though some temporary colours may be absorbed if the hair is very porous. Temporary colours remain on the hair until they are shampooed off.

Semi-permanent colours

Semi-permanent colours are available in several forms, though they are usually applied as a cream or rinse. Most are pre-mixed, but some have to be mixed before they are used, so it is important to read the manufacturer's instructions carefully.

Semi-permanent colours deposit their colour molecules in the hair cuticle, and also in the outer part of the hair cortex: the molecules are smaller than those found in temporary colours. This means that the semi-permanent colour molecules are more difficult to remove, so the colour lasts longer, gradually fading as the hair is washed. The colour lasts for between six and eight shampoos, depending upon the condition and porosity of the hair.

Semi-permanent colours are not designed to be suitable for covering large percentages of white hair.

Quasi-permanent colours

Quasi-permanent colours are nearly permanent. They last longer than semi-permanent colours, but not as long as permanent colours. (The prefix 'quasi' means 'almost but not quite'.)

This type of colour product is more effective at covering white hair than are semi-permanent colours, and can last for up to 12 weeks dependent on a number of washes. Remember that the colour effect will fade with each wash!

Permanent colours

Permanent colours, sometimes called permanent tints, are available in the form of creams and liquids, and come in a wide variety of shades and tones. They can cover white hair and naturally pigmented hair to produce natural or fashion shades, which can be very vibrant if the client so desires.

The colour molecules in permanent colours are much smaller than those found in temporary and semi-permanent colours: they pass easily into the hair cortex. Most permanent colours are mixed with hydrogen peroxide. This oxidizes the hair's natural pigments, causing them to combine with the molecules in the permanent colour product and form a chain of larger molecules which become permanently trapped in the cortex, known as polymerization.

Permanent colours stay in the hair until the hair grows out, when the hair's natural pigmentation will again become visible. This regrowth must be re-coloured if the client wishes to keep his hair the desired colour.

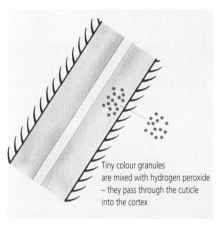

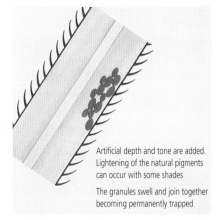

Tiny colour granules are mixed with hydrogen peroxide – they pass through the cuticle into the cortex

Artificial depth and tone are added. Lightening of the natural pigments can occur with some shades

The granules swell and join together becoming permanently trapped

Permanent hair colouring

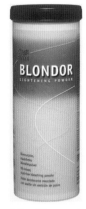

Hair lightening/bleaching product

Very Pale Yellow
Pale Yellow
Yellow Yellow
Orange Yellow
Orange
Reddish Orange
Reddish Brown
Brown
Black

Stages of lift in hair lightening using bleach based products

HEALTH & SAFETY

Manufactures' Instructions and the EU Cosmetic Products Directive
Under European Union (EU) Legislation – Directive Amendment Number 2010/4/EU the use of certain chemicals liable to cause allergic reactions is restricted in hairdressing products. Manufacturers are required to label their products to identify the presence of such chemicals and provide guidance on how the product should be used and stored, including restrictions on the use of products on those who are under 16 years of age. You must always follow these instructions carefully. Never use a product on someone under 16 if the label states, 'This product is not intended for use on persons under the age of 16'.

TIP ✓

When colouring, lightening or toning, remember to take into account the temperature of the salon. A warm room will reduce processing time, while a cold room will increase processing time.

Lightening (sometimes known as bleaching)

Lightening is the process used to make the hair colour lighter when regular hair colourants are not strong enough to be effective. Lightening products are available in the form of liquids, oils, creams, gels and powder.

Lightening products require a ready supply of oxygen to work. Mixing the lightener with the correct strength of hydrogen peroxide provides this. Lighteners are alkaline, which causes the hair shaft to swell and the cuticles to lift, allowing the lightening product to enter the hair cortex, where the oxygen reacts with the natural colour pigments, leaving them colourless.

The eumelanin pigment, which produces the colours black and brown, is the first to be affected; then the pheomelanin pigment, which gives red and yellow colours. Pheomelanin is more difficult to alter, so it becomes more noticeable as the eumelanin is lightened, sometimes making the hair appear yellow or 'brassy'. As the lightening process proceeds, the hair gradually becomes lighter until at some point it stops getting any lighter.

The actual colour that can be achieved by lightening depends on the proportions of eumelanin and pheomelanin in the hair. Some natural shades, such as light brown and blond, can simply be lightened to the correct light shade. Most dark shades, however, need a toner applied to neutralize any remaining yellow. There are special toners made specifically for lightened hair, or diluted temporary, semi-permanent or permanent colour products may be used instead.

HEALTH & SAFETY

Too much lightening/bleaching will destroy the hair structure. Do not lighten/bleach hair that is in poor condition. Always avoid overlapping sections or combing the lightening product through hair that has been previously lightened. Before starting, process a strand of hair with a strand test.

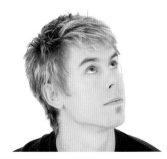

Partially lightened hair

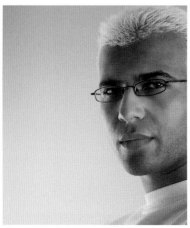

Bleached hair

Hydrogen Peroxide

In quasi-permanent, permanent, lightening and bleaching services hydrogen peroxide, also known as H_2O_2 because it consists of two molecules of hydrogen to two molecules of oxygen, is used as the oxidizing agent that stimulates processing. Hydrogen peroxide is a reactive substance that easily releases oxygen molecules, which when mixed with the hairdressing product reacts with chemicals in the product to create the effect required. Hydrogen peroxide is commonly available in four different strengths:

H_2O_2 Strengths	Used for
10 vol (3%)	Ensuring darkest depth of colour. Refreshing faded areas.
20 vol (6%)	Achieving lift up to 1 shade on base shades of 5 and higher
30 vol (9%)	Achieving lift up to 3 shades on base shades of 5 and higher
40 vol (12%)	Achieving lift up to 5 shades on base shades of 5 and higher

Make sure that the manufacturer's instructions for the product you are using are followed accurately – both the correct strength and ratio of hydrogen peroxide to colour product are important. This may be shown as 2:1, meaning two parts of hydrogen peroxide are required to one part of colour product, or 1:1, meaning one part of hydrogen peroxide is required to one part of colour product.

TIP ✓

Sometimes it might be necessary to dilute higher strengths of hydrogen peroxide for a particular colour. This can be achieved by working out what ratio of water should be added to the hydrogen peroxide, for example: to make 6 per cent (20 vol) from 12 per cent (40 vol) calculate the difference as a fraction: $\frac{6}{12} = \frac{1}{2}$ (or $\frac{20}{40} = \frac{2}{4} = \frac{1}{2}$). Thus, one part of water should be added to one part of H_2O_2.

HEALTH & SAFETY

Take care not use too strong a solution of peroxide. Strong solutions can easily damage the hair structure and burn the skin. Avoid the bleach coming into contact with your own or your client's skin.

TIP ✓

Make sure that you replace the top firmly after dispensing hydrogen peroxide as its effectiveness will decrease if left open to the air. Never return unused hydrogen peroxide to the original container as this will cause the contents to deteriorate; it should be poured down the sink and flushed away with fresh water.

HEALTH & SAFETY

Always be careful when handling hydrogen peroxide. It is a harmful irritant. Follow the manufacturer's instruction carefully.

Consultation for colouring men's hair

Most of the principles and techniques for colouring are the same for both men's and women's hair. What differs in men's colouring is how the techniques are used to create the effects and looks that men like.

The choice of correct colouring method, product and processing time for each client relies on careful consideration of many different factors. Here are some of the critical factors that must be considered when colouring hair.

- ◆ Identify the client's requirements; then advise them on suitable styles, colouring methods and products.

- ◆ Look carefully for signs of broken skin or any abnormalities on the skin or hair. Remember that these might be contra-indications!

- ◆ Determine the hair type and hair characteristics.

- ◆ Determine the current depth and tone of the client's hair; is this colour natural or artificial?

◆ Consider the client's current style and haircut, together with your client's age and lifestyle.

◆ If the client is a regular colouring client, refer to their record card for details of previous work.

◆ Determine the condition of the hair. Has it been previously chemically treated? Is the hair dry, damaged or porous?

◆ Carry out tests, as required.

It may help you to read CHAPTER 4, 'Client care for men' for more information on consultation.

HEALTH & SAFETY

You must carry out a thorough consultation to ensure that you identify any adverse conditions of the hair or skin. It is particularly important to establish whether a suspected infection or infestation is present, to check for an allergic reaction to para dyes, and to check whether the skin is inflamed, cut or grazed. If any of these conditions is present, you must not colour the hair.

Remember that for any client, having one's hair coloured is a major decision. For a man it can be especially so. Always discuss your client's requirements with them and establish why they want their hair coloured and what they are expecting. Before commencing work, determine whether temporary, semi-permanent, quasi-permanent or permanent colouring is the correct solution for their needs.

ACTIVITY: CASE STUDY – WALK-IN CLIENT: ADJIT

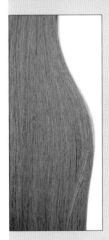

A new walk-in client is requesting a permanent colour. He is 45 years old and says he is "too young to go grey". He adds, "I have given up trying to hide it and want a permanent solution." During the consultation you see this colour hair. What action should be taken regarding the client?

TIP ✓

Treat the hair gently after permanent colouring and especially after bleaching, particularly when drying it into style.

TIP ✓

This chapter is intended to introduce the barber to hair colouring services and illustrate how these might be introduced into the barber's shop. More detailed technical information on hair colouring, for both men and women, particularly regarding solving hair colour problems, known as colour correction is provided in other books within the Cengage Learning series. **Ensure** you have all the required skills and understanding of hair coloring to be competent, or are suitably supervised **before** providing these services.

TIP ✓

Make sure that you accurately record details of the client's skin test, previous colouring services and any contraindications, especially any client history of allergic reactions. You should record the client's actual responses and ask them to sign these as confirmation. Remember, colouring services must not be carried out if a **contraindication** is present.

KEY DEFINITION

Contraindication: The presence of a condition or factor that indicates a particular service or treatment should not be carried out.

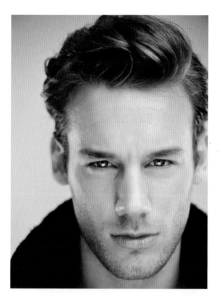

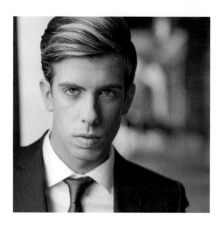

Carefully explain what is involved in the type of colouring selected. Describe the benefits that your client can expect, and what aftercare will be required. Here are some important things for you to cover:

◆ Your client may not be familiar with the type and range of colouring products that are available, so you will need to explain the benefits and features of each of them to them.

◆ Advise your client of the time colouring takes and the costs that are involved. Before you begin work, make sure that they agree the course of action to be taken and check that there is no misunderstanding.

◆ Make sure your client knows how long each type of colour lasts, especially if the results will be permanent!

◆ Make sure that you prepare a record card for each client and note all details of the service accurately for future reference.

◆ After the colour, advise the client on how to manage their hair at home. The advice will differ depending upon the type of colour used. Hair that has been permanently coloured, and especially hair that has been lightened/bleached, will require careful handling and conditioning. Some manufacturers provide aftercare information leaflets that you can give to clients.

ACTIVITY: CASE STUDY – WALK-IN CLIENT: DAVE

This new walk-in client is considering adding some colour. He says this is 'to liven up my natural mousey colour', which you know is better defined as a depth of 6 with cool ash tones. Dave has never had a hair colour before and is concerned about it being too noticeable and being permanent. During the consultation he tells you that he occasionally has eczema. Dave is sure that he doesn't want anything too noticeable.

What action should be taken regarding the client?

Colouring in men's hairdressing

Men are often unaware of the benefits that colouring can bring, so they do not consider colouring services. Sometimes men are deterred from having their hair coloured because the colouring results they see displayed appear too feminine. At other times it is the service itself that acts as a deterrent, as some men find the colouring process embarrassing, particularly if it is carried out in full view of those passing by the salon.

Here are some examples of how you can introduce men to the benefits of colouring and encourage them to consider colouring services when these are the best solution for their requirements.

◆ Describe how colouring can provide added depth, tone and texture to enhance your client's new haircut or make his old hairstyle more interesting.

◆ Display examples of how colouring has been used in men's hairdressing and especially those that illustrate how colouring can create and enhance masculine looks. Use examples of such looks to support the client consultation.

◆ Wherever possible, avoid using brightly coloured capes and gowns, as these may embarrass the client.

◆ Carry out colouring services in areas of the salon designed for that purpose, and not in areas where other clients are only having haircutting services. Do not seat colouring clients where they can be seen by people passing by.

Lee Stafford

❝ Adding great, tasteful colour to a guy's haircut can make it sing, as well as putting some extra cash in your pocket! ❞

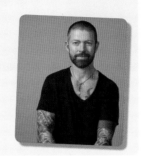

Examples of colouring in men's hairdressing

Most men who have their hair coloured prefer the results to appear natural. Indeed, most men's colouring is carried out to enhance the haircut, and the colouring effects are often quite subtle. Full head colouring is sometimes used, but partial hair colouring, such as highlights or lowlights, is more popular with most men.

A wide range of techniques and equipment may be used to partially colour hair, including wrapping hair in caps, foil or other packages, or simply applying the product onto the selected section of hair with a brush, comb foil or other implement.

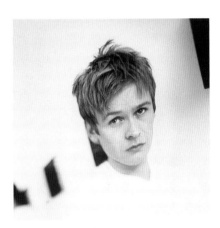

Partial colouring is particularly useful for defining the movement and texture within a haircut, and is often preferred by clients who have longer hair on the top and short hair at the back and sides, especially for styles that are dressed straight back on the top. Colouring can also break up solid shapes, making the hair appear more disconnected and so more interesting.

Men generally want their hair to look as natural as possible, so vibrant coloured effects are not often required, but remember to consider what the client says, as an extreme look might be their goal!. You will always need to take account of the requirements of each individual client.

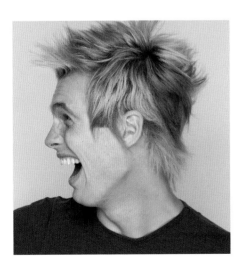

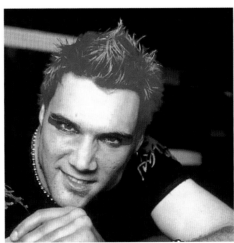

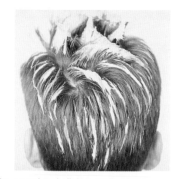

Tipping enhances texture through the top

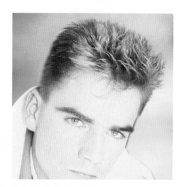

The completed slicing application

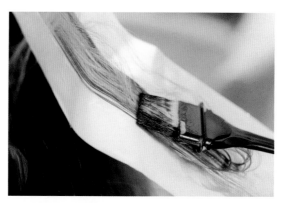

Partial lightening/bleaching

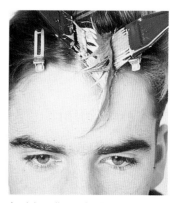

Applying slices of colour to a selected section of hair

The following examples show how colouring can be used to enhance some common looks. In each case the colours may be lighter or darker than the client's natural base to create either highlights or lowlights. The actual choice of colour is dependent on the requirements of each client.

Tipping

Tipping is good for creating textured effects and accentuating movement within the look. It can be applied with great accuracy so that only very specific parts of the hair are coloured.

Weaving and Slicing

Slicing is good for defining movement on layered hair.

Stippling and slices

Stippling is a development of the slicing technique. It is good for enhancing textured effects in disconnected haircuts, and for defining movement.

The finished slicing effect

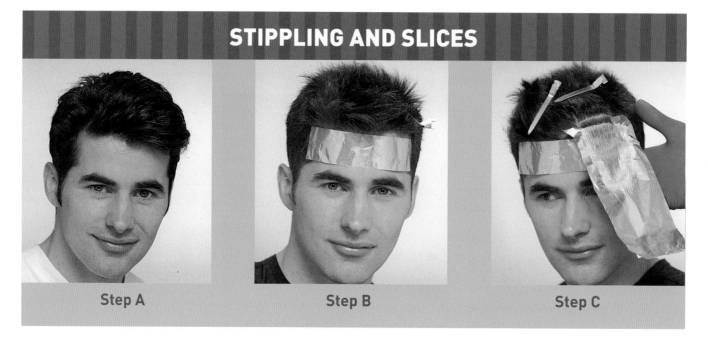

STIPPLING AND SLICES

Step A

Step B

Step C

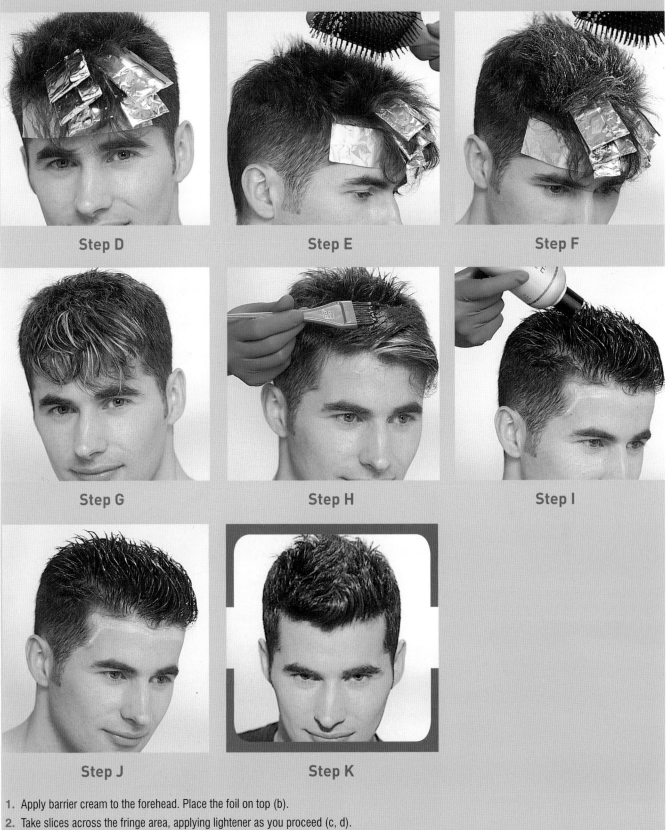

Step D

Step E

Step F

Step G

Step H

Step I

Step J

Step K

1. Apply barrier cream to the forehead. Place the foil on top (b).
2. Take slices across the fringe area, applying lightener as you proceed (c, d).
3. To achieve the stippling effect, apply the lightener to a paddle brush, and brush it onto the hair (e, f).
   Do not overdo this, or the effects will be too solid, unless this is the effect being sought!

(Continued)

STIPPLING AND SLICES (*Continued*)

4. Allow the lightener to develop, then remove it by shampooing (g).
5. Using a brush, apply the colourant to the pre-lightened hair (h).
6. Apply colourant to the rest of the head, straight from the bottle (i).
7. Allow the product to develop (j).
8. Shampoo, condition and style the hair, as required (k).

Polishing

Polishing – sometimes called shoeshine colour – is often used to create movement and texture through the ends of short layered hair.

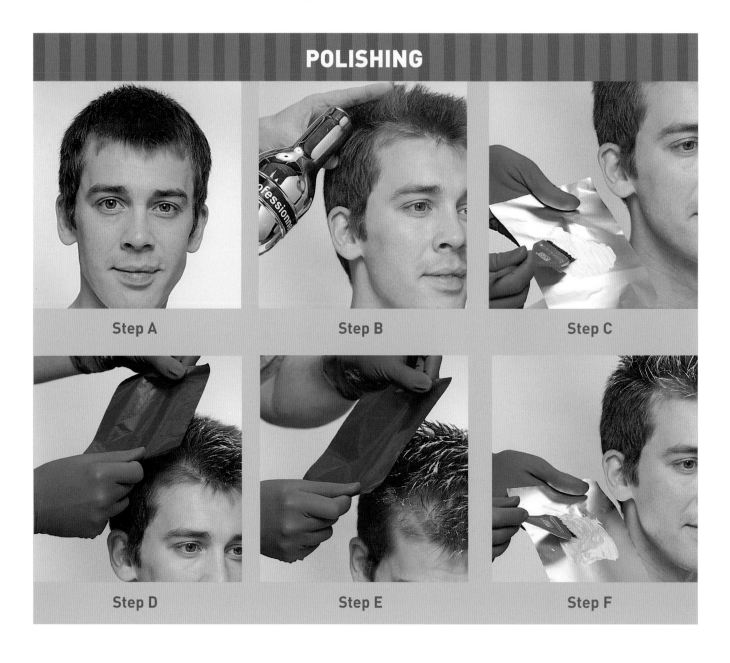

POLISHING

| Step A | Step B | Step C |
| Step D | Step E | Step F |

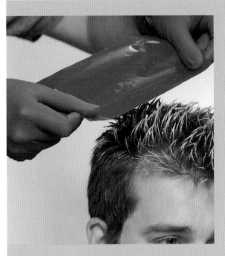
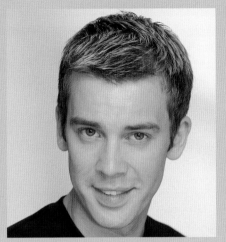
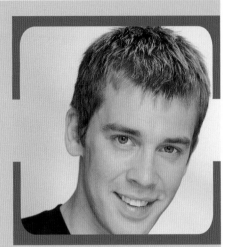

Step G   Step H

1. Mist the hair lightly with hairspray, and blow-dry it to make the hair stand up (b).
2. Apply the first colour to a foil, using a brush (c).
3. Lightly wipe the foil across the hair, to apply colour to the ends only (d).
4. Continue applying colour over the whole of the top of the head (e).
5. Apply the second colour to the foil (f).
6. Apply the second colour, as before (g).
7. Allow the product to develop, then shampoo, condition and style the hair, as required (h).

Block Colouring

Block colouring is used to create bolder, more defined effects and can include multiple colours.

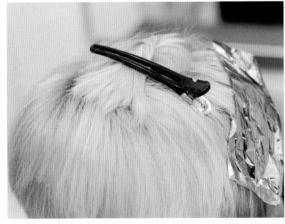

Sectioning for block colouring

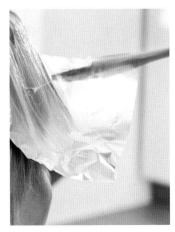

Application of block colour

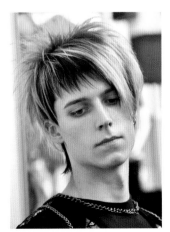

Finished effect

TIP ✓

Remember, when removing permanent and high-lift colour products after their development it is important to **emulsify** the product to ensure they are effectively removed. This is achieved using rotary and friction massage movements and working the product into the moistened hair. This action lifts the excess colour from the hair and scalp where they are suspended in an **emulsion** that can be rinsed away.

It may help you to read CHAPTER 5, 'Shampooing and conditioning men's hair' for more information on shampooing and conditioning techniques.

Health and safety

It is important to consider health and safety when colouring hair because of the risks associated with using chemicals and the risk of damaging the skin. Here are some important health and safety factors that you must consider when providing colouring services.

Avoid infection

It may help you to read CHAPTER 2, 'Health and safety in the barber's shop' for more information on working safely in the barber's shop.

◆ If the client has any cuts or abrasions on his head, or you suspect that an infection or infestation is present, you must not carry out the colouring service.

◆ Use only clean tools and equipment.

◆ Work safely with chemicals.

◆ Always handle, use and store chemicals with care, and in accordance with the manufacturers' instructions.

◆ Protect your hands when using chemicals.

◆ Follow the manufacturers' instructions for testing, particularly for skin testing and incompatibility testing.

◆ Keep accurate records of skin test results and your consultation with clients for colouring services. Ask clients to check and sign their responses to confirm they are correct.

◆ Dispose of used chemicals in accordance with the manufacturers' instructions, salon policy, and local authority regulations.

◆ Check your salon's COSHH list of hazards to find out how to use products carefully.

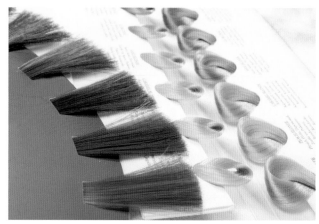

ICC hair swatches

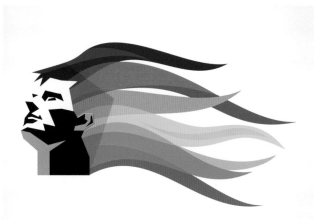

Bold advertising can help increase colour services

Be prepared for accidents

◆ Make sure that you know the whereabouts of your salon's first-aid kit.

◆ Keep yourself up-to-date with your salon's first-aid and accident procedures.

◆ Take care not to splash colouring products onto the client's skin or clothes, or surrounding areas.

IMAGE GALLERY

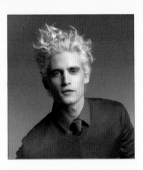

Visit the online image gallery on this book's accompanying website to see inspirational hair colouring images.

BRINGING IT ALL TOGETHER

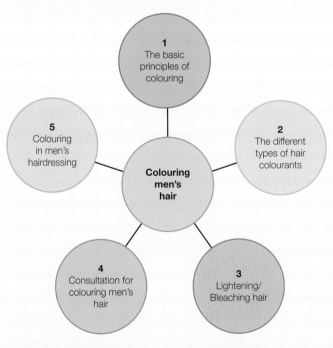

- 1 The basic principles of colouring
- Colouring men's hair
- 5 Colouring in men's hairdressing
- 2 The different types of hair colourants
- 4 Consultation for colouring men's hair
- 3 Lightening/Bleaching hair

Summary

1 The process of colouring hair is mostly the same for men and women. Some products differ, usually in their perfume and packaging but it is the techniques and the effects desired that are most different.

2 The colour we see is the part of the colour spectrum reflected back by the object viewed.

3 The natural hair colour, depth and tone is determined by the amount of eumelanin and pheomelanin present in the hair.

4 The International Colour Chart (ICC) is used in professional hairdressing to determine and record the natural depth and tone and target shade and tone of hair colour.

5 There are two basic types of hair colourant: vegetable and mineral.

6 Metallic dyes are incompatible with hydrogen peroxide.

7 Hairdressing colouring products can cause allergic reactions that can be severe.

8 Always follow the manufacturer's instructions for skin testing to avoid problems through allergic reactions to para dyes and other chemicals in colourants. Skin testing before using a new hair colouring product is essential.

9 Some products are restricted and cannot be used on those under the age of 16 – the manufacturer's instructions must be carefully followed in all cases.

10 Semi-permanent products produce effects that will fade but the effects of permanent products will remain until the hair grows out.

11 The lightening process using bleach must be timed and carefully monitored to achieve the correct colour. The chemical reaction will continue and the hair colour may become too light and the hair damaged.

12 Partial colouring is often more suitable for defining texture and movement in men's looks.

13 Polishing is a good technique for creating textured effects on short layered hair.

14 Always handle and store colouring products following the manufacturer's instructions – make sure you know the product's COSHH requirements.

15 Always wear gloves and other PPE when handling and using colouring products to avoid any allergic reaction and contact dermatitis.

Activities

1 Visit local barber's shops, unisex and women's salons, and use the Internet to research colouring in men's and women's hairdressing. Find out what types of colours and effects are most popular for each. Compare your findings to identify how men use colouring services and consider how this information might help your barber's shop offer colouring services. You can then make recommendations to your manager. This activity may be combined with the similar activity in the additional online material, 'Perming men's hair'.

2 Use the Internet and magazines to find images that show how colouring is used in men's hairdressing. Produce a style book that can be used during consultation with the clients in your salon. Remember to get permission from your manager first. This activity may be combined with the similar activity in the additional online material, 'Perming men's hair'.

3 Practise your colouring techniques on a mannequin head or block until you can work quickly and neatly. Only then should you process the colour to become familiar with the effects. Make sure you do this and are sufficiently skilled and knowledgeable in colouring hair before you work on clients. Check with your manager or supervisor first.

4 Make a list of all the information you think should be recorded about clients relating to colouring services. Research the different record cards available at local wholesalers and use the Internet to compare them with your list. Design a new record card that includes all the most relevant information. Compare this against your salon's record card and note any differences. Recommend any improvements to your manager and be prepared to explain your reasons. This activity may be combined with the similar activity in the additional online material, 'Perming men's hair'.

Check your knowledge

1 Why do we see a red object as being red?

2 What is the correct name of the natural pigment in the hair?

  a. Granules

  b. Pigments

  c. Melanin

  d. Cuticles

3 What effect can artificial light have on how we see colours?

4 Describe the International Colour Chart.

5 Which colour is opposite red on the colour circle?

  a. Blue

  b. Green

  c. Yellow

  d. Purple

6 Why is it important to carry out a skin test before certain colouring services?

7 What are the reasons for carrying out an incompatibility test?

8 What are the changes that take place in the hair structure during the permanent colouring process?

9 How long do quasi-permanent colours last?

10 List two types of temporary colourant.

11 Describe the changes that take place in the hair structure during the lightening process.

12 List two types of lightening products used in hairdressing.

13 State the most commonly used oxidant in colouring.

14 List seven factors that must be considered when colouring hair.

15 List three ways of encouraging men to take up colouring services.

16 State one technique that is suitable for enhancing textured effects in men's haircuts.

17 What action should be taken if the results of a skin test are positive?

18 How should you dispose of used colouring chemicals?

19 Which of the following is the correct ratio of water to dilute 12 per cent hydrogen peroxide and make 3 per cent?

   a. One part water to three parts hydrogen peroxide
   b. Two parts water to two parts hydrogen peroxide
   c. Three parts water to one part hydrogen peroxide
   d. One part water to one part hydrogen peroxide

20 What are the age restrictions on the provision of colouring services?

10 Creating basic patterns in hair

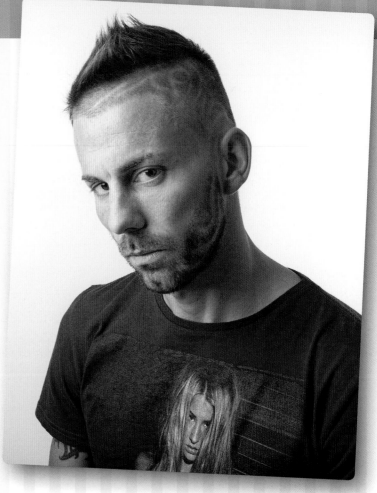

QUALIFICATION SIGNPOSTING

This chapter will help your studies of the following qualifications:

❖ Level 2 NVQ Awards and Diploma in Barbering.
❖ City & Guilds VRQ Level 2 Award, Certificate and Diploma in Barbering.
❖ ITEC Level 2 VRQ Awards and Diplomas in Barbering and Men's Hairdressing.
❖ VTCT Level 2 VRQ Certificates and Diplomas in Barbering and Barbering Studies.

LEARNING OBJECTIVES

In this chapter you will learn:

◆ How to design basic patterns in hair using curved and straight lines.

◆ The factors that must be considered when creating basic patterns in hair.

◆ The cutting techniques used to create basic patterns in hair.

◆ How to work safely when cutting basic patterns in hair.

◆ About aftercare for basic patterns in hair.

For further information on the qualifications covered by this chapter see the qualification mapping grid at the front of the book.

INTRODUCTION

In the 1960s and 1970s some men, and boys, wore short haircuts that were personalized by the addition of lines cut, or channeled into the hair. Sometimes these lines created simple partings to make the look more interesting, especially on African hair (Type K4), or perhaps to disguise a small scar. Others were more elaborate though. One of the most popular was the 'tennis ball crew cut', where all of the hair was cut to about 10 mm in length and a curved tramline was added to make the head resemble a tennis ball.

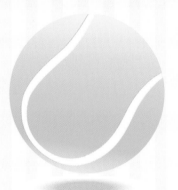

Today the addition of curved and straight lines to the haircut has become the even more popular and distinct service of 'creating patterns in hair', sometimes also referred to as 'hair tattooing'. These lines range from simple notching in eyebrows and sideburns to looks were the lines are worked together into intricate shapes that create highly personalized looks. In this chapter we will be looking at the techniques used for creating basic **linear** patterns in hair and will be covering the following topics:

❖ Factors to be considered when creating curved and straight line patterns in hair.

❖ Basic design principles – including shape, scale, proportion and position.

❖ Cutting techniques – including channelling, notching and tramlines.

❖ Cutting procedures.

❖ Aftercare.

❖ Notes on health and safety.

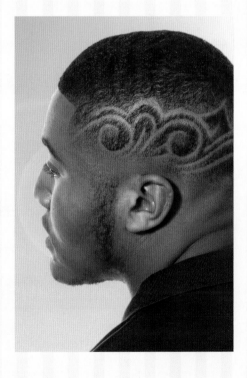

KEY DEFINITION

Linear design: A one-dimensional design that only uses lines.

Before reading this chapter it may help you to read CHAPTER 7, 'Cutting men's hair using basic techniques' and CHAPTER 11, 'Advanced men's hair cutting'.

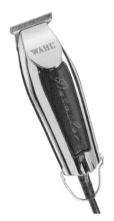

T-liner blade detailer trimmers

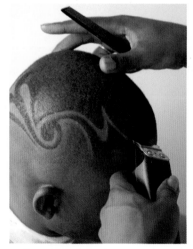

Channelling with 'T-liner blade' trimmers

It may help you to read CHAPTER 4, 'Client care for men' for more detailed information on consultation before reading this section.

Factors to be considered when creating curved and straight patterns in hair

Many similarities exist in the procedures used to create regular haircuts and create haircuts with patterns. The same cutting techniques can be used for most of the work required and some of the basic haircut shapes produced are the same. The head and face shape, hair density, adverse hair and skin conditions and other factors still have to be fully considered. But differences do exist in the consultation required and in some of the techniques used.

DON'T BE TEMPTED

Make sure you accurately establish the features and size of the pattern the client wants and then 'meet the client's brief'. Don't be tempted to add lines or features to the design that are not in their brief. Unexpected changes in patterns can be very obvious and are not likely to be welcomed!

HEALTH & SAFETY

You must carry out a thorough consultation to ensure that you identify any adverse conditions of the hair or skin that may be present. It is particularly important to establish whether a suspected infection or infestation is present, as are contraindications that would prevent you from cutting the hair.

The work regularly requires cutting techniques to be combined and adapted to take account of both the client's wishes and the many factors that affect the creation of the new pattern. The client consultation is essential in determining the right pattern for each client.

TIP

Hair growth patterns must be identified because they determine the shapes that can be created and the techniques that you should use. The movement created by the hair growth pattern can become a feature and be incorporated into the pattern to create a particular effect.

Consultation

Before you can create the pattern, or design a new pattern where there is an opportunity for the pattern to be changed, you must carry out a thorough consultation to consider factors including the client's wishes, face shape and existing haircut. Here is a reminder of some of the critical factors that must be considered when designing and creating patterns in hair:

◆ Accurately establish what the client wants.

◆ Determine why they wish to have a pattern in their hair.

◆ Look for signs of broken skin, abnormalities on the skin or any unusual features or hair growth patterns.

◆ What is the hair type – type S1, W2, C3 or K4?

◆ What are the hair characteristics –

  ◆ Is the hair fine, medium or coarse?

◆   Is the growth dense or sparse?

◆   Does the density of growth vary around the head – does the client have male pattern alopecia, as this will significantly limit the extent of the pattern?

◆ Determine the client's face shape.

◆ Determine the existing and required length and shape of their hairstyle.

> **TIP** ✓
>
> Remember to look for variations in the density of growth when planning the pattern. The pattern may have to be adapted in some areas to cover very sparse growth or a scar. Remember that some small scars can be 'hidden in full view' by incorporating them into the pattern, but always check with the client first.

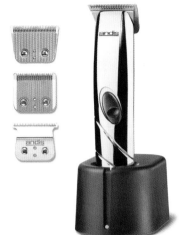

See **CHAPTER 4** pages 60–62 for full details on hair types and classifications.

Face shape, features and haircut length The client's face shape and features must be considered when choosing the most suitable haircut and pattern. The principles applied to choosing the right shape and length of haircut for different face shapes is explained fully in Chapter 7, 'Cutting men's hair using basic techniques' and they also apply here. But a particular concern when creating patterns in hair is the existing and required length of the haircut.

The length of the client's existing haircut is an important factor because some patterns cannot be achieved if the hair is too short as the line created would not be visible. Longer haircuts with layers beyond around 4 cm in length can of course be shortened to lengths suitable for creating patterns, but clients who wish to keep their hair layers longer than this should be discouraged from including patterns in these areas. Patterns may be included in other shorter areas though, such as in the front, back or sides even though the layers in the crown area are longer. Longer layers are usually less suitable for creating patterns because the hair tends to cover the pattern and the effect can appear unbalanced. The exception is in **disconnected** haircuts where the contrast between short and long is the desired effect.

Shorter, layered haircuts between 5 mm and 2 cm are usually best for linear patterns and geometrical shapes. On hair shorter than 5 mm good graphical or geometric shapes can be created.

> **KEY DEFINITION**
>
> Disconnected haircut: The layers between two areas of the head are not blended together in order to produce a clear contrast in hair length.

Disconnected work is covered in more detail in **CHAPTER 11**, 'Advanced men's haircutting'.

> **TIP** ✓
>
> On clients with male pattern baldness closer cut haircuts usually work best as the foundation for the pattern because they appear more evenly balanced. But, remember that the extent of the pattern will be more limited.

ERIK LANDER **Education Director, Habia**

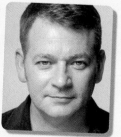

❝ Cutting a pattern in your client's hair is a great way of personalizing their haircut, making them happy and a great advert of your barbering skills and those of your barbers' shop. ❞

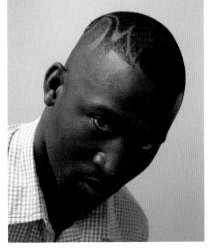

Channelling

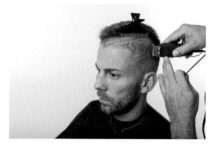

Channelling a disconnected look

A 1D shape – a line

Advanced pattern work includes additional design features such as perspective, 3D and pictorial effects and is covered in CHAPTER 15, 'Design and create patterns in hair'.

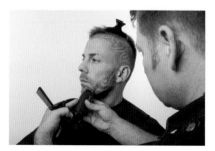

Llinear pattern on head and face

Basic design principles

The basic principles used when creating linear patterns in hair are:

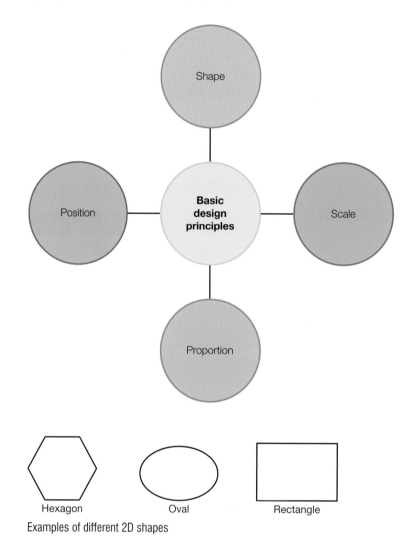

Examples of different 2D shapes

Hexagon   Oval   Rectangle

Shape

Shape generally describes a **two-dimensional** or 2D object. A **one-dimensional** shape is simply a line. A pattern made only of lines is called a linear pattern. This type of pattern is the focus of this chapter. Lines come in many different varieties – fine lines, thick lines, broken lines, etc. In complex patterns lines are used to determine precise limits on the space between objects within the pattern. In linear patterns the lines themselves are the main feature.

When creating linear patterns in hair, the lines are created using either a freehand technique with electric clippers, trimmers or scissors, or by following the outline of a stencil, which may have been designed by the barber or purchased ready-made.

Scale

Usually the objects that inspire designs are bigger or smaller than the size of pattern we wish to create. This means the design of the object must be enlarged or reduced and we use scale to help us do this. Scale is a number system that allows us to establish the relative dimensions of objects and designs. In this way an object that is 20 cm × 10 cm can be reduced to half its original size by dividing each measurement by two, making the new size 10 cm × 5 cm. This design would be a 1:2 scale replica of the original object.

> **TIP** ✓
>
> To ensure that the lines of the pattern are cut accurately when using freehand techniques place the thumb of one hand on the line of one object within the design. Stand back at arm's length, or looking in the mirror, slide the other thumb to the position of the new line until both thumbs appear level. Memorize the position of the thumbs. Now cut the new line to the correct position and length. This method can be easily adapted to establish the width of lines and so obtain accuracy.

The barber must establish the dimensions of the area where the pattern is to be sited and use scale to design patterns that fit effectively within these dimensions. This can be achieved when using freehand techniques by using estimation and imagining a grid across the area for the design; imagine placing transparent graph paper over the head, similar to the composition grid on page 194. Features of the pattern are estimated in size and reduced or enlarged to fit within each square of the imaginary grid until the pattern is complete. It will be shown that this imaginary grid is also useful in proportion. A more scientific method is to produce a stencil, which can be measured and cut accurately before being placed on the head to check for size and position before the line is traced onto the head.

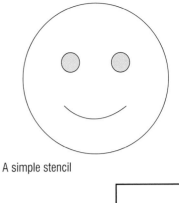

A simple stencil

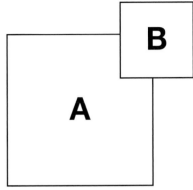

Scale: Box B is 1:4 scale replica of Box A

Proportion

Proportion is similar to scale in that it describes the relative size of one shape or object within a design to the size of another shape or object. It is often referred to by ratios, e.g. we might say that the logo is three times larger than the word in a particular design – a ratio of 3:1. Proportion is important because it helps establish **aesthetically** pleasing compositions.

> **KEY DEFINITION**
>
> Aesthetically: An artistic composition that is visually appealing.

Since ancient times mathematicians and artists have known that a specific ratio of proportion achieves the most pleasing visual effects. This is known as the 'Golden Proportion' or 'Golden Ratio'. Two objects will meet this golden ratio if their ratio is the same as the ratio of their sum to the larger of the two quantities, e.g. if **rectangle 1**, which has a longer side (a) and shorter side (b), is placed adjacent to **square 1** with sides of length (a) it will produce a similar 'golden rectangle', **rectangle 2**, with longer side (a) + (b) and shorter side (a).

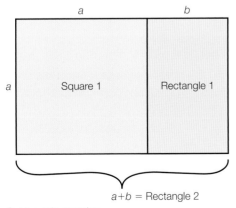

Golden ratio equation

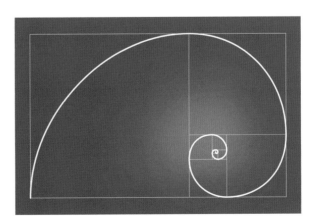

Fibonacci Spiral

The golden ratio will become more important in advanced pattern work that includes perspective, 3D and pictorial effects, which are covered in **CHAPTER 15**, 'Design and create patterns in hair'.

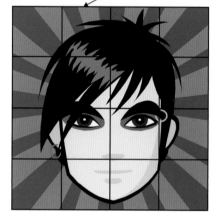

Composition grid

This might seem complicated but **geometry** can help us apply the golden ratio visually by using the 'fibonacci spiral', sometimes called the 'golden spiral'. This is created by drawing circular arcs connecting the opposite corners of objects within the composition.

When an artist is sketching, their work can be divided into squares, or the grid described earlier in the paragraph on scale. The golden spiral can be traced lightly within these squares to help set out proportion within the composition. The squares and the golden spiral can be erased or covered over and will not be visible when the sketch is completed. When creating patterns in hair this composition grid has to be imagined because it cannot be erased easily from the hair and would be visible in the final pattern.

The golden spiral is then imagined within the squares of the grid, connecting the opposite corners of objects, or in this chapter, the lines you want to place in the **composition**. The size and location of each line is determined by considering different positions along the imaginary golden spiral.

Remember, when creating basic patterns in hair the dimensions of the head and extent the hair covers the head are the main factors determining proportion, as making the lines within a pattern too big may look out of proportion with the size of the head. Proportion also establishes whether patterns should go over a partial or full head.

TIP ✓

Remember in linear patterns both the proportion of each line to other lines in the pattern and the overall size of the pattern to the clients head and face shape must be considered. Make sure that the combination produces the most effective composition to meet the client's brief.

Position

Position, or placing, is important to ensure that the pattern is symmetrically placed on the head, unless the design requires an **asymmetric** design, though here too position is still important. Many factors and hair characteristics affect the positioning of patterns in hair, such as hair growth patterns, hair density and proportion. When using freehand techniques the correct position can be established by placing one thumb on the head at arm's length, or by looking in the mirror, and moving the thumb around until it appears to be in the correct place. Stencils may be placed directly on the head and similarly moved around until they appear correct.

Inspiration for the pattern

Ideas for the pattern can come from many different sources. Magazines, trade shows and exhibitions are often helpful. Competitions are also good places to see and develop ideas. Popular patterns often include both straight and curved lines in tribal and cultural themes.

TIP ✓

Remember to consider any facial hair in the pattern. The sideburns, moustache, beard and eyebrows can all be features within the pattern. Most often it is simple notching and tramlines that are used in facial hair patterns.

Here are some important things to remember about designing patterns in hair:

◆ The overall outline of the pattern should usually be cut to appear symmetrical, unless the look is to be asymmetric. Do not just use the ears to determine the position of the pattern, as they are not usually placed level themselves.

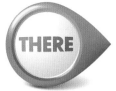
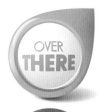
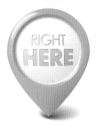

Position – choosing where to place the design can be a challenge!

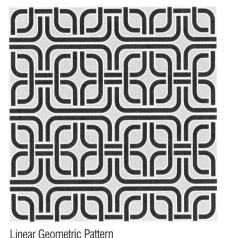

Linear Geometric Pattern

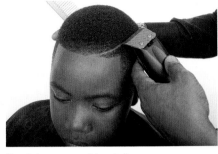

Tramlining – more elaborate lines are known as channelling

◆ Pay particular attention to where the haircut meets any beard and ensure that they blend together, as required. Think of the haircut and moustache and/or beard as being integrated parts of one style.

TIP ✓

Remember, you should always follow your barber's shop policy for working on those under 16 years old, or on those who appear vulnerable. This is especially important when creating patterns as the distinctive effects are often popular with younger people but might not be welcomed by their parents or guardians – check first if you are unsure.

Cutting techniques

Many cutting techniques, such as scissors-over-comb, clippers-over-comb and freehand are used when creating the foundation haircut for the pattern. These are explained fully in Chapter 7, 'Cutting men's hair using basic techniques'. But there are some techniques that are used especially in creating the pattern itself. These are explained in the following sections.

Read CHAPTER 7, 'Cutting men's hair using basic techniques' for more information on techniques used in the foundation haircut for the pattern.

Channelling

Channelling is the technique used to create complex lines within the pattern. It is performed with electric clippers or trimmers. The edge of the blades are placed end on to the scalp in order to remove the hair in narrow lines. Close cutting fixed blades, such as on balding clippers, or the shortest setting on adjustable blades are usually used.

Accompanying video available for channelling technique. Please scan this QR code.

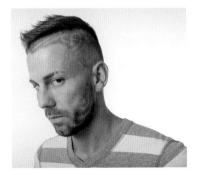

Channelling and a notched eyebrow

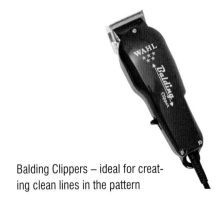

Balding Clippers – ideal for creating clean lines in the pattern

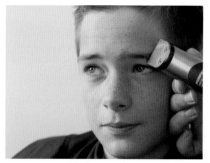

Notching the eyebrow – remember to ask the client to close their eyes first!

Notching

The notching technique is used to create short straight notches in the hair pattern. It is often used in isolation such as on the eyebrows and is performed with electric clippers, trimmers or T-blade/T-liner trimmers. The edge of the blades are placed end on to the scalp in order to remove the hair in narrow lines that can then be widened to create the width of required notch.

Tramlines or tramlining

Tramlines are a form of channeling where the simplest lines are created. These are also created with electric clippers or trimmers used with the edge of the blades end on against the scalp.

Accompanying video available for tramlining technique. Please scan this QR code.

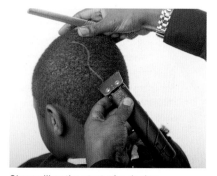

Channelling the start of a design

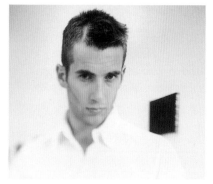

A simple tramlined parting

HEALTH & SAFETY

Extra care is needed when using clippers and trimmers in close contact with the skin when creating patterns. Check that the blades are correctly aligned before use, as a protruding cutting blade might easily cut the scalp. Always use light pressure and controlled gentle movements, as the blade can quickly and easily remove too much hair if not used correctly. Make sure the blades remain cool to touch.

ACTIVITY: CASE STUDY – MARKUS

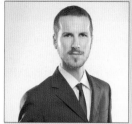

Markus is a regular client in your barber's shop. He wants a tribal themed pattern in the nape area. What pattern would meet Markus's brief?

HEALTH & SAFETY

Always sanitize clipper and trimmer blades before use on each client. Use sanitizing cleansing wipes and sprays – the sprays also help to cool and lubricate the blades during use.

Cutting procedures

Many different cutting procedures may be followed to cut men's hair. Individual barbers will usually decide where to start and which cutting techniques to use, mostly according to personal preference. The following examples show how some basic patterns in hair can be achieved.

SIMPLE LINEAR PATTERN WITH FADED OUTLINES

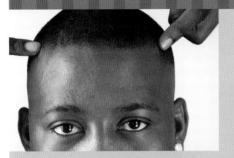

Step A

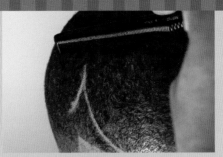

Step B

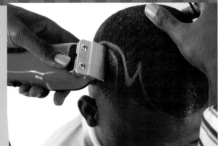

Step C

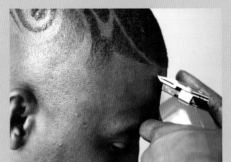

Step D

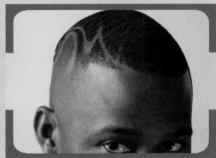

Step E

Step F

1. Cut the hair to the length required to create a foundation for the pattern. In this case a number 1 comb attachment is used.
2. Establish the position of the pattern on the chosen area of the head. The relative size and location can be estimated using the fingers (a).
3. Start at the front of the pattern and use channelling to outline the first line according to the chosen scale and proportion (b).
4. Add additional lines, as required working methodically across to one side of the pattern (c).
5. Return to the centre and repeat step 4 working towards the back.
6. Stand back from the client or refer to the mirror regularly to check that the pattern is developing correctly.
7. Remove any unwanted hair from inside the lines, as required. The hair outside the pattern may be removed or faded to enhance the pattern if required (d).
8. If necessary, shave inside the lines and the areas outside the outlines (see Chapter 12, Shaving services). In this work a 'balding blade' clippers is used to achieve a similarly close finish (e).
9. Remove all hair clippings from the pattern and client. Some clients enjoy the soothing effects of talcum powder or Aloe Vera based gels or cream on the skin within the pattern. Make sure that the client is not sensitive to such products before use. Always follow the manufacturer's instructions!
10. Styling gel or wax can be added to enhance definition, if required (f).

DON'T BE TEMPTED   X

As a professional barber your first obligation is to work safely and ensure the comfort of your client. Don't be tempted to forget about the client's comfort whilst you are enthusiastically concentrating on creating the pattern. Remember that clippers and trimmers can become quite warm in use, especially during the more intricate work when creating patterns in hair – make sure they are always comfortable to touch. You must also think of the position of the client's head, and your own position, and make sure comfort is maintained, especially as the work may require the client to sit still for a long period of time. Take a short break if needed to let the client and you change position and rest.

HEALTH & SAFETY

Remove excess hair cuttings from the client's face, neck and working area at regular intervals to ensure the client is comfortable.

Accompanying video available for creating a linear pattern. Please scan this QR code.

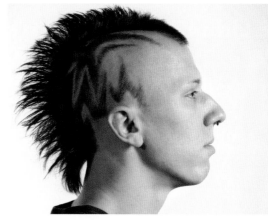

A highly personalized linear pattern

Accompanying video available for creating a tribal pattern. Please scan this QR code.

TRIBAL LINEAR PATTERN

Step A

Step B

Step C

Step D

Step E

Step F

Step G

1. Cut the hair to the length required to create a foundation for the pattern. This will be a textured disconnected look (a).

2. Establish the position of the centre of the pattern on the chosen area of the head. Start in the middle of the pattern and use channelling to outline the first line. This tribal pattern will arc around the temple and into the beard (b).

3. Add additional lines, as required working methodically across to one side of the pattern (c).

4. Stand back from the client or refer to the mirror regularly to check that the pattern is developing correctly.

5. Extend the pattern into the facial hair, if required (d).

6. Keep building up the pattern by adding lines until the design achieves the client's brief (e).

7. Remove any unwanted hair from inside the lines, as required, with a balding blade clipper (f).

8. Shave the areas inside the lines if required (see Chapter 12, Shaving services).

9. Remove all hair clippings from the pattern and client. Apply talcum powder or Aloe Vera based gels or cream to soothe the skin within the pattern, if required by the client. Make sure you always follow the manufacturer's instructions.

10. Styling gel or wax can be added to enhance definition, if required (g).

USING A SIMPLE STENCIL

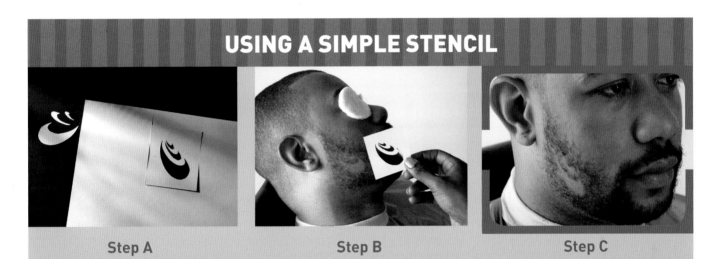

Step A   Step B   Step C

1. Create a stencil, or choose a commercial stencil that meets the requirement for design, scale and proportion in the pattern (a).

2. Cut the hair to the length required to create a foundation for the pattern.

3. Establish the position of the centre of the pattern on the chosen area of the head and place the centre of the stencil at this point.

4. Adjust the position of the stencil until it appears correct and transfer the design onto the hair by dusting the stencil with a little talc (a light application of hairspray first can help the talc stick to the hair). Alternatively, use a temporary hair colour spray or trace the outline of the stencil using T-liners (b).

5. Use channelling to remove the hair from within the outline made by the stencil.

6. Additional lines can be added, as required by moving the stencil to new positions to build up the pattern, or simple patterns can be easily created.

7. A simple linear stencil pattern (c).

TIP ✓

Cleaner lines and outlines can be achieved by cutting the hair with either close-cutting clippers or trimmers, such as balding blade clippers, T-liners or an electric razor. The hair may also be removed completely by shaving with a razor but great care is needed. Normally the close results achieved with balding blades are suitable for the lines within the pattern – wet shaving within these lines is not advised.

It may help you to read CHAPTER 12, 'Shaving services' for more information on shaving to produce the cleanest outlines.

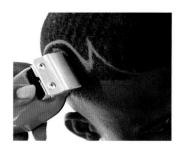

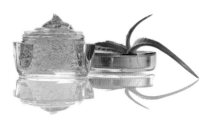

It may help you to read **CHAPTER 2**, 'Health and safety in the barber's shop' for general information on working safely in the barber's shop.

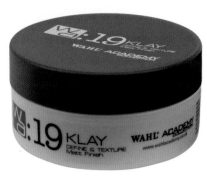

Soothing Aloe Vera Gel

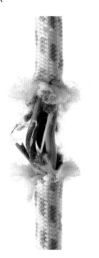

Finishing wax

Frayed cable

Aftercare

It is important that you inform your client of how to look after their new pattern and haircut before they leave the barber's shop. This should include the following:

◆ Recommend when the client should book the next appointment – remember that in shorter styles the haircut will need re-styling sooner as the new hair growth is likely to quickly equal the length of the actual haircut. This would soon be noticeable. Unwanted hair outside the haircut perimeter would also soon be visible and will need removing. In shorter styles appointments should generally be for every 2 to 4 weeks. However, where the haircut includes a pattern the client will need to visit sooner if they wish the pattern to remain distinct, as over time the pattern will fade.

◆ The client should shampoo and cleanse their hair according to the hair length, hair and scalp condition and their lifestyle.

◆ Which products can help the client maintain the overall style; particularly those such as gel and wax that can help define the pattern by smoothing the hair outside the pattern lines. Some clients also enjoy the soothing effects of gel or cream, such as Aloe Vera gel on the skin within the pattern. Consider retailing such products in your barber's shop!

Health and safety

It is important to consider health and safety when creating patterns in hair because of the risks associated with using electricity and the risk of burning the scalp or cutting the skin. Here are some important health and safety factors that you must consider when providing hair cutting services:

◆ If the client has any cuts or abrasions on his face or head, or you suspect that an infection or infestation is present, the work must not be carried out as these are contraindications.

◆ Pay special attention to hygiene when cutting hair because of the risk of cross-infection through open cuts.

◆ Protect the client's eyes from hairs with tissues or cotton wool pads when cutting dense coarse facial hair. Keep your own face away from your work; consider wearing safety glasses for protection, if required.

◆ *Never* place cutting tools in pockets.

◆ A fixed-blade razor must always be *sterilized* before each use.

◆ A new blade must always be used for each new client when using a detachable-blade open razor.

◆ Used razor blades, called sharps, must be disposed of correctly in accordance with your salon policy. Soiled disposable materials should be placed in sealed plastic bags for removal.

◆ Electrical equipment must always be handled and used with care in accordance with the manufacturer's instructions.

◆ *Never* use or place electric clippers or other electrical equipment near water.

◆ *Do not* go near electrical equipment that is lying in water – isolate the mains power first.

◆ Visually check that electrical equipment is safe to use before commencing work – check that the cable has not frayed or been pulled and that the plug is not loose.

◆ Pay attention to the position of cables when using and storing electrical equipment.

◆ *Never* overload sockets by plugging too many items of electrical equipment into the same socket.

◆ Follow the manufacturer's instructions for the care of your clippers – ensure that you clean and lubricate the blades regularly to avoid damage. Make sure that the blades are correctly aligned before and during use.

◆ Only use clean tools and equipment.

◆ Make sure that you know the whereabouts of your salon's first-aid kit. Keep yourself up-to-date with your salon's first-aid and accident procedures.

◆ Electrical equipment must be regularly tested, called Portable Appliance Testing (PAT) and given a certificate of testing to confirm that it is safe for use. Your salon owner will ensure that this is carried out, as required.

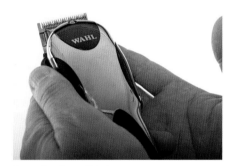

Correctly aligned blades

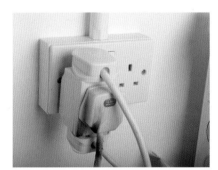

Overloaded plug socket

IMAGE GALLERY

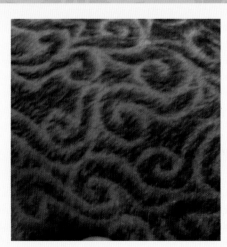

A linear paisley pattern

Visit the online image gallery on this book's accompanying website to see other inspirational hair patterns and hair tattoos.

BRINGING IT ALL TOGETHER

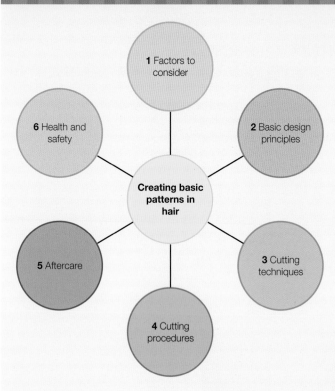

1 Factors to consider

2 Basic design principles

3 Cutting techniques

4 Cutting procedures

5 Aftercare

6 Health and safety

Creating basic patterns in hair

7 Popular patterns often include both straight and curved lines in tribal and cultural themes.

8 Channelling and tramlining are the main techniques used to create complex lines within the pattern.

9 Notching is often used to create isolated lines such as on the eyebrows and in beards and moustaches.

10 Remember that clippers and trimmers can become quite warm in use, especially during the more intricate work when creating patterns in hair. Take care not to burn your client's scalp!

Activities

1 Search the internet to research ideas for different linear patterns. Use the information to create a style book that you and your colleagues can then use in consultations with clients in your barber's shop.

2 Create a simple straight line and curved line stencil to help when creating linear patterns.

3 Research the availability of commercial stencils for linear patterns. Share the information with your manager and colleagues and consider whether your barber's shop should obtain any.

Summary

1 Many similarities exist in the procedures used to create regular haircuts and create haircuts with patterns.

2 The movement created by the hair growth pattern can become a feature and be incorporated into the pattern to create a particular effect.

3 Patterns may have to be adapted in some areas to cover very sparse growth or a scar.

4 Small scars can be 'hidden in full view' by incorporating them into a pattern.

5 A one-dimensional shape is simply a line. A pattern made only of lines is called a linear pattern.

6 Proportion is important because it helps establish pleasing compositions. The golden ratio will help determine the correct proportion for lines in the pattern and can be applied visually with the golden spiral. The size of the head and extent of the hair growth have dimensions that must be considered proportionally within the design.

Check your knowledge

1 Why is it important to accurately establish the type, location and size of pattern to be created?

2 Explain how male pattern alopecia might affect the choice of pattern?

3 Why is it important to consider hair growth patterns when creating linear patterns in hair?

4 Why should hair length be considered when cutting patterns in hair?

5 Describe the principle of proportion using examples from linear hair patterns.

6 Which of the following correctly describe an asymmetric pattern?

a. A pattern that is equal length on both sides
b. A pattern that is longer on one side than the other
c. A pattern that is wider at the nape than at the crown
d. A pattern that is symmetrical when viewed from all sides

7   Describe how scale is used to decide on the size of pattern to be created.

8   Why can hair density affect the position of a pattern?

9   Which of the following statements are correct:

   a. A linear pattern consists only of lines
   b. A linear pattern includes both lines and shapes
   c. A linear pattern is mostly 1D shapes with some 2D shapes
   d. A linear pattern only includes one-dimensional shapes

10   How can facial hair affect the design of a pattern?

11   How do tramlines differ from channelling?

12   Explain how stencils are used to create patterns?

13   Describe how to maintain high standards of hygiene for using clippers and trimmers.

14   Explain why electrical testing certificates are important.

15   Which of the following statements are correct:

   a. 'T-liner' trimmers are best for notching
   b. Balding blades cut as close as a wet shave
   c. Disconnected haircuts are not suitable for patterns in hair
   d. Haircuts between 5 mm and 2 cm are usually best for linear patterns

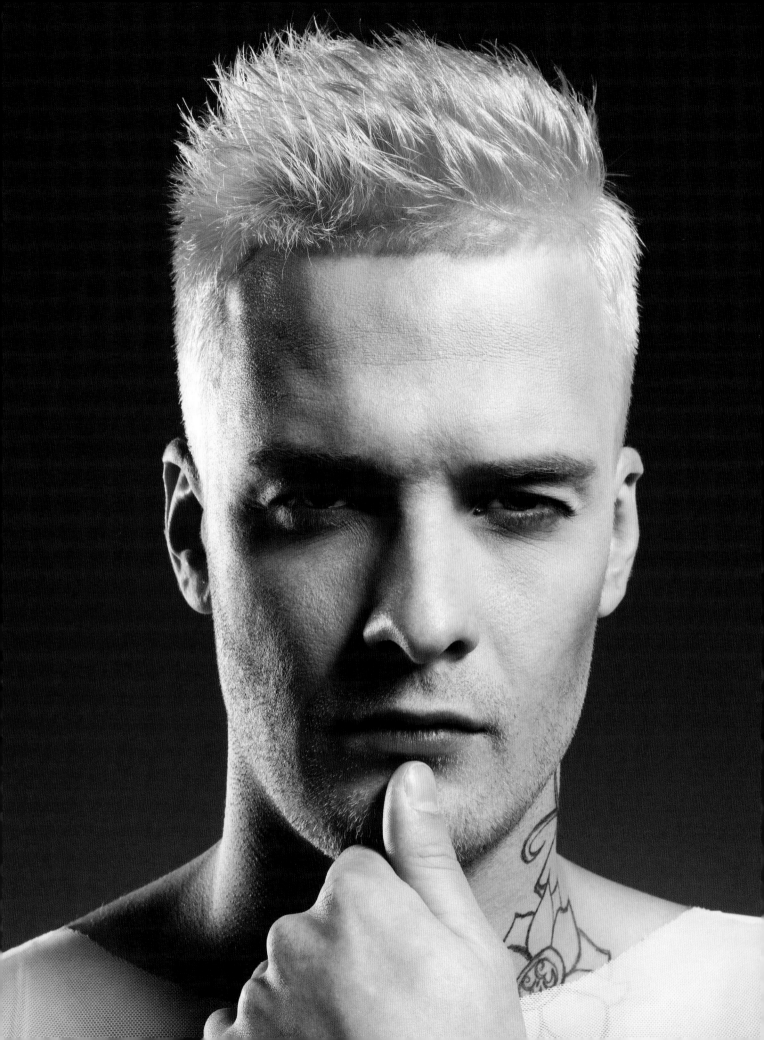

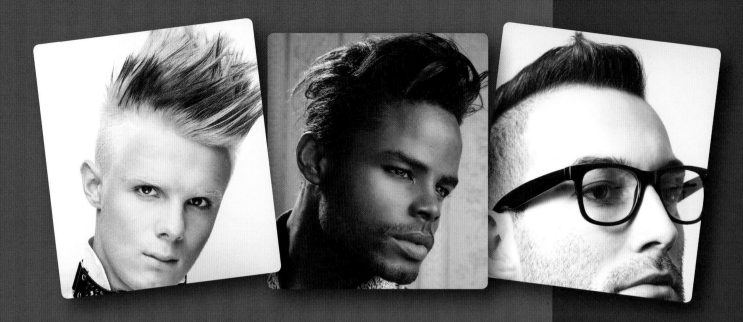

PART THREE

Advanced Menswork

Part 3 of this book covers the advanced skills and knowledge required of the senior barber: advanced men's hair cutting, shaving services, face massage and designing and creating facial hair shapes and patterns in hair. The topics covered include, consultation for advanced menswork, combining advanced cutting techniques and the significant anatomy and health and safety considerations for professional shaving and face massage. The principles of design are explained to help in designing and creating facial hair shapes and patterns in hair. There is also an additional online chapter covering specialist hair and scalp treatments.

11 Advanced men's hair cutting

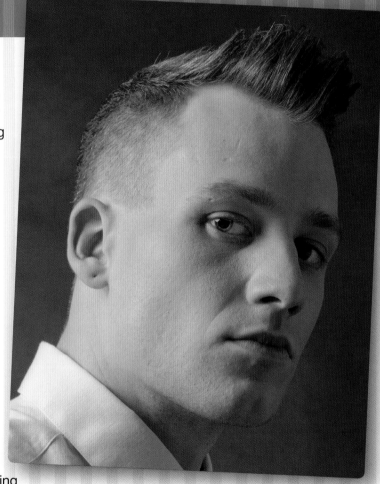

QUALIFICATION SIGNPOSTING

This chapter will help your studies of the following qualifications:

❖ Level 3 NVQ Awards and Diploma in Barbering.
❖ City & Guilds VRQ Level 3 Award, Certificate and Diploma in Barbering.
❖ ITEC Level 3 VRQ Award, Certificate and Diplomas in Barbering and Men's Hairdressing.
❖ VTCT Level 3 VRQ Certificates and Diplomas in Barbering and Barbering Studies.

LEARNING OBJECTIVES

In this chapter you will learn:

◆ The factors to be considered when creating a variety of men's looks – including how barbering principles apply in advanced men's work.

◆ The advanced cutting techniques – including tapering, texturizing and disconnecting.

◆ About advanced cutting procedures.

◆ About aftercare advice.

◆ The health and safety requirements for cutting hair.

For further information on the qualifications covered by this chapter see the qualification mapping grid at the front of the book.

INTRODUCTION

All haircuts should be personalized to best suit each client's features and give them a more individual style or look. The haircut forms the basis of all these looks and for all the subsequent styling of the hair. Many advanced men's haircuts rely intensely on accurate cutting techniques and on an accurate finish. Other advanced haircuts demand techniques that produce highly textured effects that do not appear to conform to traditional lines and accuracy. Sometimes a perfect taper is required; yet other times it is the contrast of disconnection that works best. Today's barber must have all these advanced men's hair cutting techniques at their disposal in order to create the variety of highly personalized looks that many men wear today.

In this chapter we will be looking at the techniques the barber uses for advanced men's hair cutting and will be covering the following topics:

❖ Factors to be considered when creating a variety of men's looks – including barbering principles in advanced men's work.

❖ Advanced cutting techniques – including tapering, texturizing and disconnecting.

❖ Advanced cutting procedures.

❖ Aftercare advice.

❖ Notes on health and safety.

Before reading this chapter it may help you to read CHAPTER 7, 'Cutting men's hair using basic techniques', as this provides an introduction to all the tools and methods of working assumed as being understood in advanced work.

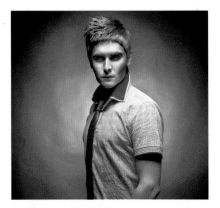

KEY DEFINITION

Asymmetric cut: When the different sides of a haircut are not identical, e.g. one side is longer or fuller than the other.

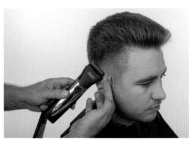

Cutting outlines

It may help you to read CHAPTER 4, 'Client care for men' for more detailed information on consultation before reading this section.

Factors to be considered when creating a variety of men's looks

As we discovered earlier in this book, it is the haircut that forms the basis for all good hairdressing. This is especially so when creating advanced men's looks, as many of these looks would be difficult or impossible for the client to achieve without 'a good cut' as the foundation.

There are many similarities between basic and more advanced men's hair cutting. Often the same cutting techniques are used and some of the looks produced have styling features that are similar to their more basic versions. Factors including facial hair, dense hair growth on the neck, the hair type and hair characteristics – for example male pattern alopecia (baldness) and other adverse hair and scalp conditions still have to be fully considered. Taller, less full or leaner shapes are also usually more flattering on men requiring advanced looks. But differences do exist in the overall complexity of the looks that are required and the methods that are used to achieve them.

Barbering principles In advanced work you will see that the barbering principles learnt earlier about shape and form are often followed more loosely. For example: some fashionable advanced looks appear to work best by being taller and fuller; in some an **asymmetric** rather than symmetrical effect works best; and in others the key barbering principle of not cutting into the natural hairline can be overlooked to achieve a specific style feature. Longer hairstyles are often produced when creating a variety of looks. This longer men's work is sometimes referred to as 'men's hairdressing', apparently making a distinction from barbering, as certain barbering principles, such as outlining and traditional neckline shapes appear less relevant to the look being created. Even so, remember that all men's hairdressing should still consider and apply barbering principles to the relevant features of the haircut, for example in longer square layered looks the layers are common in all hairdressing but the masculine features, such as sideburns and neck hair should still be cut following the barbering principles.

DON'T BE TEMPTED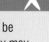

Barbering principles are often approached more flexibly in advanced work but don't be tempted to overlook them without first considering how they should be applied. They may need adapting, but barbering principles are still evident in the best work, even in extreme looks. Make sure your work is the same; otherwise the resulting haircut will appear to be absent of true barbering skills!

Advanced work regularly requires cutting techniques to be combined and adapted to take account of both the client's wishes and the many factors that affect the creation of the look. The client consultation is again most essential in choosing and personalizing the right look for each client; indeed it is more important here where the look to be created is often more extreme.

Consultation

Remember – a successful haircut will always begin with a thorough consultation! You must always make time to discuss the client's requirements and expectations with them, whether they are a new or regular client. Here is a reminder of some of the critical factors that must be considered when cutting men's hair:

◆ Identify the client's requirements then give them advice on suitable looks and agree the final effect to be achieved.

◆ Look for signs of broken skin or any abnormalities on the skin or hair – make sure there are no contraindications present as they would prevent you from carrying out the work.

◆ What is the hair type – type S1, W2, C3 or K4 (sometimes called VC4)?

◆ what are the hair characteristics –

  ◆ Is the hair fine, medium or coarse?

  ◆ Is the growth dense or sparse?

  ◆ Does the density of growth vary around the head – does the client have male pattern alopecia?

◆ Is the client wearing an added hairpiece?

◆ Does the client have a beard or moustache? Would styling of the facial hair, including the sideburns and eyebrows enhance the look?

◆ Determine the features of the client's head, face and body – is the client wearing spectacles or a hearing aid?

◆ Establish the age of the client.

◆ Consider the client's lifestyle – how might their occupation affect the look that can be created?

◆ Consider the style requirements of any artificial colour that has been, or will be used to determine how the haircut and colour can compliment each other. Is there a **cross selling** opportunity?

◆ Would perming help the client achieve a desired look – is this a cross selling opportunity?

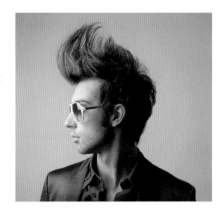

See **CHAPTER 4** pages 60–62 for full details on hair types and classifications

KEY DEFINITION

Cross selling: Recommending an additional product or service that might be beneficial to the product or service being requested.

HEALTH & SAFETY

You must carry out a thorough consultation to ensure that you identify any adverse conditions of the hair or skin that may be present. It is particularly important to establish whether a suspected infection or infestation is present, as these are contraindications that would prevent you from cutting the hair.

Cutting outlines

Many men have dense hair growth that grows outside the natural hairline, particularly on the face and in the nape areas. In shorter layered looks, the barbering principles are most prevalent and the haircut should always be outlined and the unwanted hair from outside the haircut outline removed or it will appear untidy and unfinished. In longer fashionable styles it can seem less important to outline, as the longer hair may cover the hairline. Unwanted hair outside the outline should still be removed though, as for example the client may fasten their hair up in a ponytail and expose the hairline.

Some outlines are cut to give a natural appearance, whilst others are created with lines so that they are obvious, and yet others are faded so that no outline is visible at all, such as the skin fade that is popular with some African-Caribbean men. The outline of a haircut is usually most noticeable in the nape, where it is known as the neckline.

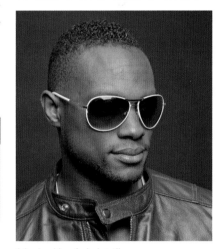

A look with a faded outline

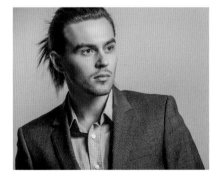

Barbering principles should be followed even on longer looks

It may help you to read **CHAPTER 7**, 'Cutting men's hair using basic techniques' page 113 for further information on traditional neckline shapes.

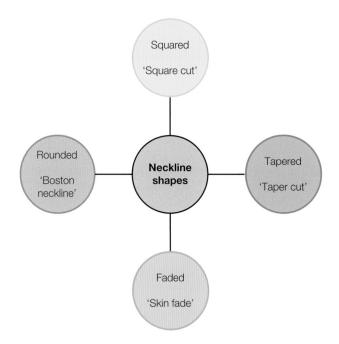

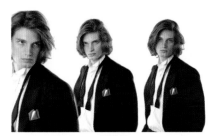

Longer styles often have natural necklines

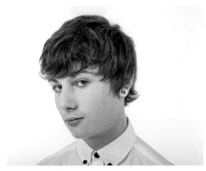

Natural neckline

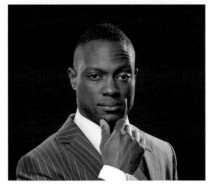

Faded outlines and neckline

It may help you to read **CHAPTER 15**, 'Design and create patterns in hair' to see how a hair pattern, sometimes called a hair tattoo, might be included in the advanced look.

Neckline shapes These are important in men's hairdressing because the natural neck hairline is usually less well defined, as hair often grows densely on the neck. There are three traditional neckline shapes that suit most men's looks and one of these is likely to be suitable for most short layered advanced men's looks:

- ◆ *Squared neckline shapes* – sometimes known as a 'square cut'.
- ◆ *Tapered neckline shapes* – sometimes known as a 'taper cut'.
- ◆ *Rounded neckline shapes* – sometimes known as a 'Boston neckline'.

There are two additional neckline shapes used in advanced work:

- ◆ The natural neckline.
- ◆ The fade, skin fade, or faded neckline.

The natural neckline does not have any distinct shape and usually appears on longer styles, although the neckline might be longer than other interior areas of the haircut. It is usually slightly rounded in shape. The fade is similar to the taper cut but cut much closer so that the hair fades into the skin with no perceptible weight line.

Neckline shapes can also be cut to appear more or less natural. The correct shape and effect will meet the client's wishes and take account of the overall look and the hair growth patterns in the nape area. Longer looks below the height of a typical shirt collar usually do have a more rounded neckline shape than normally found in men's hairdressing. But

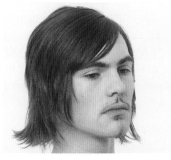

A contemporary rounded neckline

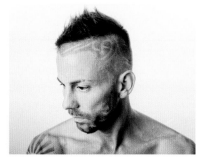

Hair patterns often require cutting into the natural hairline

heavy rounded outlines are still best avoided. Layered and textured effects usually work better, as these create movement and reduce the weight of the outline.

Stronger and more extreme looks often have styling details that are more radical. Strong, less natural outlines may be features of these types of look and in such cases the outlines can be cut to almost anywhere, or even incorporated into elaborate patterns and designs. Likewise, such radical details can be added to facial hair, including beards, moustaches and eyebrows to make effective contributions to the overall look required.

As you can see, in the same way as the principles of shape and form discussed earlier, the principles of outlining in advanced work can also be applied more loosely to achieve the correct look!

Here are some important things to remember about outlining advanced men's haircuts:

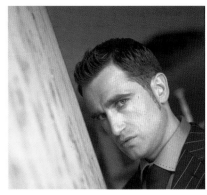

It may help you to read CHAPTER 14, 'Designing facial hair shapes' to see how a moustache or beard should be considered as part of the look.

◆ On most men, especially with short layered looks, the haircut must still be outlined or it will appear untidy and unfinished.

◆ Follow the natural hairline wherever possible, particularly when outlining shorter haircuts. Avoid making unnecessary cuts into the natural hairline, especially around the ears and at the sides of the nape, unless the look requires these more radical and less natural effects.

◆ Many outlines appear more natural if they are gently tapered, particularly on shorter styles, in the nape and at the bottom of the sideburns.

Cutting sideburns

Sideburns are important in most men's haircuts. Usually men want sideburn shapes that are less prominent, with the emphasis on creating a natural balanced look that matches their haircut. In fashionable advanced looks sideburns are often styled into longer shapes, sometimes into points and other more elaborate designs. In each case the face shape and hairstyle should be used to determine the correct choice of sideburn shape for each client. Here are some important things to remember about cutting sideburns:

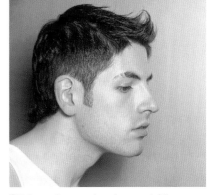

Sideburns are an important style feature

◆ Most men's haircuts are improved by having sideburns. Sideburns help to balance the haircut and create an attractive masculine frame to the face.

◆ Avoid cutting the length of the sideburns higher than the top of the ear and into the hairline unless the look requires these more radical and less natural effects.

◆ Sideburns should usually be cut level, unless the look is to be asymmetric. Do not use the ears to determine the level of the sideburns, as they are not usually placed level themselves.

◆ Pay particular attention to where the haircut meets the sideburns and ensure that they blend together.

◆ Think of the haircut and sideburns as being integrated parts of one style.

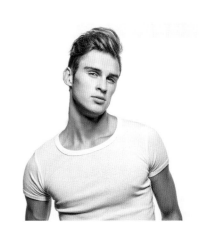

Sideburn shape and eyebrow notching enhance this contemporary look

TIP ✓

To ensure that the sideburns are cut level place the thumb of each hand high on each sideburn. Whilst looking in the mirror slide one thumb down until the desired length is reached. Slide the other thumb down until both thumbs are level. Memorize the position of the thumbs; you can use a position on each ear as a point of reference. Now cut each sideburn to the correct length. This method can be easily adapted to establish the width of the sideburns and so obtain symmetrical shapes, even in the most elaborate sideburn designs.

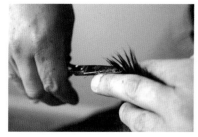

Club cutting

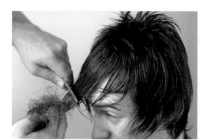

Tapering

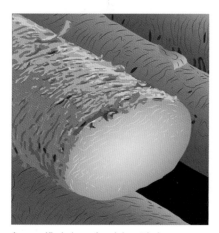

A magnified view of a club cut hair

Advanced cutting techniques

Many cutting techniques, such as scissors-over-comb and clippers-over-comb are used in both men's basic hair cutting and men's advanced hair cutting. But differences do exist in the way that the techniques are used and in the different effects that they achieve. There are some techniques, however, which are only really used in more advanced work and these are explained in the next section.

Tapering

Tapering is used to cut the hair so that it tapers to a point, unlike the blunt end created when club cutting (the images below show the different effect of club cutting and taper cutting on the hair shaft). This helps to achieve a more natural finish that is desired in many styles, as the hair ends normally grow to have a naturally tapered end – they do not naturally have blunt cut ends. However, remember that blunt cut ends are useful for styles where a defined weight line is the intended effect.

Both unwanted weight and length may be removed with tapering techniques. It is particularly useful for blending in heavier sections of the hair, as the weight at the ends in these sections can be reduced without affecting the hair length. This helps further to recreate the natural tapered effect that arises due to the normal hair growth pattern. Not only is each hair naturally tapered but in every square centimetre of scalp hairs will be at different stages of the hair growth cycle and hence at different lengths. The means that the ends of the section of hair are not all at the same length and the section becomes less dense towards the ends. A tapered effect is the result. Remember that sometimes a tapered effect is not required; indeed hair usually needs cutting to recreate more defined sections that have 'grown out', but the skilled barber understands how and where tapering should be used.

Here are some methods that are commonly used in tapering men's hair.

◆ **Scissor tapering** (sometimes called slide cutting, slice cutting or slithering) – is carried out on dry hair. It is achieved by moving the open scissor blades backwards and forwards along the hair section in a slithering, sliding movement. The blades are gently opened and closed a small amount during the movement to remove the required amount of hair. The blades must not be completely closed or the section of hair will be cut straight through!

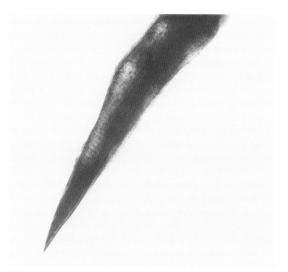

A magnified view of a taper or razor cut hair

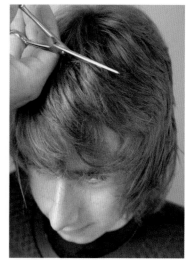

Slicing

◆ **Razor tapering** – sometimes just called 'razor cutting', is only used on wet hair. It is achieved by placing the razor on the hair section at an angle of about 30° and then making gentle slicing movements as the razor cuts the hair. On shorter hair the section to be cut should be combed through until the comb is at least 3 cm away from the hairline. The comb is then kept in this position and the razor is placed at the correct angle on the hair about 2–3 cm down from the comb. The hair is then cut using gentle slicing movements with the razor. The razor and comb should move down the section together, remaining about 2–3 cm apart throughout.

◆ **Razoring** (shaving) – is sometimes used to create clean outlines and emphasize a haircut shape. It is performed with a razor, which may be either an open razor or a safety razor. Disposable-blade razors should be used by professional barbers because they are more hygienic. Electric razors are also sometimes used.

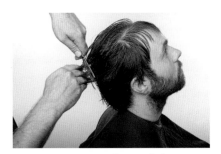

Razor tapering – sometimes called razor cutting

Accompanying video available for razor tapering. Please scan this QR code.

TIP ✓

Great care must be taken when razor tapering or cutting. Do not razor cut the hair too near to the hairline or roots, as the hair will stick up and be very difficult to style. Always use gentle cutting actions and small movements, as the razor can quickly and easily remove too much hair if not used correctly.

Texturizing

Texturizing techniques are used to break up a solid mass of hair and create a more random movement and texture. Many different cutting techniques can be used to produce the varying lengths of hair that create the 'textured' effect. Most often freehand pointing, chipping, slicing and chopping actions with the scissors will produce the required effects. The razor can also be used to achieve similar effects. The hair is usually cut in the middle third of the section and towards the ends, as cutting too near the roots will make the short hairs stick out. Short layered haircuts are often texturized through the top to disconnect the shape and create a sensation of movement and energy. Freehand texturizing techniques are often used in advanced work as these are able to create random effects exactly where the barber wishes.

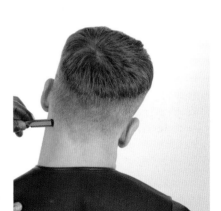

Shaving outlines

HEALTH & SAFETY

Razors have very sharp blades and must always be treated with care and respect. Keep the handle closed or cover the blade when not in use and especially when carrying or passing them. *Never* place a razor in your pockets and always keep them out of the reach of children.

Accompanying video available for texturizing. Please scan this QR code.

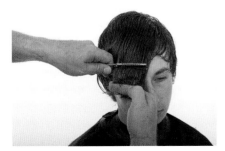

Razor tapering

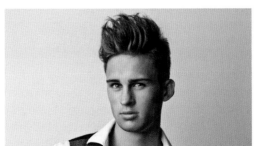

Textured effects through the top

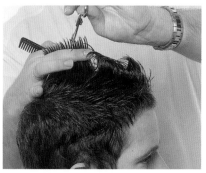

Pointcutting

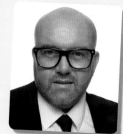

SIMON SHAW European Artistic Director at Wahl (UK) Ltd.

 Texturizing the haircut is often the sign of advanced work – it breaks up solid shapes and frees the hair, creating softer and more natural looks. Scissors or clippers, with or without blades; the skilled barber knows how to turn on the texturizing magic to make a good haircut, a great haircut!

Disconnecting

Traditionally the skilled barber has sought to make all his work appear even and blended with no visible lines. Indeed, trainee barbers spend many hundreds, if not thousands of hours perfecting their cutting skills so the dreaded 'steps' are never visible in their work. But in modern advanced men's work the rules are different!

Here the barber seeks to use the contrast of long and short, solid or textured, thinned or thick, and sometimes all three to achieve striking and highly personalized looks.

The technique relies on other haircutting skills, such as scissors and clippers-over-comb, thinning, tapering and texturizing to remove hair from specific areas whilst leaving length, weight and/or a solid shape in the adjacent areas.

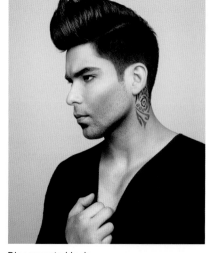

Disconnected look

TIP

Disconnecting will sometimes require that hair sections that are to be left longer or fuller are held out of the way whilst the shorter areas are cut. Clips may be used to hold this hair away from the working area whilst you work – remember though, avoid using brightly coloured clips!

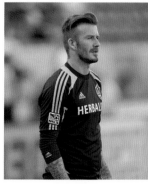

A famous disconnected look

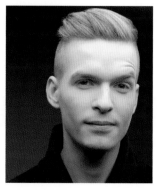

Disconnected look

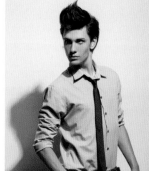

Longer disconnected look

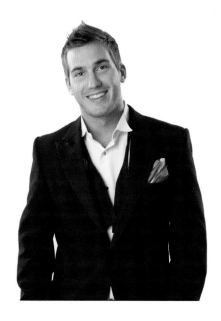

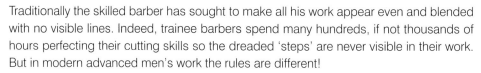

Cutting procedures

Many different cutting procedures may be followed to cut men's hair. Individual barbers will usually decide where to start and which cutting techniques to use mostly according to personal preference. In advanced cutting it is the barber's creativity and individualism that comes to the fore. The range of basic and advanced skills at their disposal enables them to choose the best technique for a specific task within the haircut. This is the key to advanced work! Many cutting techniques can achieve similar effects and the advanced barber will combine and adapt these, as necessary, to achieve the required results. The best procedure remains one that allows the barber to work accurately and efficiently throughout the whole haircut. The following examples show how some advanced men's looks can be achieved.

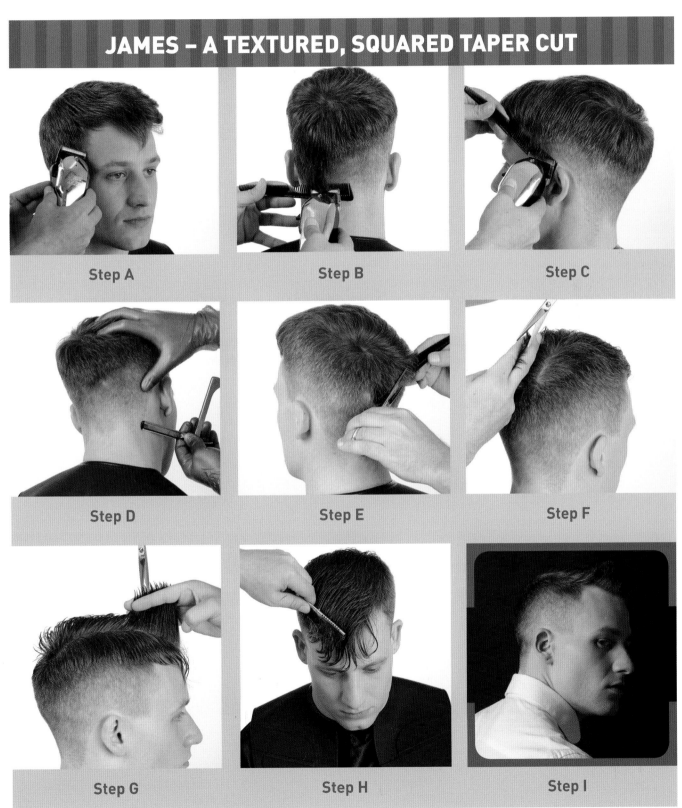

JAMES – A TEXTURED, SQUARED TAPER CUT

Step A

Step B

Step C

Step D

Step E

Step F

Step G

Step H

Step I

(Continued)

JAMES – A TEXTURED, SQUARED TAPER CUT (*Continued*)

1. Start at one side and using clippers-over-comb cut the side to length. Scissors-over-comb could be used instead (a).
2. Continue cutting through to the back area (b).
3. Continue round and repeat on the other side (c).
4. To create the cleanest look the area outside the outlines can be shaved. Remember, gloves should be worn (d).
5. Using scissors-over-comb blend the sections into the top around the crown area. Do not work too far forward as the front section will be **disconnected** (e).
6. Point cut the top to length – point cutting will create texture behind the front where weight and length will be increased (f).
7. Work forward from the crown holding the sections at about 40-45° to the head, increasing length towards the front (g). Point cutting continues to add texture. Crosscheck to ensure panels and sections are accurate.
8. Razor cut towards the front – this will increase the texture, length and weight difference towards the front leave a more solid front shape (h).
9. The finished look (i).

KEY DEFINITION

Disconnected haircut: The layers between two areas of the head are not blended together in order to produce a clear contrast in hair length, weight or form.

DON'T BE TEMPTED   X

As a professional barber your first obligation is to work safely and ensure the comfort of your client. Don't be tempted to forget about the client's comfort whilst you are enthusiastically concentrating on creating that fantastic look! Remember, you must think of the hair cuttings and position of the client's head, and your own position, and make sure comfort is maintained.

ACTIVITY: CASE STUDY – SHANE

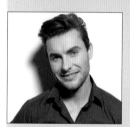

Shane is a 23-year-old new client in your barber's shop. He is off to South America backpacking for a gap year before starting work as a lawyer and sees this as his chance to have a more radical haircut. He requests that you restyle his hair into a short modern look but wants three ideas to choose from. What three looks would you suggest?

ANDREA – A RAZOR CUT, HIGHLY TEXTURED NATURAL NECKLINE LOOK

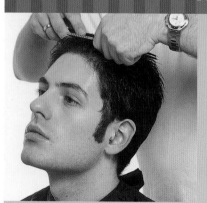

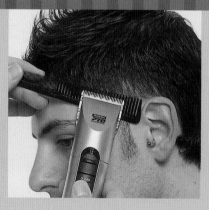

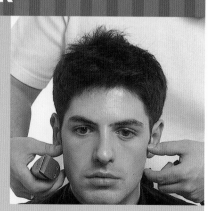

| Step A | Step B | Step C |

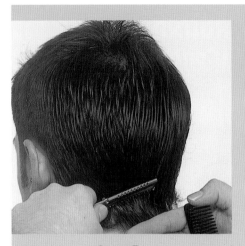

Step D

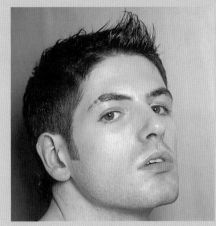

Step E

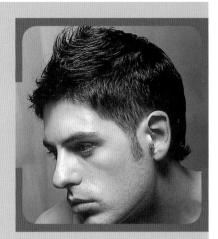

Step F

1. With the hair wet, comb it back and razor cut to reduce weight through the front section (a).

2. Continue this through to the crown area.

3. Move to one side and reduce the length using clippers-over-comb (b).

4. Increase the length towards the back by increasing the angle of the comb out from the cutting line created at the side. Make sure that the cut blends through without an obvious step in length.

5. Repeat steps 3 and 4 on the other side.

6. Check that the sideburns are level and cut them to the required length and shape (c).

7. Leave the hair longer in the nape and to the natural hairline at the sides of the neck, but remove unwanted hair outside this outline.

8. Make sure that the hair is wet at the back and use a razor tapering technique towards the nape to reduce weight and create texture. Remove small strands of hair around the bottom to break up the outline (d).

9. One eyebrow can be channelled to create notches for added detail, if required (e).

10. Shave the areas outside the haircut outlines, if required (see Chapter 12, Shaving services).

11. Blow-dry into shape and finish the look with wax or gel to add definition (f).

CRAIG – RAZOR CUT, TAPERED, ROUNDED NECKLINE – A VERSATILE LOOK!

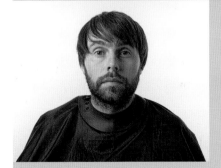

Step A

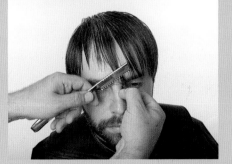

Step B

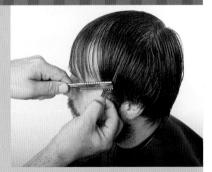

Step C

(continued)

CRAIG – RAZOR CUT, TAPERED, ROUNDED NECKLINE – A VERSATILE LOOK! (*Continued*)

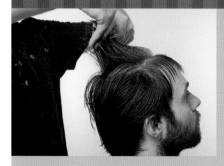
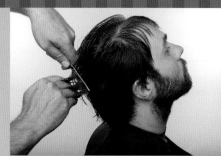
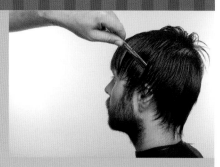

Step D   **Step E**   **Step F**

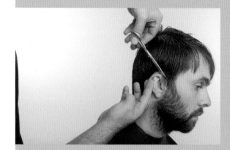
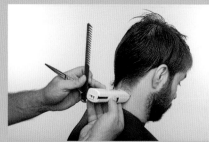
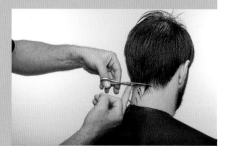

Step G   **Step H**   **Step I**

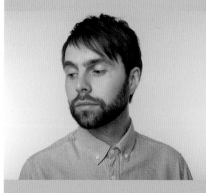
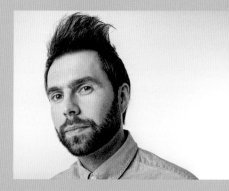
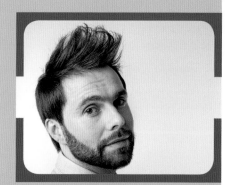

Step J   **Step K**   **Step L**

1. Gown and prepare your client (a).
2. With the hair wet, razor cut the front using a slicing movement – the aim is to reduce length and break up the solid shape creating texture (b).
3. Continue into the sides (c).
4. Comb the hair back extending away from the front and razor cut to reduce weight and create texture. Extending the hair away from the front will retain length at the front as this hair is traveling further before being cut (d).
5. Continue this through to the crown area and through the sides (e).
6. Move to one side and gently razor cut following the line you want the cut to follow. Gentle movements are required to remove just the correct amount of weight. *Note: here a razor with a guard is used (commonly called a hair shaper). If using a razor without a guard extra care is needed and you should use a comb as a guide, as described in 'razor tapering' earlier in this chapter* (f).
7. Scissors-over-comb can be used to graduate the outline area before the outlines are cut (g).
8. Taper the nape outline and remove unwanted hair outside this outline (h).
9. Cut the neckline to the correct length – remember a rounded neckline is cut square first and then only the corners are gently rounded. This shape works well on Craig due to the nape whorls (i).

10. The facial hair was then cut (see Chapter 6, Cutting facial hair using basic techniques). Areas outside the haircut outlines can be shaved, if required (see Chapter 12, Shaving services).

11. Blow-dry into shape and finish the look with gel to add definition – range of final looks are possible! (j), (k) and (l).

TIP ✓

Remember, when determining the correct height for the neckline you should consider the length of the neck, the position of the ears, the head shape and the length of the hair. If the neckline is too low on a short neck it will make the neck appear shorter, whilst if it is too short on a long neck it will make the neck appear longer.

Accompanying video available for razor cut. Please scan this QR code.

STEVE H – 'THE PYRAMID' – GRADUATED AND TEXTURED, TAPERED NECKLINE LOOK

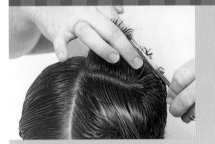

Step A

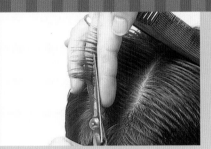

Step B

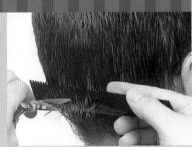

Step C

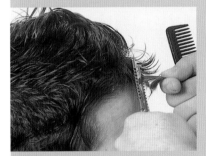

Step D

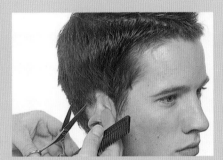

Step E

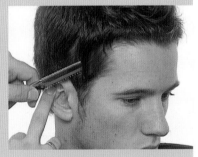

Step F

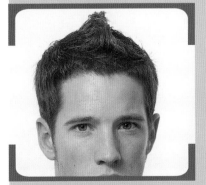

Step G

(continued)

STEVE H – 'THE PYRAMID' – GRADUATED AND TEXTURED, TAPERED NECKLINE LOOK (*Continued*)

(colour used to emphasize the cut)

1. First create the basic haircut shape, the hair must be wet. Section the hair in two by making a parting from the crown to the front. Make a second parting from ear to ear across the top of the head. Take a section parallel to this parting at the crown and hold it at 90° to the head then cut it to length using the scissors-over-fingers technique. Make sure you cut the section at 45° with the highest point in the middle of the head and the lowest at the length required at the sides – imagine the highest point of the pyramid sits in front of the crown (a).

2. Take a section down the centre of the head and cut this at 45° with the longest point at the crown and shortest at the front (b).

3. Take a section parallel to section 1 and cut this to the guidelines created by both the first and central sections. Continue taking sections parallel to this first section and cutting to the guidelines working down the panel to the front hairline.

4. Transfer the guideline down onto the side and back of the head by taking vertical sections. Continue cutting these sections to the required length. *Note:* The hair length may be graduated to remove weight around the ears by angling the cut across the section or by using scissors-over-comb, as required (c).

5. Razor cut the front hairline to add texture and definition (d).

6. Point cut the top to break up the solid form and enhance movement.

7. Use scissors-over-comb to graduate the bottom of the back and sides, and then outline the sideburns, around the ears and down the sides of the nape with the tips of your scissors (e).

8. Cut the neckline to the shape required by the look and remove the unwanted hair from outside the outlines.

9. Freehand razor cutting, using just the toe of the razor is used to create more texture through the sides (f).

10. Shave the areas outside the haircut outlines, if required (see Chapter 12, Shaving services).

11. The shape is blow-dried and finished with gel or wax to add definition (g).

KRIS – DISCONNECTED FADE CUT (INCLUDING TRIBAL PATTERN)

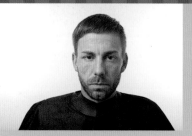

Step A

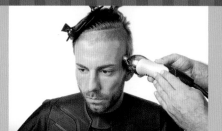

Step B

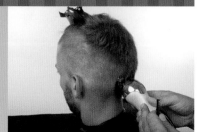

Step C

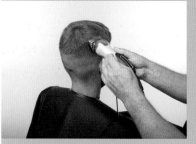

Step D

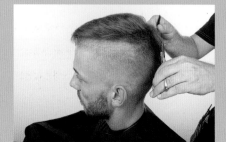

Step E

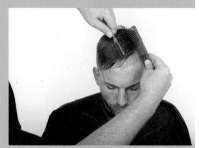

Step F

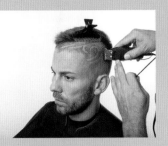

Step G

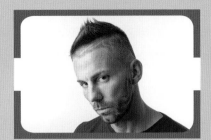

Step H

1. Gown and prepare your client (a).

2. Separate the hair sections where the disconnection will occur and secure this hair away from the working area. Using clippers-over-comb, and ensuring the clippers are on their longest setting (an attachment can be used in longer styles) and are placed flat against the neck in the nape, push the clippers slowly up the head in a *smooth continuous movement* until you reach the disconnected area (b).

3. Keep the clipper blades flat against the scalp until you reach the point at which any graduation to a longer length is required. Then in a smooth *rocking* movement *pivot* the clippers away from the head to increase length and produce the shape required (c).

4. Continue across the crown and into the other side (d).

5. Further blending of the graduation is completed using scissors-over-comb – in this look the model's right-hand side is not disconnected (e).

6. Razor cut the top – creating texture and reducing length, as required (f).

7. Point cut the top to break up the solid form and enhance texture and movement.

8. The pattern is then created (see Chapters 10, Creating basic patterns in hair and 15, Design and create patterns in hair) and the facial hair is cut (see Chapters 6, Cutting facial hair using basic techniques and 14, Designing facial hair shapes), as required (g).

9. Areas outside the haircut outlines can be shaved, if required (see Chapter 12, Shaving services).

10. Blow-dry into shape and finish the look with wax to add definition (h).

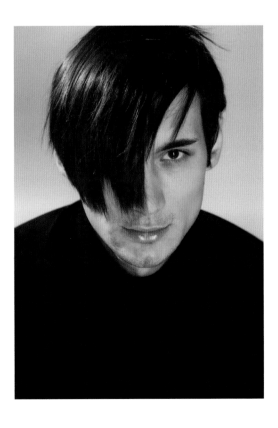

Accompanying video available for fade cut. Please scan this QR code.

Remember, it may help you to read CHAPTER 2, 'Health and safety in the barber's shop' for general information on working safely in the barber's shop.

Accompanying video available for 'point and razor cut'. Please scan this QR code.

FRANKIE – POINT AND RAZOR CUT, TEXTURED NATURAL NECKLINE LOOK

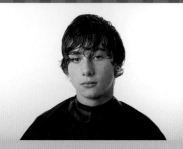

Step A

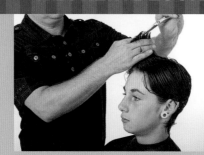

Step B

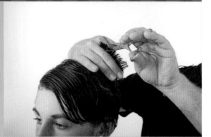

Step C

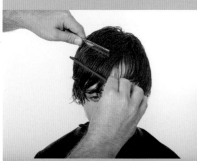

Step D

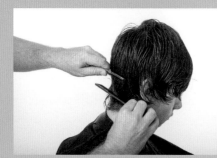

Step E

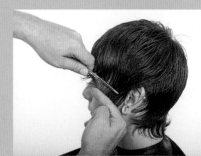

Step F

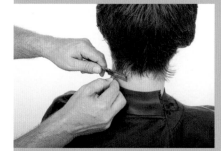

Step G

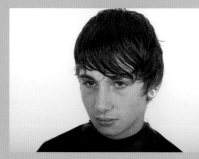

Step H

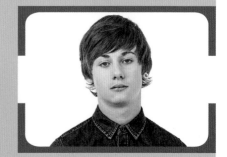

Step I

1. Gown and prepare your client. *Note: Frankie has a range of piercings in his ears. You should ask the client if these can be removed whilst you complete the work. If this is not possible you must take extra care whilst working – remember to work away from the piercing wherever possible, and always make sure you know where the piercing is before combing or cutting the hair in the adjacent areas!* (a).

2. Point cut the top to the desired length (b).

3. Continue across the head to the crown and into the sides (c).

4. Razor cut the top – creating texture and reducing length, as required (d).

5. Razor cut the back, increasing the tapering into the nape area so that the length and weight reduces as the work gets nearer to the neckline (e).

6. Repeat the razor tapering around the sides and towards the front – note the care taken around Frankie's ear piercings! (f).

7. Finish the natural neckline shape using gentle slicing movements. Areas outside the haircut outlines can be shaved, if required (see Chapter 12, Shaving services) or balding blade trimmers can be used (g).

8. The finished textured cut (h).

9. Blow-dry into shape and finish the look with wax to add definition (i).

MARK – TEXTURIZED CUT USING TEXTURE BLADE, FLICK AND SMACK TECHNIQUE

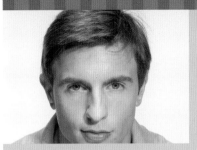

Step A

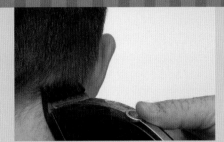

Step B

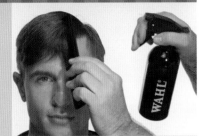

Step C

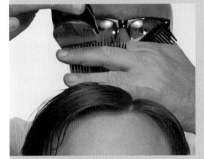

Step D

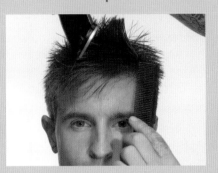

Step E

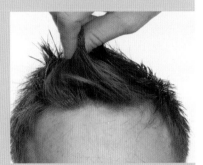

Step F

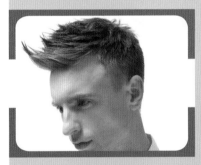

Step G

Accompnaying video available for Wahl flick and smack technique. Please scan this QR code.

1. Comb hair. Use grade 3 (9 mm) attachment at the sides and temple area to take down the length. Use in an upwards pivoting motion. Clippers-over-comb can be used, if preferred (a).
2. Repeat on the other side.
3. At the back, continue to clip through the back area to connect the sides, still on a guard 3 (b).
4. Turn the clippers upside down to blend in, going over the same sections but in a downwards motion this time.
5. Spray the hair with water and comb through (c).
6. Add layers by clubbing over the fingers using the clippers; section the hair into 1" sections. Point the clipper downwards and towards you and take it across the hair, following through with the guard line (d).
7. Complete the top then split the hair in half and blend into the side sections using clippers-over-comb.
8. Once the layers are cut to a desired length, add on the texture blade and use the 'flick 'n' smack' technique to add texture to the haircut (e).
9. Blow-dry the hair, pointing the nozzle up into the roots to ends to create height and volume at the roots.
10. Use Klay to show off the texture (f).
11. Go back in with the clippers to define the temple, sides and back sections, still on a guard 3.
12. Use a trimmer to outline the edges. Shave the areas outside the haircut outlines, if required (see Chapter 12, Shaving services) (g).

Steve – a sculpted close skin fade A full step-by-step sequence of a basic skin fade haircut is included in Chapter 7 'Cutting men's hair using basic techniques'. A sculpted skin fade is cut using the same techniques but is more technical as the length is increased to sculpt the top. Here is how it is done:

1 The hair is cut at the back and sides using the clippers set to the longest setting or with a size 1 blade.

2 Ensure that the clippers are placed flat against the neck, just below the neckline. Using a *smooth continuous movement*, push the clippers slowly up the head, keeping them flat against the scalp until you reach the occipital bone. In a smooth *rocking* movement *pivot* the clippers away from the head to produce the shape required.

3 Move to the adjacent panel of hair and repeat the process as before, making sure the panels are connected. Keep working around the head.

4 Move to one side of the head. Note the required length for any sideburns that may be present, ensure they are level and cut them to shape.

5 The neckline and outline must now be tapered to create a natural effect so that the hair appears to fade. Set the clippers to cut at the shortest setting, or use a size 000 or balding blade. Hold the clipper blade directly against the scalp. Pivoting the clippers away in a smooth rocking movement blends and fades the neckline.

6 At the centre panel of hair at the back of the head blend the hair where the top of the taper meets the hair on the top of the head. Move across the head working on small sections and ensure that each panel is connected to blend the two areas together to create an even, continuous effect without any weight lines.

7 Move across the head following the direction of hair growth and ensure that each panel of hair is connected.

8 The front hairline is then shaped with the clippers.

9 Channelling with the clippers may now be used to create lines, shapes and designs, if required.

10 Scissors or clippers-over-comb and freehand cutting techniques are then used to shape the top. Make sure that you use even tension throughout the cut, as hair pulled out further and cut will shrink back and leave a hole later.

11 Shave the areas outside the haircut outlines, if required (see Chapter 12, Shaving services).

12 Finish the look with wax to smooth and define the curl movement.

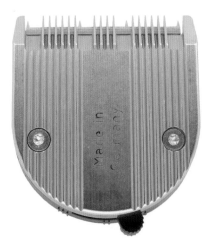

Texture blade

Flattops

At one time flattop haircuts were popular in many barber's shops. Sometimes they were cut very close and faded and were popular with men in the emergency services and

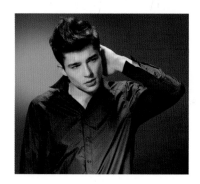

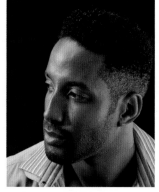

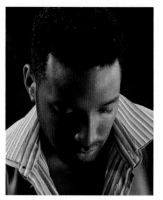

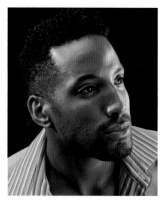

Finished skin fade looks   Finished skin fade looks   Finished skin fade looks

armed forces, as they were easy to care for but with added styling details compared to other looks, for example the 'buzz cut' or 'crew cut'.

Flattops were commonly regarded as one of the most technical and demanding haircuts in the skilled barber's repertoire. Very precise scissors and clippers-over-comb skills were needed to create the flat, square shape on a rounded head. Symmetry was essential through all 360° views. The top had to be perfectly horizontal and the sides perfectly vertical when the client's head was in its normal sitting or walking position. Some looks included square corners where the top and sides meet, whilst in others these corners were gently rounded.

Flattops are still are an advanced haircut if cut using only scissors and clippers-over-comb skills without any flattop devices; what might be called a 'hand cut flattop'. Flattop devices often include large flat surfaces and/or spirit levels, such as the 'Flat-topper Comb' and are designed to help the newer barber achieve the required even and level shape.

Flattops have been worn by several celebrities and have been in and out of fashion, but they are becoming popular again – not only for men as some women also enjoy wearing this distinctive look.

Today, flattops are often longer and more flexible so they can be dressed conservatively when required but into their true flattop shape at other times.

Sometimes flattops are disconnected rather than graduated so that the flatter, square shape is seen yet the sides and top do not blend. The key is to know how to create the flat, square shape; the skilled barber can then adapt the techniques to create the looks that client's today desire. Here is a method used to create a contemporary flattop:

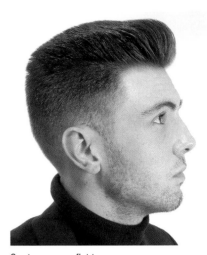

Contemporary flat top

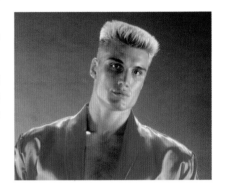

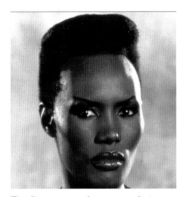

The flattop sometimes appeals to women – barber's might consider such work

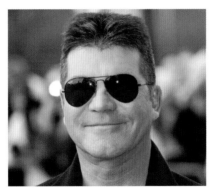

Variations of flattop have appealed to many people

RODGER – A 'HAND CUT' CONTEMPORARY LONGER FLATTOP

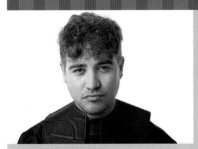

Step A

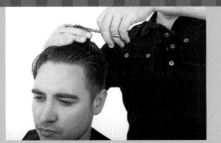

Step B

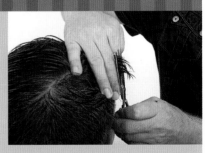

Step C

(continued)

RODGER – A 'HAND CUT' CONTEMPORARY LONGER FLATTOP
(*Continued*)

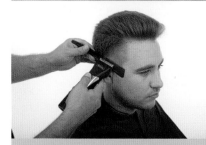

Step D

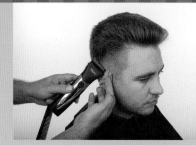

Step E

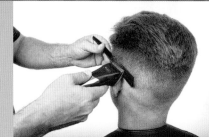

Step F

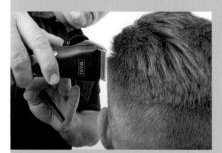

Step G

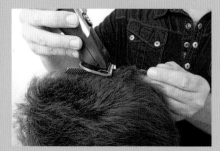

Step H

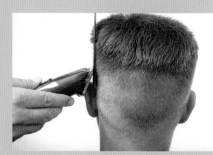

Step I

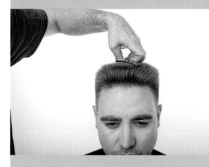

Step J

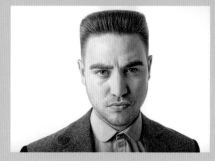

Step K

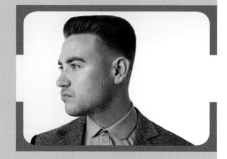

Step L

1. Gown and prepare the client (a).

2. Club cut the top to the basic desired length (b).

3. Continue across the head and into the sides – this is just preparing the basic shape (c).

4. Dry the hair into the basic shape. Clippers-over-comb is used to cut the sides and back to the correct length – remember to keep checking the mirror and from different angles to make sure a level and square shape is created (d).

5. Taper and outline as you work around the head – keep checking that the level square shape is developing (e).

6. Continue around the back of the head and across the other side. Note that the neckline has been tapered to a fade too! (f).

7. Freehand clipper work is used to build the square shape (g).

8. Clippers-over-comb is then used across the top. Reduce the length to that required by the look. Keep building a square flat shape – remember to keep checking for symmetry; use the mirror regularly and stand back from your work often! (h).

9. The corners are created using clippers-over-comb – use the straight surface of the comb to help build the level square shape (i).

10. Precise freehand scissors work and clippers work is used to perfect the finish (j).

11. Blow-dry into shape and finish the look with wax to add definition (k).

The routine for a traditional short 'hand-cut' flattop

1 Cut the back and sides to about 1 cm or shorter in length using clippers-over-comb or scissors-over-comb techniques. Avoid tapering the bottom of the sides too much. The shape created should appear square and symmetrical when viewed in the mirror. Be careful not to cut into the hair on top of the head at this stage.

2 Move to one side of the head. Note the required length for any sideburns, ensure they are level and cut them to the correct length and shape.

3 The neckline and edge of the outline must now be gently tapered to create a natural look.

4 Wet the top of the hair then dry it straight back into a rough flattop shape. You may need to reduce the overall length of the top first if it is longer than about 5 cm. Start at the crown and use scissors-over-comb or clippers-over-comb techniques to blend the crown area into the hair at the back of the head. This shape can be rounded, as the squared corner shape should begin from the area above the back of the ears.

5 Cut the hair in the central panel to the same length working forwards from the crown. This is the shortest area on top, as the hair length will need to increase to retain the flat shape where the head slopes down towards the sides and front. At the front make sure that your comb stays horizontal – do not let it turn to 90° to follow the shape of the head where it slopes down.

6 Move to the adjacent panel at one side and cut the hair straight across and away from the central guideline in the crown area. Again, here too you must keep the comb horizontal and not let it turn to 90°. The shape you are trying to create is a squared corner. Continue this process along the panel until the head slopes away near the front when you cut to the front guideline. Repeat this on the other side.

7 Take a vertical section at one side above the back of the ear and cut the hair straight up, ensuring that the squared corner shape is retained. Continue this around each side until the squared shape is achieved. You may need to re-wet and blow-dry the hair into the flattop shape again before final cutting to make sure all the hairs are lying in their correct positions.

8 Using the previous techniques and freehand cutting, move across the head working on small sections and ensure that each panel is connected to create an even, continuous effect without any lines.

9 Finish the look with a little wax or hairspray, if required.

Accompanying video available for 'hand cut' contemporary longer look flattop. Please scan this QR code.

> **TIP** ✓
>
> Flattops can be cut at many different lengths – you simply adjust the length of the sides and crown area and cut the top to suit. Traditional flattops were often very short.

Aftercare

Your client will need to know how to look after their new haircut before they leave the barbers' shop. This should include the following:

◆ Recommend when the client should book the next appointment – remember that in faded and other short looks the hair will need restyling sooner as the new hair growth will quickly be longer than the length of the actual haircut and soon be noticeable. Hair outside the haircut perimeter would also be visible and will need removing. In the shortest styles appointments should generally be for every 4 weeks or less. In longer styles 4 to 6 weeks might be acceptable. However, where the haircut includes a pattern the client will need to visit sooner if they wish the pattern to remain distinct.

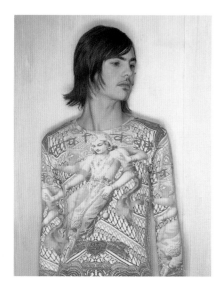

- The client should shampoo their hair according to the hair length, hair and scalp condition and their lifestyle.

- Which products can help the client maintain the overall style; particularly those such as gel and wax that can help define the pattern by smoothing the hair outside the pattern lines. Consider retailing such products in your barber's shop!

Health and safety

It is important to consider health and safety when cutting hair because of the risks associated with using electricity and the risk of cutting the skin. Here are some important health and safety factors that you must consider when providing hair-cutting services:

- If the client has any cuts or abrasions on their head, or you suspect that an infection or infestation is present the haircut must not be carried out – remember these are known as contraindications.

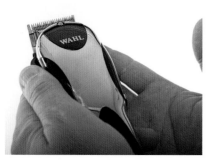

It may help you to read **CHAPTER 2**, 'Health and safety in the barber's shop' for general information on working safely in the barber's shop.

- Pay special attention to hygiene when cutting hair because of the risk of cross-infection through open cuts.

- Open and safety razors have very sharp blades and must always be handled and used with great care.

- Always close the handle to protect the blade of an open razor when it is not being used or when it is being carried.

- *Never* place razors or scissors or other cutting tools in pockets.

- A fixed-blade razor must always be *sterilized* before each use.

- A new blade must always be used for each new client when using a detachable-blade open razor – this type of razor should now be used in professional barber's shops!

- Used razor blades, called sharps, must be disposed of correctly in accordance with your salon policy. Soiled disposable materials should be placed in sealed plastic bags for removal.

- Electrical equipment must always be handled and used with care in accordance with the manufacturer's instructions.

- *Never* use or place electric clippers or other electrical equipment near water.

- *Do not* go near electrical equipment that is lying in water – isolate the mains power first.

- Visually check that electrical equipment is safe to use before commencing work – check that the cable has not frayed or been pulled and that the plug is not loose.

- Pay attention to the position of cables when using and storing electrical equipment.

- *Never* overload sockets by plugging too many items of electrical equipment into the same socket.

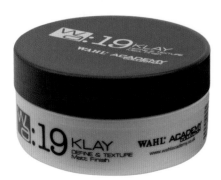

Finishing Klay for defining the style and adding texture

- Follow the manufacturer's instructions for the care of your scissors and clippers – ensure that you clean and lubricate the blades regularly to avoid damage.

- Keep your working area and the barber's shop hygienically clean. Clear away hair cuttings to prevent slip hazards.

- Only use clean tools and equipment – use alcoholic wipes and sprays to keep clippers clean and disinfected between each client.

- If the client's skin is cut whilst you are cutting his hair stay calm and explain what has happened. Follow your salon's first-aid and accident procedures.

Checking for correctly aligned blades

◆ If you cut your own skin whilst you are cutting the client's hair stay calm and explain what has happened. Follow your salon's first-aid and accident procedures.

◆ If the cut is more serious seek medical attention as soon as possible.

◆ Make sure that you know the whereabouts of your salon's first-aid kit. Keep yourself up-to-date with your salon's first-aid and accident procedures.

◆ Electrical equipment must be regularly tested and given a certificate of testing to confirm that it is safe for use. Your salon owner will ensure that this is carried out, as required.

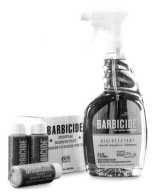

Sanitizing products

IMAGE GALLERY

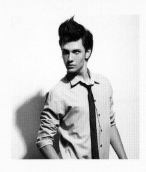

Visit the online image gallery on this book's accompanying website to see other inspirational men's haircuts.

BRINGING IT ALL TOGETHER

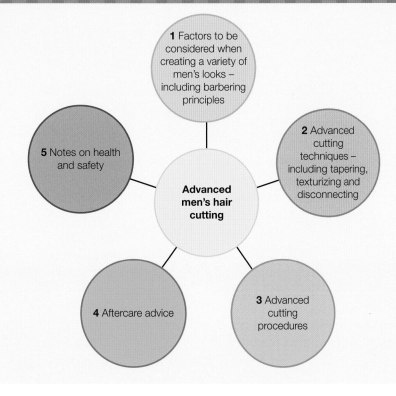

Summary

1 In advanced work the barbering principles about shape and form are often followed more loosely. Even so, remember that all men's hairdressing should still consider and apply barbering principles to the relevant features of the haircut, for example in longer square layered looks the layers are common in all hairdressing but the masculine features, such as sideburns and neck hair should still be cut following the barbering principles.

Advanced work regularly requires cutting techniques to be combined and adapted to take account of both the client's wishes and the many factors that affect the creation of the look.

Remember – a successful haircut will always begin with a thorough consultation.

There are two additional neckline shapes used in advanced work: the natural neckline; the fade, skin fade or faded neckline.

2 Tapering is used to cut the hair so that it tapers to a point, unlike the blunt end created when club cutting. This helps to achieve a more natural finish that is desired in many styles. Scissor tapering (sometimes called slide cutting, slice cutting or slithering) – is carried out on dry hair. Razor tapering – sometimes just called 'razor cutting', is only used on wet hair. Razoring (shaving) – is sometimes used to create clean outlines and emphasize a haircut shape. Texturizing techniques are used to break up a solid mass of hair and create a more random movement and texture.

Disconnecting is a technique where the layers between two areas of the head are not blended together in order to produce a clear contrast in hair length, weight or form.

3 Individual barbers will usually decide where to start and which cutting techniques to use mostly according to personal preference. In advanced cutting it is the barber's creativity and individualism that comes to the fore. The key to advanced work is understanding that many cutting techniques can achieve similar effects and the advanced barber will combine and adapt these, as necessary, to achieve the required results.

As a professional barber your first obligation is to work safely and ensure the comfort of your client. Don't be tempted to forget about the client's comfort whilst you are enthusiastically concentrating on creating that fantastic look!

If you client has piercings ask if these can be removed whilst you complete the work. If this is not possible you must take extra care whilst working – remember to work away from the piercing wherever possible, and always make sure you know where the piercing is before combing or cutting the hair in the adjacent areas.

Flattops are an advanced haircut if cut using only scissors and clippers-over-comb skills without any flattop devices; what might be called a 'hand cut flattop'. Flattop devices often include large flat surfaces and/or spirit levels, such as the 'Flat-topper Comb' and are designed to help achieve the required even and level shape.

4 Remember to advise your client when their next appointment should be made; in the shortest styles appointments should generally be for every 4 weeks or less. In longer styles 4 to 6 weeks might be acceptable.

5 If the client has any cuts or abrasions on their head, or you suspect that an infection or infestation is present the haircut must not be carried out – remember these are known as contraindications.

Never place razors or scissors or other cutting tools in pockets.

Follow the manufacturer's instructions for the care of your scissors and clippers – ensure that you clean and lubricate the blades regularly to avoid damage.

Make sure that you know the whereabouts of your salon's first-aid kit. Keep yourself up-to-date with your salon's first-aid and accident procedures.

Activities

1 Obtain three hair cuttings over 10 cm in length. Carefully club cut one, cutting straight across; taper cut the second and razor cut the third (take great care whilst cutting!). Compare how the different techniques affect the distribution of weight and movement in the hair cutting.

2 Whilst creating haircuts, try using different texturizing techniques and note the effects they produce. Take photographs of the effects (remember to obtain the client's permission first) and make notes. You can then use these to help you explain the techniques to your junior colleagues.

3 Organize a photo shoot in your barber's shop with other colleagues. Create your best work and use the resulting images to publicize your salon, create style choices to show clients, or submit them to magazines for wider coverage of your work. Remember to get permission from the clients/models and your manager first.

Check your knowledge

1 Compare and state the key differences regarding shape and form when producing advanced men's looks to producing basic men's looks.

2 State how techniques are used differently when undertaking advanced cutting.

3 Why is it important to consider hair type when cutting hair?

4 Why should hair colour be considered when cutting hair?

5 Which one of the following is the least important reason for considering neckline shapes in men's hairdressing?

   a. Speed of working
   b. Maintaining the haircut look for longer
   c. Creating a masculine shape
   d. Keeping the neckline off the client's shirt collar

6 When might it be appropriate to cut into a natural outline?

7 List three points that should be considered when designing sideburn shapes.

8 What is the alternative name for scissor tapering?

9 Which of the following statements are correct?

   a. Club cutting makes the ends of the hair shaft blunt
   b. Tapering makes the ends of the hair shaft angled to a point
   c. Club cutting a hair section held at 90° to the head will decrease the weight line
   d. Tapering a hair section will decrease weight towards the ends of that section

10 Which cutting technique(s) should be carried out on wet hair and not carried out on dry hair?

11 When might razoring be used in hair cutting?

12 Describe two texturizing techniques.

13 Describe how channelling can be used to emphasize a haircut.

14 Describe a skin fade haircut.

15 Describe how to maintain high standards of hygiene for using electric clippers.

16 What actions should you take if you were to cut your client whilst cutting his hair?

12 Shaving services

QUALIFICATION SIGNPOSTING

This chapter will help your studies of the following qualifications and units:

❖ Level 1 NVQ Certificate in Hairdressing and Barbering.
❖ Level 3 NVQ Diploma in Barbering.
❖ City & Guilds Level 3 VRQ Diploma in Barbering

LEARNING OBJECTIVES

In this chapter you will learn:

◆ Why professional shaving declined in the barber's shop and how shaving is becoming more popular in the barber's shop today.

◆ Wet and dry shaving methods.

◆ Consultation prior to shaving.

◆ Preparation for shaving.

◆ How to prepare and use shaving materials – products, tools and equipment.

◆ How to prepare – applying hot towels and lather.

◆ The shaving techniques and shaving procedure.

◆ How to finish the shave.

◆ The common shaving problems and how to resolve them.

◆ Health and safety.

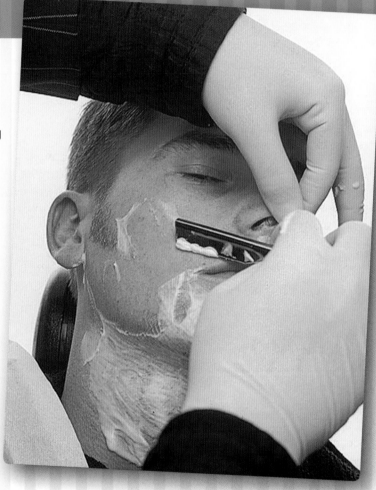

For further information on the qualifications covered by this chapter see the qualification mapping grid at the front of the book.

INTRODUCTION

At one time shaving was one of the barber's most popular services, but the introduction of the safety razor and the electric shaver has led to its decline. More recently there has been renewed interest in shaving as a service, particularly in city centre salons that offer a full range of services to the busy professional or traveller.

This chapter looks at the techniques used for shaving and covers the following topics:

❖ The decline of shaving in the barber's shop.

❖ Shaving in the barber's shop today.

❖ Wet and dry shaving methods.

❖ Consultation prior to shaving.

❖ Preparation for shaving.

❖ Shaving materials – products, tools and equipment.

❖ Preparing razors for use – including setting and stropping fixed-blade razors.

❖ Beard preparation – applying hot towels and lather.

❖ Shaving techniques.

❖ A shaving procedure.

❖ Finishing the shave.

❖ Common shaving problems.

❖ Health and safety.

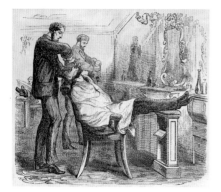

Traditional shaving

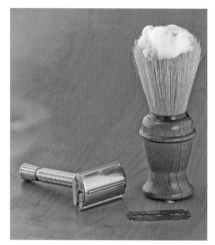

Traditional safety razor and shaving brush used by the self shaver

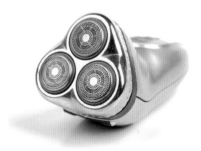

Electric shaver

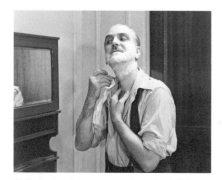

Self-shaving became popular after 1930s

The professional shave

The decline of shaving in the barber's shop

For over 2000 years men have visited the barber's shop regularly for shaving. Indeed, until just a few decades ago many men would visit the barber's shop *daily* for their shave.

At that time shaving was performed with an open, fixed-blade razor, commonly known as a cut-throat razor, which needed regular care to keep it in good working order. Shaving oneself with this type of razor was difficult, time-consuming and often uncomfortable. A shave in the barber's shop, however, was pleasant and relaxing: the barber would perform a face massage, or facial, as part of the service.

The introduction of the safety razor in about 1905 and the introduction of electric shavers in the 1930s made shaving at home much easier.

More and more men started shaving themselves and the 'self-shaver' became a feature of modern society. Demand for the 'professional shave' declined further in the 1970s when disposable razors were introduced and the barber's art of shaving was in real danger of being lost.

Shaving in the barber's shop today

The 'self-shaver' is not a completely new phenomenon: self-shavers have existed for hundreds of years. It is the *number* of self-shavers that has had the greatest impact on shaving as a barber's shop service.

Today most men choose to shave because it suits their personal image, or their business or hygiene requirements; shaving is an important part of their personal daily grooming routine. The barber cannot hope to change this, but he can design his services to match his client's shaving routine and experiences. Many men welcome professional advice and information on shaving, particularly if these can help them overcome common shaving problems. Shaving products, equipment and skin care products are also in constant demand by the self-shaver. Men must still get their hair cut and for this most visit the salon. Today the opportunities clearly exist for the barber to introduce his clients to shaving services.

Here are some ideas to consider if you are interested in providing shaving services:

- Offer shaving (and face massage) services for special occasions such as weddings.

- Offer shampooing, blow-drying and shaving services to travellers and other busy men.

- Offer instructions on how to shave effectively, this is a service welcomed by many clients but particularly by younger men who are just finding they need to shave for the first time.

- Provide advice on shaving problems. For example, many men have difficulty shaving their sideburns level – they use their ears to judge the balance, but on most people the ears are not level. You can show them how to do this correctly. You can also discuss ways of avoiding razor burn, blood spotting and so on.

- Provide advice on products. It will help if you also stock these products and can achieve retail sales for your barber's shop!

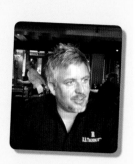

GARY MACHIN Barber and Director
of 'Roger's Barber Shops'

Nearly all men who don't choose to wear a beard need
to shave every day. This need offers the barber's shop great
opportunities to develop shaving services as part of their business.
Don't overlook this potential – get the edge and hone up your
shaving skills.

Shaving

The purpose of shaving is to remove the visible part of the hair and leave the skin smooth to touch. This is achieved by means of a razor or some other tool that cuts the hair close to the skin. A good shave is achieved without irritating the skin. Both men and women regularly practise shaving but here we will only consider its use on men within the salon.

The professional shave is used to remove unwanted hair from the face and neck. It may be used to outline moustaches, beards, sideburns and necklines or to remove all visible beard hair.

Wet and dry shaving methods

A shave may be achieved by either wet or dry methods.

Dry shaving Dry shaving uses an electric shaver, which may be powered by disposable or rechargeable batteries, or by mains electricity.

There are many different types of electric shaver, but typically they all consist of a number of sharp cutting blades that move rapidly to cut the hair when power is applied. The blades move behind a very thin flexible guard, which both protects the skin and positions the hairs for optimum cutting.

Electric shavers are mostly used by the self-shaver, and are particularly suitable for the busy professional or traveller. They are easy to carry and can be used with ease in almost any location, especially if powered by batteries. However, they are less suitable for use in the salon, as they are more difficult to sterilize effectively, do not provide such a close shave and are unlikely to achieve the desired superior service experience.

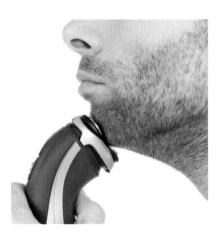

Dry shaving

DON'T BE TEMPTED X

Dry shaving does not refer to using a razor intended for wet shaving purposes without lather as this would pull the hair and skin and be very uncomfortable! Don't be tempted to use such a razor dry!

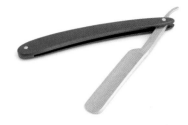

Open fixed blade cutthroat razor – hollow ground

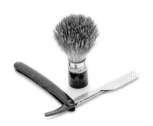

Open detachable blade razor

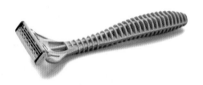

Modern disposable blade razor – type is mostly for self-shaving

It may help you to read CHAPTER 4, 'Client care for men' for more detailed information on consultation before reading this section.

See CHAPTER 4 pages 60–62 for full details on hair types and classifications.

Wet shaving Wet shaving is the method of shaving traditionally used in the salon. It is achieved by means of a razor, which can either be an open ('cut-throat') razor or a safety razor.

In wet shaving the area to be shaved is prepared by the application of lather, gel or shaving oil prior to shaving. The hairs are then removed with a razor while they are still wet.

The open razor comprises a very sharp steel blade which is protected by a hinged cover when not in use. Safety razors have guards that limit how far the blade edge protrudes, often such razors have a thin guard entirely covering the blade, which both protects the skin and positions the blade and hair for optimum cutting. Several different types of safety razor are available: some are totally disposable, whilst others have a detachable blade that is easily replaced when a new blade is required.

Consultation prior to shaving

Consultation is an essential part of any hairdressing service, and is particularly important when shaving because of the risks associated with the use of razors.

Time must always be given to discussing the client's requirements with them. It is essential that careful consideration be given to each of the following factors before any lather is applied to the face.

HEALTH & SAFETY

A thorough consultation will ensure that you identify any adverse conditions of the hair or skin that may be present. It is particularly important to establish whether a suspected infection or infestation is present: these are contraindications that would prevent you from carrying out the shave.

You must establish:

◆ What does the client want – does he want a close shave?

◆ Do they have a moustache, a beard or sideburns? If so, do they wish to keep them?

◆ Look for signs of broken skin, abnormalities on the skin, and any unusual beard growth patterns.

◆ What is the facial hair type – type S1, W2, C3 or K4?

◆ What are the facial hair characteristics –

    ◆ Is the beard hair fine, medium or coarse?

    ◆ Is the beard growth dense or sparse?

    ◆ Does the density of beard growth vary around the face?

The facial hair characteristics, hair type and facial features significantly affect the way you carry out the shave. The following are the most important:

◆ Hair growth patterns.

◆ Hair texture.

◆ Density of the beard.

◆ Hair type.

◆ The facial features.

Hair growth patterns

Hair growth patterns are the ways in which individual hairs or a section of the beard may grow in a particular direction. Hair growth patterns must be identified, and the 'first time over' shave should always be carried out *following* the direction of the hair growth. (Shaving *against* the hair growth at the start of the shave would cause the razor to drag, and would be very uncomfortable for the client.)

> **TIP** ✓
>
> The 'first time over' shave should always be carried out *following* the direction of hair growth. Often shaving against the growth is not required and should only be used when a closer shave is required.

If the client requests a close shave, shaving against the direction of growth may be performed during the 'second time over' shave. Care should be taken not to shave the hair *too* close, however, as this would irritate the skin and might cause 'ingrown hairs', particularly on men with type C or type K (curly and very curly/kinky hair). Ingrown hairs can become infected and may lead to conditions such as impetigo or folliculitis.

Some clients have very strong hair growth patterns in their beard, such as hair whorls. In such cases, shave by following the direction of hair growth around the whorl.

> **TIP** ✓
>
> Ask your client whether there are any areas he finds difficult to shave. Each client is usually an expert when it comes to identifying problem areas on his own face!

Texture

As with all hair, the texture of hair in a beard can be fine, medium or coarse. Fine hair is easy to shave, as it creates little resistance to the razor. Coarse hair can be very difficult to shave and requires much more lather and massaging to **soften the beard** before shaving. Young men usually have fine facial hair, but as men get older their facial hair often becomes much coarser.

> **TIP** ✓
>
> Very dense and coarse beards should be steamed with a hot towel and well lathered before shaving: the steam and lather help to soften the beard. The lather should be massaged into the beard for a few minutes and then reapplied before commencing the shave.

Density

Hair density means the amount of hair that grows in a given area of skin. This is important to consider in shaving as the density of the growth may make it necessary to carry out a 'second time over' shave.

Young men often have sparse facial hair growth, but this becomes denser as they get older. Some men have very dense beard growth, often called 'blue beards' as the density of growth gives the skin a blue tinge which remains even after shaving. Men with very dense beards may have to shave twice a day to keep a clean-shaven appearance. Not surprisingly, they may decide to stop shaving and grow beards.

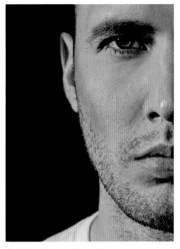

Facial hair growth pattern

> **KEY DEFINITION**
>
> Softened beard: Facial hair that has been steamed with hot towels so that the cuticles open and moisture and lather enter to increase the elasticity of the hair.

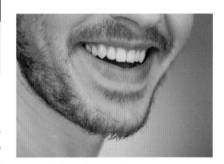

Sparse facial hair growth

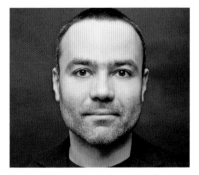

Dense facial hair growth – a blue beard

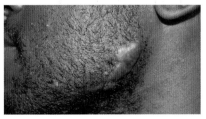

Keloids

KEY DEFINITION

Keloids: Scarring around an injury due to overgrowths of fibrous skin tissue.

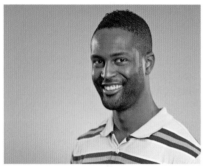

Dense Type 4 facial hair growth

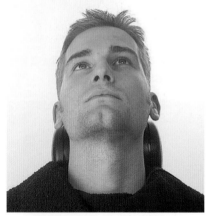

The prepared client before lathering

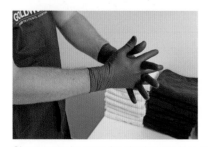

Gloves must be worn for shaving services to meet infection control requirements

Hair types

Chapter 4 describes the differences between the main classifications of hair type and should be read before reading this section. The hair type requires different considerations when shaving, as follows:

◆ Type S1 – a and b are generally easier to shave but type c can be more difficult depending upon the density of growth. Dense type S1c will require more steaming and lather to soften the beard.

◆ Type W2 – a and b are again generally easier to shave but type c can be more difficult depending upon the density of growth.

◆ Type C3 – a and b types are increasingly more difficult particularly if growth density is high. Some clients with type C3 hair avoid shaving as the hair is prone to growing into the skin if cut short.

◆ Type K4 – a and b types are difficult to shave as the hair is often curled in the skin making the surface bumpy. Men with type K4 hair, especially 4c avoid shaving, particularly if the growth is dense as this hair type often grows into the skin if cut too short.

Facial features

To prevent damage to the skin it is important to identify and consider the client's facial features. Careful note should be made of the following:

◆ The mouth.

◆ The width of the top lip.

◆ The nose.

◆ The shape of the jaw and chin.

◆ Any unusual features, such as moles, dimples, scarring or piercings.

The prepared client

1 Carry out your consultation with the client. Look for signs of broken skin, abnormalities on the skin, and unusual beard growth patterns.

2 Agree with your client the methods of shaving that you will use.

3 Before you begin work, gather together all the materials, products, tools and equipment you will require.

4 Position the client in a reclining chair with support for their head. Use a clean paper towel over the headrest.

5 Gown the client, remembering to use a neck strip and place a clean towel across their chest, tucked in at the neck. Place a clean paper towel over the towel and across their shoulder (from the client's neck towards your body).

6 Your hands and nails should be clean: let your client see that you have washed them. Make sure that the razor has been prepared correctly. Show your client that you have sterilized the razor or that you are fitting a new blade – make it clear that you use high standards of hygiene in your work.

Shaving materials, products, tools and equipment

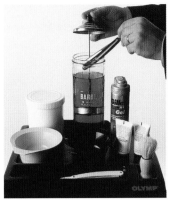

Shaving equipment must be sterilized and sanitized before each use

Materials

Required materials include the following. First, you will need hot and cool towels. Unless they are specially supplied pre-packed for shaving, these should be sterilized. You will also need a roll of tissue paper, for wiping used lather from the razor.

In case of any accidents, you must have access to first-aid materials. For small nicks or cuts you will need styptic liquid or powder. You may use a styptic pencil, but only once – you must use a fresh one for each new client to minimize the risk of cross-infection. To avoid the risk of cross-infection, you should wear gloves.

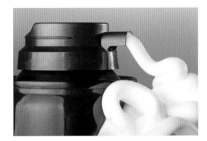

Shaving foam

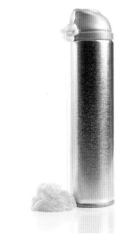

Products

To carry out the shave you will need shaving soaps, foam or gel, for lathering the face, or shaving oil, to ensure that the face and beard is adequately lubricated.

To finish you may need products such as aftershave lotions, aftershave balms, moisturisers and talcum powder. Each has a specific purpose: aftershave lotions act as an astringent that closes the skin pores and helps to prevent infection, although this can sting. Most are perfumed; balms contain moiturisers that calm the skin; talcum powder is used to calm the skin and reduce shine.

Shaving gel

Tools

Open razors Open razors are usually used in barbering. They have either a fixed blade, which must be sharpened or set, or a detachable blade, which is disposable. Open razors, also known as 'cut-throat' razors, have a hinged handle that closes to protect the blade when not in use.

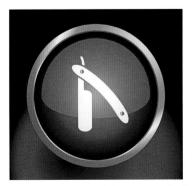

Bold advertising can help promote shaving services

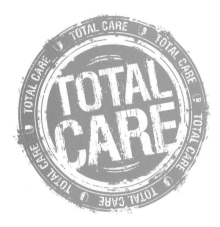

HEALTH & SAFETY

◆ Open razors have very sharp blades: they must always be treated with the greatest of care and respect. Keep the handle closed to cover the blade when not in use and especially when carrying or passing the razor. Never place a razor in your pocket. Always keep razors out of the reach of children.

◆ When passing an open razor, the handle must always be closed. In addition, wrap your hand around it to prevent it from opening accidentally. Pass the razor with the tang facing away from you and towards the other person.

Fixed-blade razors Fixed-blade razors can be either 'hollow-ground' or 'solid-ground'. They were the preferred choice of traditional barbers for many years, but are more difficult to use commercially because they have to be sterilized before use on each client.

HEALTH & SAFETY

You should not use fixed-blade open razors in professional shaving today due to the difficulties in achieving full sterilization of the razor between clients. It is easier and highly recommended to use disposable-blade open razors that have new sterile blades for each client.

HEALTH & SAFETY

◆ It is highly recommended to use disposable-blade open razors in the barber's shop. If a fixed-blade razor is preferred, a different fixed-blade razor should be kept for each client's personal use: the razor should be used on no-one else. Remember that fixed-blade razors must *always* be effectively sterilized before each use.

◆ Before using a fixed-blade razor for shaving, check your local bye-laws. In many areas the use of fixed-blade razors is prohibited. (Your local council will be able to help you.)

◆ *Remember*: It is good practice to use disposable-blade open razors for professional shaving services.

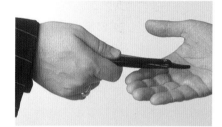

(a) Correct: tang facing away

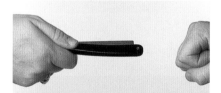

(b) Incorrect – blade is facing the recipients hand and could open to cut them whilst being passed

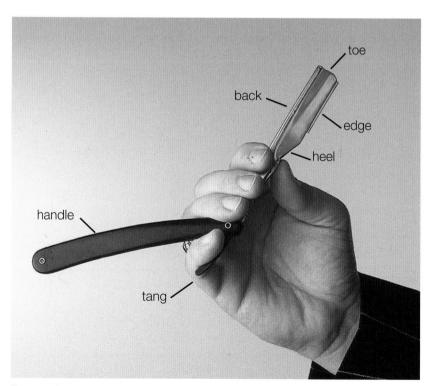

Features of an open type razor

TIP ✓

Fully disposable razors are sometimes used in the salon, but they are usually designed for home use by the self-shaver, and are not as effective for the professional shave.

Hollow-ground razors may be of either German or English origin. They have a concave appearance when viewed end-on, and are made of hardened steel. The steel undergoes a special heat treatment called tempering, which gives the razor the correct degree of hardness to produce a good cutting edge. Hollow-ground razors are usually 'hard-tempered', which makes them more difficult to sharpen (set), but the sharp edge lasts longer. Hollow-ground razors are light and have a particular feel that is much preferred by most barbers, especially when carrying out shaving. They are less suitable for cutting hair.

Solid-ground or French razors have a wedge-shaped blade that is much heavier and more rigid than the hollow-ground razor. They too are made of hardened steel and are usually 'soft-tempered', which makes them easier to sharpen, but the sharp edge does not last as long. Due to their greater weight and rigidity they are suitable for cutting hair, but they are difficult to use when shaving.

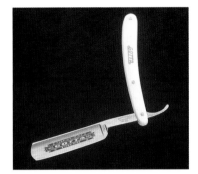

A hollow-ground razor – notice the concave blade

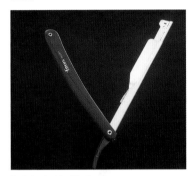

A detachable-blade razor

DON'T BE TEMPTED ✗

Don't be tempted to pass an open razor to someone else toe first. The blade can easily open and a serious injury might happen. Always pass the razor tang first.

Detachable-blade razors Detachable-blade razors are the preferred choice for professional shaving today because they are more hygienic than fixed-blade razors. They are designed to be very similar to a hollow-ground razor but they have disposable blades, which are easily replaced. Some detachable-blade razors come with special dispensers that store new blades and help attach them without their being handled.

The hair shaper is a type of detachable-blade razor that has a removable guard over the blade. These are not really suitable for shaving as the toe of the blade forms a point which can easily cut the skin when in use. However, they are good for haircutting because the guard can be left in place to help control the amount of hair being removed.

Equipment

The client should be seated in an adjustable chair, which can be positioned so that the client can recline comfortably while he is being shaved. It should have a headrest, and the height of the chair should be adjusted so that you do not have to bend uncomfortably whilst working.

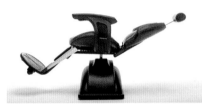

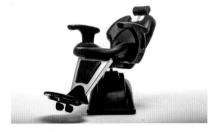

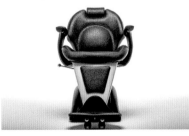

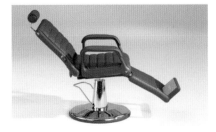

HEALTH & SAFETY

Remember to lock the chair before the client sits down and again whilst carrying out the shave so that it does not swivel and cause accidents.

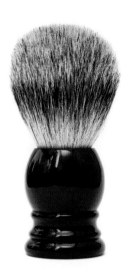

Shaving brush

A hone and strop will be required if you intend using fixed-blade razors. You also need a shaving brush and a shaving mug or bowl, particularly if you intend to use shaving soaps. The shaving brush and mug must be cleaned thoroughly in disinfectant and sterilized between clients. This is often difficult to do commercially, and it is easier to keep a personal brush and mug for each client.

Preparing razors for use

Setting fixed-blade razors

Hollow-ground and solid-ground razors have to be sharpened or set to keep them in good working order. The process of setting a razor is commonly called honing, as the razor is sharpened on a hone.

Honing is a process that requires a great deal of skill to ensure that the edge of the razor is set correctly. The edge of a razor has a number of very fine teeth cut into it that have a saw-like appearance if viewed under a microscope. The teeth make the razor sharp. The process of honing sets new teeth into the edge of the razor and realigns any older teeth that remain.

The razor edge may easily be damaged or over-honed during honing so the razor should be tested frequently to determine the degree of sharpness. The simplest way to test the razor's edge is to place it *very carefully* and *lightly* on a moistened thumbnail. Slowly draw the nail along a little from the heel to the toe of the razor: if the razor tugs the nail with a smooth and steady grip, the edge is sharp.

Hones

Various types of hones are available for sharpening razors. They usually consist of a rectangular block of abrasive material, which because it is harder than steel cuts the edge of the razor. Most barbers have a preferred choice of hone, acquired through years of experience.

Hones can be divided into three main groups, depending on what they are made of: natural, synthetic and combination.

Natural hones come from naturally occurring rock formations. They usually have to be lubricated with water or lather before use, and have a slow cutting action that produces a very fine and long-lasting edge. Water hones, which come from Germany, and Belgian hones are two popular varieties of natural hone.

Synthetic hones are man-made and can be used either wet or dry. Their cutting action is much faster than that of natural hones and they can produce a good cutting edge in less time. It is particularly important to test the razor edge regularly when using a synthetic hone, as it is very easy to over-hone a razor with a hone that cuts quickly! A carborundum hone is a popular type of synthetic hone.

Combination hones are the preferred choice of many barbers. They have two working sides: one side is a natural hone, the other a synthetic hone. The synthetic side is used to quickly cut a new edge on the razor. The natural side is then used to produce a very fine and long-lasting finished edge.

THE METHOD OF SETTING HOLLOW-GROUND RAZORS

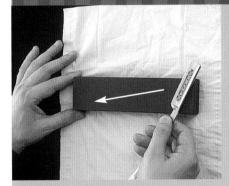

Step A

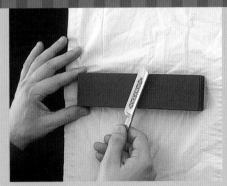

Step B

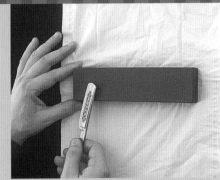

Step C

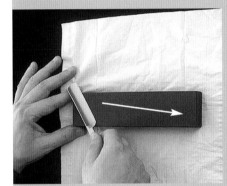

Step D

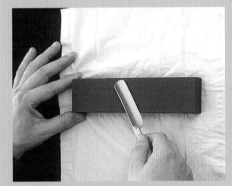

Step E

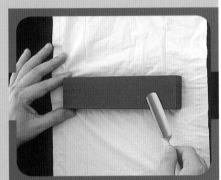

Step F

1. Lubricate the hone with water, lather or oil, as recommended by the manufacturer.

2. Place the razor flat on the hone, with the edge facing towards the middle (a).

3. Using light pressure, slide the blade across the hone, moving diagonally from the heel to toe (b).

4. Rotate the razor between the thumb and forefinger whilst keeping the back of the razor on the hone – keep rotating until the razor edge is pointing straight up.

5. Using no pressure push the razor up the hone away from your body until the heel is level with the bottom edge of the hone (c).

6. Continue rotating the razor, as before, to make the blade lie flat with its edge again facing the middle of the hone (d).

7. Slide the blade back across the hone, moving diagonally from heel to toe (e, f).

8. Repeat these movements several times.

9. Every few strokes of the hone, test the development of the edge by gently and carefully placing the razor edge on a moistened thumbnail. Slowly draw the nail along a little from the heel to the toe of the razor: if the razor tugs the nail with a smooth and steady grip the edge is sharp.

Stropping fixed-blade razors

The razor strop is used to give the razor a smooth 'whetted' edge. Stropping a razor does not cut into the steel, as honing does; instead, it cleans or polishes the edge, depending on which side of the strop is used. There are two main types of strop available: hanging strops (sometimes known as German strops), and French strops.

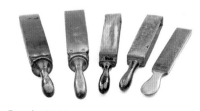

French strops

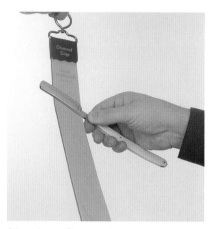

A hanging or German strop

> **TIP** ✓
>
> Remember, the canvas side of the strop should be used first, as this cleans the edge of the blade. This must always be followed with the leather side to polish it and produce a smooth whetted edge.

Hanging strops are usually combination strops that consist of canvas on one side and leather on the other. As their name implies, they are designed to hang from a swivel attached to one end (as illustrated below). Hanging strops are mostly used for stropping hollow-ground razors and are preferred by most barbers. French strops are usually made of wood and covered, again with canvas on one side and leather on the other. They are mainly used for stropping solid-ground razors and are less common.

New strops usually have to be 'broken in' before they will work effectively. Breaking in should be carried out following the manufacturer's recommendations. A method frequently used involves rubbing pumice stone across the surface to make the strop smooth. Stiff lather is then rubbed in repeatedly. Finally, and after some time, a smooth bottle or glass is rubbed over the strop until a very smooth surface is achieved.

The *canvas* side of a strop is used to clean the razor's edge and realign the cutting teeth, which become unaligned when the razor is used. The strop's effect is similar to mild honing, so a freshly honed razor should not be stropped using the canvas side. The *leather* side of a strop is made of cowhide, horsehide or imitation leather. Horsehide strops are usually of higher quality and are more expensive. The leather side polishes the edge to create a smooth finish, which is commonly called a whetted edge. This is achieved when all the very fine teeth on the razor edge are clean and aligned in the direction of the shaving stroke.

> **TIP** ✓
>
> A lot of practise is required to be able to strop a razor quickly and effectively. It is a good idea to practise with an old razor on an old strop. Make the movements slowly at first – increase the speed only when you become more proficient.

The method of stropping razors   The action used for stropping is similar to the action used in honing, but the razor is moved with *the back facing the direction of movement.* (Moving the razor with the edge facing the direction of movement would both cut the strop and damage the razor!)

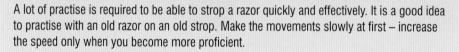

THE METHOD OF STROPPING RAZORS

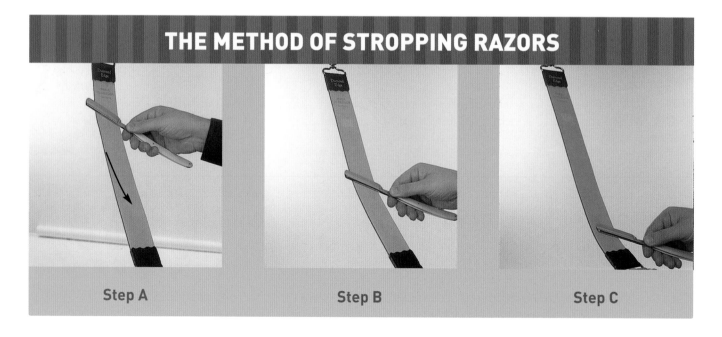

Step A   Step B   Step C

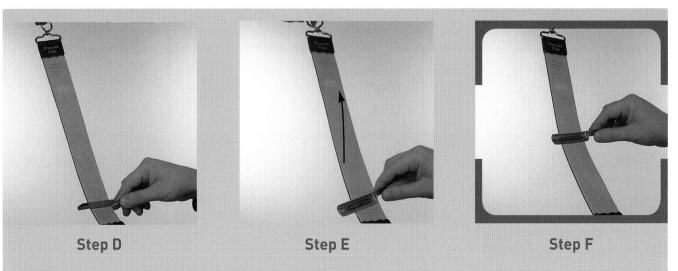

Step D   Step E   Step F

1. Place the razor flat on the strop with the back facing towards the middle (a).
2. Using light pressure, slide the blade across the strop, moving diagonally from the heel to toe (b).
3. Rotate the razor between the thumb and forefinger, keeping the back of the razor on the strop – keep rotating until the razor edge is pointing straight up (c).
4. Using no pressure, push the razor across the strop away from your body until the heel is level with the edge of the strop (d).
5. Continue rotating the razor as before, until the blade lies flat with its back again facing the middle of the strop.
6. Slide the blade back across the strop, moving diagonally from heel to toe (e).
7. Slide the razor back to position (a) and repeat these movements several times.

DON'T BE TEMPTED

Don't be tempted to hone or strop a detachable-blade razor. It is unnecessary and likely to harm the razor, hone and strop and possibly yourself too!

HEALTH & SAFETY

Always sterilize fixed-blade razors after stropping.

TIP   ✓

Show your client that you have sterilized the fixed-blade razor, or that you are fitting a new blade to a detachable-blade razor. Making it clear that you have high standards of hygiene in your work will give clients confidence.

It may help you to read CHAPTER 2, 'Health and safety in the barber's shop' for general information on working safely and hygienically in the barber's shop.

Detachable-blade razors

Used blades (known as sharps) must be removed carefully and disposed of in a suitable container. The razor must then be thoroughly washed in disinfectant.

Preparing the beard

HEALTH & SAFETY

Remember: A new disposable blade must be fitted for each client.

Ensure that the client's face and beard are visibly clean. Long beard growth that is to be removed should be disentangled as necessary, and the excess hair removed with scissors and clippers before starting the shave.

A beard must be softened before shaving is attempted. Softening the beard is achieved through the application of hot towels and lather.

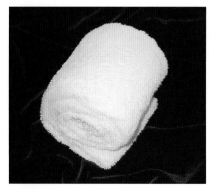

A rolled-up towel retains heat

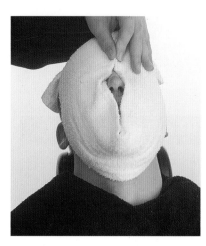

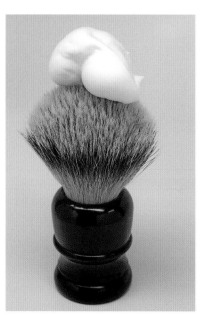

Applying hot towels

Hot towels steam the face and help in these ways:

- They remove dirt.

- They soften the hair cuticle.

- They lubricate the face, by stimulating the oil-producing glands.

- They relax the muscles, making shaving easier.

- They relax the client.

You must use *clean* towels. Some barbers use pre-packed towels, which are specially supplied ready-sterilized.

Hot towels are prepared in a steamer or by soaking them in hot water. Wring out the towel until it is nearly dry, and then roll it up so that it retains its heat while you carry it to the client.

Unroll the towel and wrap it around the client's face, being careful not to cover the nose, so that the client can breathe. Allow the towel to cool.

The cool towel should be replaced by a second (and if necessary a third) hot towel, which should be left on while you prepare the lather.

When using hot towels, remember the following important points:

- Always use clean towels for each new client.

- Prepare and apply the towels as quickly as possible but be sure to work safely – the quicker you are the more effective they will be.

- Avoid covering the client's nose.

- The towels should be nearly dry when they are applied.

- Remove the last hot towel before it becomes too cold – lather should be applied to a warm face!

Lathering

Effective lathering is essential to a good shave. Lathering is used:

- To remove dirt.

- To soften the hair.

- To lift individual hairs so that they stand erect from the skin for cutting.

- To lubricate the face so that the razor glides more easily.

Traditionally the method used to produce a rich lather was to vigorously work a shaving brush into a bar of shaving soap and a shaving mug containing warm water. 'Working up' a good lather was necessary, as the consistency of the lather was critical to the success of the shave. The lather had to be slightly watery at first to hydrate the skin and stop the lather from drying out too quickly. The stiffness of the lather was then increased to hold the hairs erect and provide adequate lubrication for the razor.

Modern shaving products are designed to produce instant lather. They contain conditioners to help protect the face and to stop the lather from drying out too quickly. Some are in the form of gels and oils which do not produce lather but have the same effect. Shaving soaps are still available for those who wish to use them – they work well but require more preparation – so it is purely a personal choice.

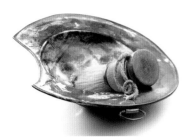

Traditional shaving brush and bowl

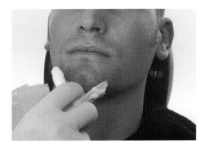

Spread the brush with your finger to make a cupping shape around the chin

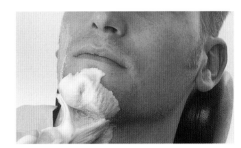

Work the lather into the beard using circular upward movements with the brush

Traditional lather has to be applied with a shaving brush, but modern products can be applied easily without the need for brushes or bowls. The use of the shaving brush does have additional benefits, though: the circular, upward motion used when applying the lather helps to work the lather into the beard and make the hairs stand erect.

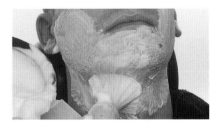

Ensure the beard is evenly covered

Here are some important points to bear in mind when applying lather:

- The lather should be applied immediately after the last hot towel has been removed.

- The lather should be applied starting under the tip of the chin (a).

- It is best applied with a lathering brush in an upward, circular motion which rotates in small circles over the face (b, c).

- The top lip is best lathered with a splayed brush, obtained by placing the index finger in the centre of the bristles (d). This avoids any lather going up the client's nose or into their mouth.

- On dense or coarse beards, the lather should be massaged into the beard for a few minutes with three fingers of either hand, and then reapplied with the brush.

- Do not let the lather run or drip, or dry out before shaving.

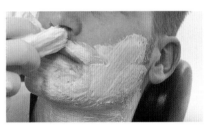

Spread the brush to create a thinner shape that will fit across the top lip

TIP ✓

Before each shaving stroke, make sure that the lather is still creamy and moist. Dry lather will not adequately lubricate the face: this will make the razor pull, causing considerable discomfort to the client. Always apply more lather first, as required.

Shaving techniques

The shaving procedure should be systematic. To be effective you require good co-ordination of both hands and the correct use of techniques. These are skills that take a lot of practise to develop.

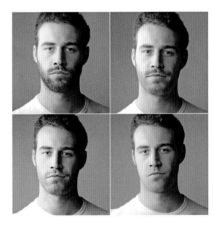

Stages of beard growth

You must be able to perform the techniques adequately *before* you try shaving anyone. A good way to practise is by shaving a lathered balloon with an old razor. (Ask someone to hold the balloon firmly for you while you do this.) If you burst the balloon, you were using too much pressure or holding the razor incorrectly. Alternatively, you could remove the blade from a detachable-blade open razor and practise with this on a model. *Make doubly sure you have removed the blade before commencing.*

This method of practising is only of use in developing 'the feel' of the razor against a delicate surface. Eventually you must make your first shaving stroke for real! You must be supervized when you do this. Work slowly and carefully, and try to remain relaxed and supple.

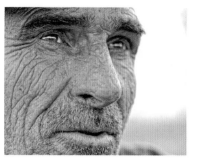

Older skin is sometimes haevily wrinkled and requires great care whilst being shaved

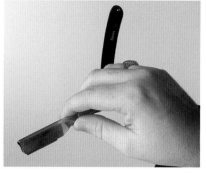

Forehand position for right-handed person

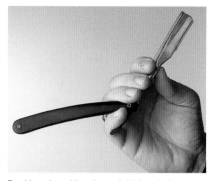

Backhand position for a right-handed person

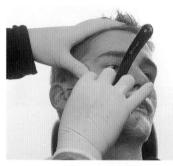

Right-hand forehand stroke

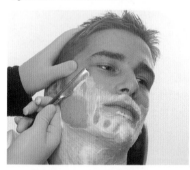

Right-hand backhand stroke

TIP ✓

Try to carry out your first shave on Type S1a or W2a hair with a sparse growth – this will create less resistance to the razor, be easier to achieve and will therefore help build your confidence.

Avoid shaving older men during your first shaves, as older skin tends to be more 'wrinkly' and less elastic. Because it usually requires more tension to make it smooth, older skin is more difficult to shave.

Holding the razor

Hold the razor in either your right or left hand, as best suits you. This hand is called your **shaving hand**. The correct way of holding the razor for a right-handed person is illustrated below. For a left-handed person the razor is simply reversed.

Tensioning the skin

Your other hand is used to tension the skin. This is called your **tensioning hand**. You must keep the fingers of this hand dry, to prevent them from slipping on the face.

The tensioning hand should be placed at the back of the razor so that you can stretch the skin under the razor before carrying out each stroke.

Shaving

The shaving stroke is performed with a single gliding movement. Try to avoid making short movements unless shaving a small area, as the razor will tend to 'pull' more and shaving will be less effective.

The forehand (sometimes called freehand) stroke is made towards you, and the backhand stroke away from you. Keep the razor at the correct cutting angle, about 40–45°, throughout the stroke. Do not apply too much pressure: the action should be light and free-moving.

Eventually you will develop a 'feel' for the correct angles and pressure to use. This feel or touch is known as the barber's hand, and when acquired it will allow you to make perfect shaves both safely and efficiently.

A shaving procedure

First time over

The shave should start on the nearest side to the barber – a right-handed barber stands on the right side of the client, a left-handed barber on the left side.

HEALTH & SAFETY

If you use shaving soap blocks and shaving brushes, you must keep a separate set for each client.

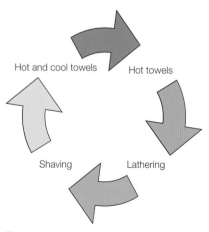

Hot and cool towels

Hot towels

Shaving

Lathering

The shaving procedure

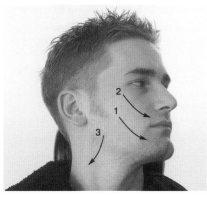

A typical pattern of shaving strokes

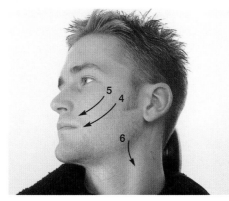

A typical pattern of shaving strokes

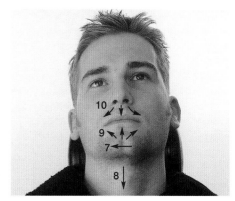

A typical pattern of shaving strokes

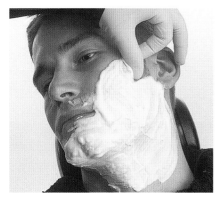

Marking the sideburns

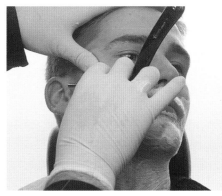

Commencing stroke 1

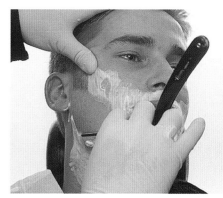

Stroke 1

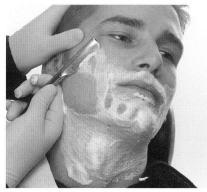

Stroke 2

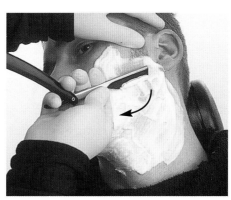

Stroke 4

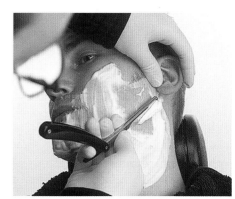

Stroke 4

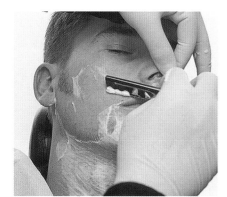

Stroke 10

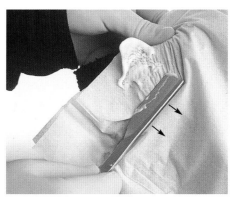

Wiping the razor – make sure you wipe directly
away from the edge of the blade

The skin must always be stretched taut before carrying out the stroke with the razor, otherwise cuts may occur and the shave will not be very close. After making sure they are level, mark the position of the sideburns by drawing your finger across the lather.

On the first-time-over shave, shaving follows the direction of beard growth in the pattern of ten strokes illustrated in the photographs on the following page. After each stroke, wipe the razor clean on the bottom of the tissue, then fold the tissue to cover the used lather. Keep wiping the razor this way until about three-quarters of the tissue length has been used, and then replace the used tissue with a new one from the roll. Make sure you dispose of the used tissue correctly.

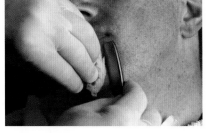

Sponge shaving

> ## TIP ✓
>
> To ensure that the sideburns are shaved level, place one finger high on each sideburn. Whilst looking in the mirror slide one finger down until the desired length is reached. Slide the other finger down until both fingers are level. Mark the position of both fingers by drawing them across the lather.

> ## HEALTH & SAFETY
>
> When wiping the razor, keep the blade flat and wipe it away from the edge. Never wipe along the blade or wrap the tissue around the blade as serious cuts would surely occur.

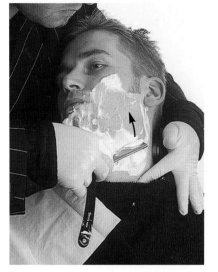

Once-over shave: shaving against the hair growth

Second time over

This shave is carried out *against* the beard growth, to get a closer shave finish. This is not always required, especially on immature or finer beards.

The second-time-over shave is usually the final shave unless the client has a very strong beard growth or a very close shave is required, in which case a sponge shave may be carried out. In the sponge shave a clean, sterilized sponge, which has been dipped in hot water, is slowly drawn across the face, closely followed by the razor. The damp sponge lubricates the face and raises the hairs into the path of the razor for close cutting. The sponge shave produces a very close shave: great care must be taken not to shave the hairs *too* close.

> ## HEALTH & SAFETY
>
> A new sponge must be used for each new client.
>
> Be very careful not to shave the hairs too close, as this would irritate the skin and could cause ingrown hairs. This is particularly likely with curly hair.

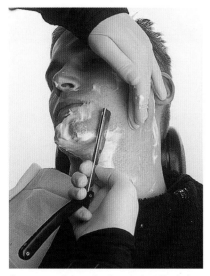

Once-over shave: shaving against the hair growth

The once-over shave

The once-over shave is the method used by experienced barbers to achieve a good even finish without having to re-lather the face and carry out a second time over. It is achieved by making a few more shaving strokes, as follows:

TIP ✓

Extra care should be taken when shaving the outlines of sideburns and moustaches. Make sure that you mark their outline by drawing your finger through the lather before shaving. Men are often very protective of their sideburn or moustache shape, and mistakes will not go unnoticed – especially right under their noses!

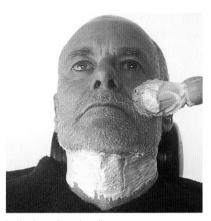

Lathering a beard outline

◆ After completing each shaving stroke, feel for remaining hair growth by running the fingers of your tensioning hand gently across the face.

◆ Where you feel hair growth remaining, gently complete a shaving stroke against the hair growth – being very careful not to shave too close.

Shaving outlines and the neck shave

Shaving is often used to prolong the clean appearance of a beard, moustache and haircut by shaving outside their outlines. For the haircut this means shaving around the neck and behind the ears.

It is performed with the same techniques used when shaving the face.

Note the following points.

◆ The client should be gowned, with the towel placed around the back of the neck.

◆ If the hair is very fine, the lather may be replaced with a little warm water.

◆ Stand to the side of the client. If you are right-handed, use a forehand stroke to shave the right side of the neck and a backhand stroke for the left side. If you are left-handed, reverse this.

◆ When shaving near the ears, protect them by folding them back gently with your tensioning hand.

◆ Finish the shave by applying a small amount of talcum powder, antiseptic or moisturiser. An aftershave lotion may be applied if the client wishes.

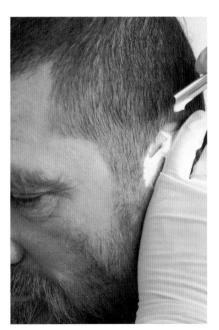

Shaving a beard outline

Finishing the shave

When the shave has been completed you may apply hot towels and carry out a face massage if your client requires this. If a face massage is not required, the face should be cleaned with a warm, damp towel or sponge, and then gently patted dry with a clean towel. Some clients enjoy the cooling and soothing effects of a cool towel: this is prepared and used just like a hot towel, but using cool water. Other clients even enjoy the bracing effects of a very cold towel, but you should ask before this is applied.

TIP ✓

If the client is having a face massage after shaving, apply a warm towel when the lather has been removed. The face should be warm and the facial muscles relaxed for face massage.

Shave outlines

Read **CHAPTER 13**, 'Face massage services' for more information on completing the shaving service with a face massage.

A small amount of talcum powder or moisturiser may be applied to soothe and smooth the skin. An aftershave lotion or aftershave balm may also be applied, if the client so desires. Aftershave *lotions* have a bracing effect on the skin – they are astringent. Aftershave *balms* are less astringent and are preferred by men who do not care for this bracing effect. Both help to close the pores of the face, reducing the risk of infection.

> **TIP**
>
> Remember to comb and style the client's hair as requested before he leaves the chair.

Common wet shaving problems

The table identifies some common wet shaving problems, possible causes and their remedies.

Problem	Possible cause	Possible remedy
Unshaven hair patches	Blunt razor Incorrect skin tension Incorrect razor angle Poor lathering	Change the blade or hone, and strop as necessary Stretch the skin smoothly before shaving Use the correct cutting angle Re-lather in the required area; re-shave uneven areas
Shave not close enough	Strong beard growth Incorrect skin tension Incorrect razor angle Poor lathering	Complete a second-time-over shave and/or a sponge shave, as necessary Stretch the skin smoothly before shaving Use the correct cutting angle Apply more lather and massage in upward moves
Shaving is painful	Blunt blade Shaving dry Shaving against the hair growth	Change the blade or hone, and strop as necessary Apply lather, water or oil Only shave *with* the hair growth on the first-time shave
Shaving rash (razor burn)	Shaving dry Shaving against the hair growth Blunt razor Shaving too close Towels too hot	Apply lather, water or oil Shave *with* the hair growth Change the blade or hone, and strop as necessary Stop shaving Remove and cool
Cuts to the skin	Blunt razor Incorrect razor angle Insufficient skin tension Too much pressure applied on razor	Change the blade or hone, and strop as necessary Use the correct cutting angle Keep the skin taut Use light shaving strokes
Hair follicles inflamed	Ingrown hairs	Refer to a doctor if infected
Bumpy skin	Ingrown hairs Acne	Advise the client to exfoliate their skin regularly to encourage the hairs to grow through and avoid shaving too close (particularly African-Caribbean men) Refer to doctor

Health and safety

Everyone in the salon has a duty to work safely and to keep the salon environment safe. This is particularly important when shaving because of the risk of cutting either the client's or your own skin, and the associated risk of cross-infection through open cuts. The following are some important factors that you must consider when providing shaving services.

It may help you to read CHAPTER 2, 'Health and safety in the barber's shop' for general information on working safely and hygienically in the barber's shop.

Supervision

◆ Always work under expert supervision until you are competent.

Consultation

◆ If the client has any cuts or abrasions on his face, or if you suspect that an infection or infestation is present, you must not carry out the shave as these are contra-indications to the shaving service.

Safety and hygiene: general

◆ Use only clean towels, tools and equipment.

◆ It is highly recommended that fixed-blade razors should no longer be used for professional shaving services. If a fixed-blade razor is used make sure it is always effectively sterilized before each use.

◆ When using a detachable-blade open razor, be sure to use a new blade for each new client and make sure that the handle and blade holder has been effectively cleaned and sterilized.

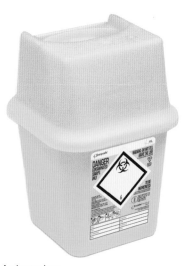

A sharps box

◆ Always wear tight-fitting, surgical-type gloves whilst carrying out shaves. Try not to carry out any shaves if you already have cuts or abrasions on your hands.

◆ Special attention must always be given to hygiene when shaving, because of the risk of cross-infection through open cuts.

Safety and hygiene: sharps

◆ The use of fixed-blade razors is sometimes prohibited by local bye-laws. Check the bye-laws in your area before offering shaving services with this type of razor.

◆ Open and safety razors have very sharp blades. They must always be handled and used with great care.

◆ Always close the handle to protect the blade of an open razor when it is not being used or when it is being carried.

◆ Never place razors or other cutting tools in your pockets.

◆ Used razor blades, like all sharps, must be disposed of correctly in accordance with your salon's policy. Soiled disposable materials should be placed in sealed plastic bags for removal.

Accidents and injuries

◆ Make sure that you know the whereabouts of your salon's first-aid kit. Keep yourself up-to-date with your salon's first-aid and accident procedures.

Styptic pencil

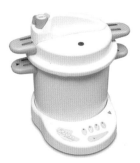
An autoclave

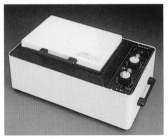
Dry head sterilising cabinet

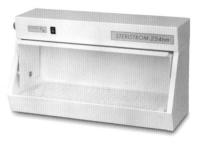
An ultraviolet ray cabinet

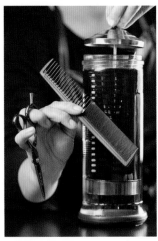
Barbicide

◆ If the client's or your own skin is nicked during shaving, the bleeding may be stopped with styptic liquids or powders. (A new styptic pencil may be used instead, but it must then be discarded correctly to minimize the risk of cross-infection: never reuse a styptic pencil.) The client should apply the styptic substance to themselves. Any soiled gowns or towels must be sealed in a plastic bag and laundered at a high temperature as soon as possible.

◆ If a more serious cut occurs, follow your salon's first-aid and accident procedures.

Methods of sterilization

Sterilization is particularly important in shaving services due to the risks associated with using razors and the potential for blood spotting.

Sterilization is the process of destroying *all* organisms, whether harmful or not. There are several methods of sterilization available, which may be divided into the following groups.

Moist heat Moist heat can be applied by boiling items in water for at least 20 minutes, or by immersing them in steam and under pressure in an autoclave.

Autoclaves are the preferred choice in many salons because they are the most effective method of sterilizing tools. Items in autoclaves reach very high temperatures, so make sure that the tools are heat-resistant: be particularly careful with plastic razor handles.

Dry heat Dry heat is applied by placing items in an oven at very high temperatures. This method is most often used to sterilize sheets and towels, and is commonly used in hospitals. Some barbers use prepacked towels which have been prepared in this way.

Ultraviolet rays Tools can be sterilized in special cabinets using ultraviolet rays. These are popular in many salons as they are easy to use.

All tools must be *cleaned* thoroughly before they are placed in the cabinet, as ultraviolet rays will not work effectively if the tools are dirty. The tools must also be turned regularly so that all surfaces are exposed to the rays (for about 30 minutes on each surface). Ultraviolet ray cabinets are good for *keeping* clean and sterile tools sterile but are less effective at achieving sterilization than an autoclave or dry heat sterilizing cabinet.

Vapours Traditionally vapours, usually formaldehyde-based were used in barber's shops to sterilize tools but concerns over this chemical means they are less often seen today. The vapours were used in cabinets and, as with ultraviolet rays, all the tools must be cleaned thoroughly before they are placed in the vapour cabinet, as the vapours cannot work effectively if the tools are too dirty. The tools must be turned regularly to ensure that all surfaces are exposed to the vapours for about 30 minutes. Similar to ultraviolet ray cabinets, vapour cabinets were known to be most effective for keeping tools sterile once they have been cleaned and sterilized.

Disinfectants Disinfectants are effective only if they are used in the correct strength. In the barber's shop, tools are often stored in jars of disinfectant: note that the disinfectant is no longer effective when it has become soiled. Follow the manufacturers' instructions to ensure that disinfectants are used correctly.

IMAGE GALLERY

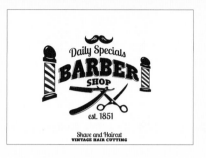

Visit the online gallery on this book's accompanying website to see other ideas for promotion shaving services.

BRINGING IT ALL TOGETHER

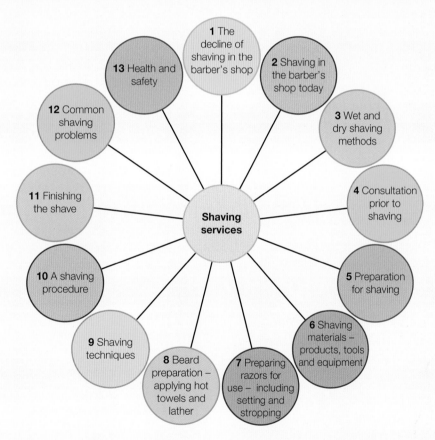

Summary

1   The introduction of the safety razor and the introduction of electric shavers made shaving at home much easier and led to the decline of barber's shop shaving services.

2   Today barbers should consider offering shampooing, blow-drying and shaving services to travellers and other busy men.

3   The purpose of shaving is to remove the visible part of the hair and leave the skin smooth to touch.

4   In wet shaving the area to be shaved is prepared by the application of lather, gel or shaving oil prior to shaving.

5   It is particularly important to establish whether a suspected infection or infestation is present: this would prevent you from carrying out the shave.

6   If the client requests a close shave, shaving against the direction of growth may be performed during the 'second-time-over' shave.

7   Fine hair is easy to shave, as it creates little resistance to the razor but very dense and coarse beards should be steamed with a hot towel and well lathered before shaving: the steam and lather help to soften the beard.

8   Facial piercings should be removed, if possible, prior to shaving unless the area around the piercing is affected by keloids.

9   Always wear gloves, to avoid the risk of cross-infection. They should be tight-fitting so that you can use the razor and tension the skin effectively during the shave.

10   Open razors are usually used in barbering. They have either a fixed-blade, which must be sharpened or set, or a detachable-blade, which is disposable.

11   You should avoid using fixed-blade open razors in professional shaving today due to the difficulties in achieving full sterilization of the razor between clients. Detachable-blade razors are the preferred choice for professional shaving today because they are more hygienic than fixed-blade razors.

12   The client should be seated in an adjustable chair, which can be positioned so that the client can recline comfortably while they are being shaved.

13   The process of setting a razor is commonly called honing, as the razor is sharpened on a hone. The razor strop is used to give the razor a smooth 'whetted' edge.

14   Modern shaving products are designed to produce instant lather. They contain conditioners to help protect the face and to stop the lather from drying out too quickly.

15   You must be able to perform the techniques adequately *before* you try shaving anyone. A good way to practise is by shaving a lathered balloon with an old razor.

16   During shaving the tensioning hand should be placed at the back of the razor so that you can stretch the skin under the razor before carrying out each stroke. The forehand (sometimes called freehand) stroke is made towards you, and the backhand stroke away from you.

17   The second-time-over shave is usually the final shave unless the client has a strong beard growth or a very close shave is required, in which case a sponge shave may be carried out.

18   When the shave has been completed you may apply hot towels and carry out a face massage if your client requires this.

19   Sterilization is the process of destroying *all* organisms, whether harmful or not.

20   The use of fixed-blade razors is sometimes prohibited by local bye-laws. Check the bye-laws in your area before offering shaving services with this type of razor.

Activities

1   Visit local barbers' shops and use the Internet to research how professional shaving services are offered today. Compare how they were offered in past times. Find out what type of clients request professional shaving services, the costs paid and whether face massage is also offered. Work out the reasons why the busiest salons are carrying out more shaving services. Consider whether your salon could do more to offer professional shaving and make recommendations to your manager. This activity may be combined with the activity in Chapter 13, 'Face massage services'.

2   Contact the local council and use the Internet to research the local bye-laws for your area. Find out whether any restrictions are placed on the use of fixed-blade razors and what other requirements relate to barbers' shops. Write up your findings and present them to your manager.

Check your knowledge

1   What are the factors that contributed to the decline of professional shaving services?

2   Explain the differences between wet and dry shaving methods.

3   Outline the importance of hair growth patterns when shaving.

4   What is the direction of shaving stroke for a first-time-over shave?

5   How should a client be prepared for shaving?

6 Which of the following statements is correct:

a. An open style razor should be passed to another person with the tang facing the other person.

b. An open style razor should never be passed to another person.

7 What is the importance of local bye-laws in relation to shaving services?

8 What type of razor is recommended for professional shaving services today?

9 What are the names of the two main types of fixed-blade razor?

10 Which of the following are key features required of a chair for use in professional shaving services.

a. The chair must recline

b. The chair must rotate

c. The chair must be height adjustable

d. The chair must have an headrest

11 Describe the correct use of a hone and strop.

12 What is the key requirement for preparing detachable-blade razors?

13 What are the purposes of hot and cool towels?

14 List four reasons for lathering prior to shaving.

15 What is the number and direction of shaving stroke for the top lip?

16 What is the direction of shaving stroke for a second-time-over shave?

17 Describe a sponge shave.

18 When would a cool towel not be applied after shaving services?

19 Why must gloves be worn when providing shaving services?

20 What actions should you take if you were to cut the client whilst shaving them?

21 What are the methods of sterilization suitable for use in barbers' shops?

13 Face massage services

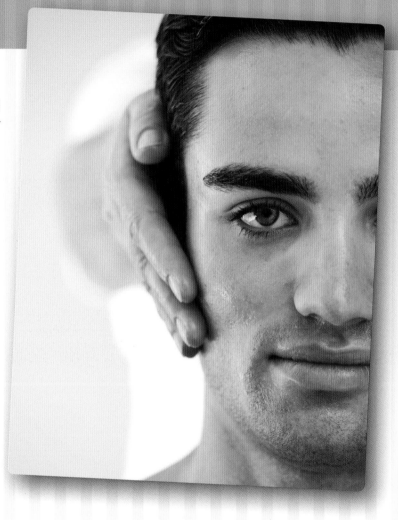

QUALIFICATION SIGNPOSTING

This chapter will help your studies of the following qualifications:

❖ Level 3 NVQ Award and Diploma in Barbering.

LEARNING OBJECTIVES

In this chapter you will learn:

◆ The face massage effects and benefits.

◆ About consultation for face massage – including anatomy.

◆ About face massage products, tools and equipment.

◆ How to prepare for face massage services.

◆ About preparing the face for massage – applying hot towels.

◆ The face massage techniques – including effleurage, petrissage, tapotement, friction and vibro massage.

◆ Face massage routines.

◆ How to finish the face massage and aftercare.

◆ The requirements for health and safety in face massage services.

For further information on the qualifications covered by this chapter see the qualification mapping grid at the front of the book.

INTRODUCTION

Many men and women enjoy the relaxing effects of a face massage or facial. At one time the face massage was a popular service in many barbers' shops, where it was often performed as part of the shaving service. The demand for face massage decreased, however, as more men started shaving at home and shaving in the barber's shop declined. More recently, though, and in common with shaving, there has been renewed interest in face massage as a service. Barbers are again offering face massage to their clients, who request a massage at the time of their regular haircut.

This chapter looks at the traditional techniques used by barbers who provide face massage. It covers the following topics:

❖ Face massage – effects and benefits.

❖ Consultation – anatomy of the face and neck.

❖ Consultation prior to face massage.

❖ Products, tools and equipment.

❖ Preparation for face massage services.

❖ Preparing the face for massage.

❖ Face massage techniques.

❖ Face massage routines.

❖ Finishing the face massage and aftercare.

❖ Health and safety.

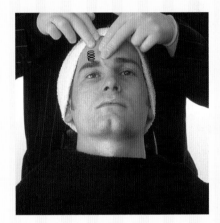

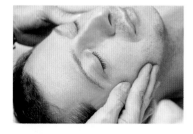

Face massage – effects and benefits

Face massage can be used to cleanse the skin and to improve its appearance, whilst providing a pleasant and enjoyable sensation for the client.

The effects and benefits of face massage include:

◆ Cleansing and softening the skin, and removing dead epidermal skin cells.

◆ Increasing the supply of blood to the skin, to nourish the skin and to promote healthy muscles and a healthy skin colour.

◆ Stimulating and toning the underlying tissues, to help break down fatty deposits, to firm the muscles and to help define the natural contours of the face.

◆ Increasing the circulation of the lymphatic system, to help remove waste products and toxins from the skin.

◆ Stimulating or soothing of the nerves, depending on the massage technique being used.

◆ Relaxing the client, both physically and psychologically, thereby helping to relieve tension.

GARY MACHIN Barber and Director of Rogers Barber Shops

" Face massage services are an intrinsic part of the shaving service in the barber's shop, but don't think that a shave must always be performed before a face massage. Maximize the business potential in your salon; promote face massage services to all your clients. Remember that face massage works equally well as part of an extended cut and blow-dry service. "

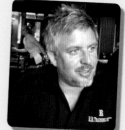

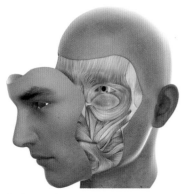

Massage cream being applied to face

The face massage is usually performed with the hands, which manipulate the soft tissues of the face and neck. Sometimes a mechanical massager, commonly called a vibro massager, is also used. A range of different massage techniques can be used to produce either stimulating or relaxing effects, depending on the client's requirements and the area to be massaged.

Consultation – anatomy of the face and neck

For safety and to be effective, anyone with an interest in providing face massage services *must* understand the basic anatomy of the face and the effects that massage has on its structures and systems. It is particularly important to know the position of the muscles and how they act, as the massage movements should generally be performed *along* the muscle and *towards its origin*. The position of the bones, nerves, blood supply and lymphatic system must all be understood, as they affect the choice of techniques and the speed and depth of pressure with which they are applied.

Understanding the anatomy of the face is essential

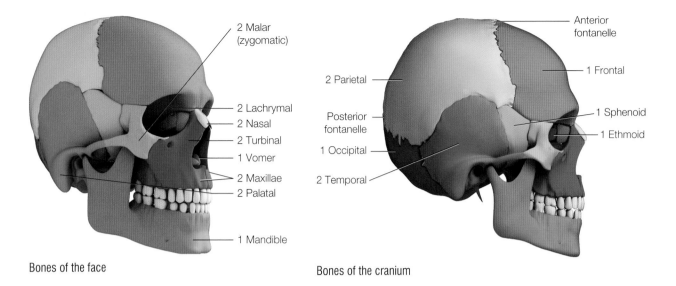

Bones of the face

Bones of the cranium

Bones

The bones are the foundation on which all the other structures and systems depend. The bones of particular interest in face massage are the maxillae, the mandible, the malar and the nasal bones. Other bones in the skull, known as the bones of the cranium, are also important in face massage, especially the frontal, the sphenoid and the temporal bones.

As you perform the face massage you will feel the bones beneath your fingers. In some areas of the face, such as on the forehead and around the eyes, the nose and the lips, there is little tissue between the bone and the surface of the skin. In these areas you must take care to choose the right massage technique and adjust both the speed and depth of pressure to avoid causing discomfort.

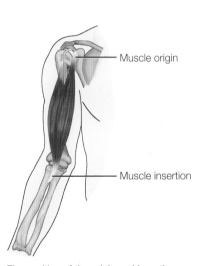

The position of the origin and insertion can be easily seen on a biceps muscle

Muscles

The muscles are an essential part of the face. They are interlinked with each other and with the bones to form an integrated system which allows you to eat, to speak, and to produce many different facial expressions.

HEALTH & SAFETY

If you wish to perform massage, it is important that you learn the position of muscles and their origins. Most massage movements are made along the muscle, *towards the origin* and *away from the point of insertion*. If you apply massage in the wrong places or in the wrong directions, you may cause the client discomfort.

Usually one end of the muscle is attached to a static bone by a strong tendon: this is called the muscle's origin. The other end is attached to a movable bone, to another muscle, or to the skin: this is called the muscle's insertion.

The main muscles of the face are:

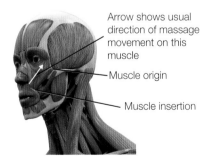

Massage movements are usually made from muscle insertion to origin

◆ *Occipital-frontalis* This muscle covers the top of the cranium. It enables you to lift the eyebrows, as when frowning.

◆ *Orbicularis oculi* These muscles surround the eyes. They help to form the eyelids and allow the eyes to close.

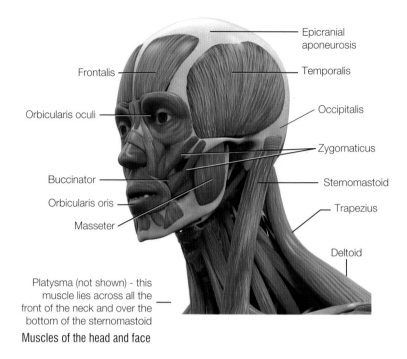

Labels:
- Epicranial aponeurosis
- Frontalis
- Temporalis
- Orbicularis oculi
- Occipitalis
- Zygomaticus
- Buccinator
- Sternomastoid
- Orbicularis oris
- Trapezius
- Masseter
- Deltoid

Platysma (not shown) - this muscle lies across all the front of the neck and over the bottom of the sternomastoid

Muscles of the head and face

◆ **Orbicularis oris** This muscle surrounds the mouth and forms the lips. It allows you to close the mouth, and also helps in speaking.

◆ **Temporalis** This muscle connects the temporal bone with the malar and mandible bones. It enables you to close the mouth and helps with chewing.

◆ **Masseter** This muscle lies between the malar and mandible bones. It helps close the jaw during chewing.

◆ **Zygomaticus** This muscle goes from the malar bones to the corners of the mouth. It allows the lip to move outwards (not shown in diagram).

◆ **Sternomastoid** This muscle runs behind the ears to the temporal bones. It helps the head rotate and bow.

◆ **Platysma** This muscle, within the front of the neck, allows you to wrinkle the skin and lower the corners of the mouth (it is not shown in the diagram to allow the underlying muscles to be seen).

◆ **Buccinator** This muscle lies between the Maxilla and mandible forming the cheek. It helps to hold the cheek to the teeth during chewing.

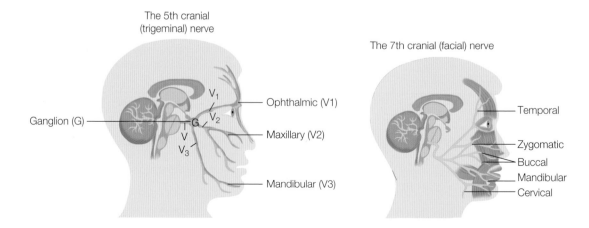

The 5th cranial (trigeminal) nerve
- Ganglion (G)
- Ophthalmic (V1)
- Maxillary (V2)
- Mandibular (V3)

The 7th cranial (facial) nerve
- Temporal
- Zygomatic
- Buccal
- Mandibular
- Cervical

Nerves

The nerves carry messages to and from the brain from and to all parts of the body.

In the face nerves carry messages to the skin, the muscles, the teeth, the nose and the mouth. The main nerves associated with the face are the 5th cranial nerve (the trigeminal nerve), which has three main branches V1, V2 and V3 and the 7th cranial nerve (the facial nerve).

Massage may be applied gently to the sites of nerve endings. During face massage, nerves may be either soothed or stimulated, depending on the technique used.

The blood supply

The heart pumps blood that has been oxygenated in the lungs through the arteries (shown as red) to nourish all areas of the body, including the face and head. The main blood supply to the face and head is through the carotid arteries, which divide into smaller arteries (arterioles) and then into many capillaries.

Eventually the capillaries join to form venules and then veins (shown as blue), which carry the blood back to the heart. The main veins from the face and head run down the sides of the neck, and are called the jugular veins.

The heart pumps the oxygen-depleted blood to the lungs where the oxygen is replaced. The blood then returns to the heart, and the process starts all over again.

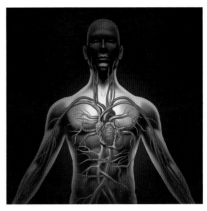

The circulatory system – the arterial system is red and the venous system is blue

TIP

Remember: the blood supply can be stimulated by the application of face massage techniques.

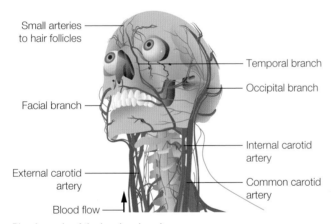

Small arteries to hair follicles

Temporal branch

Occipital branch

Facial branch

Internal carotid artery

External carotid artery

Common carotid artery

Blood flow

Blood supply of the head and neck

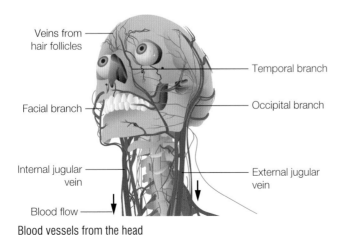

Veins from hair follicles

Temporal branch

Facial branch

Occipital branch

Internal jugular vein

External jugular vein

Blood flow

Blood vessels from the head

The lymphatic system

The structure of the lymphatic system is similar to that of the blood supply. It is made up of a network of lymph vessels, lymph nodes and lymph glands which closely follow the veins throughout the body.

Its main functions are as part of the immune system to remove bacteria, foreign matter and excess fluids from the tissues. The lymphatic system is particularly important in helping to prevent infection, and is often triggered into response when an illness strikes. You may have heard the expression 'swollen glands' – or, indeed, experienced this painful condition yourself.

Lymph is a pale yellow fluid. Unlike the blood supply, the lymphatic system contains no pump. It is the movement of the larger muscles that creates pressure within the capillaries and tissues to force lymph to move around the body.

Lymph only travels away from the tissues towards the heart, not the other way.

Like the blood supply, the lymphatic system can be stimulated by the application of face massage techniques. Massage can help to promote the flow of lymph from the face and towards the lymph nodes, thereby removing waste products and toxins from the facial tissues.

The Lymphatic System

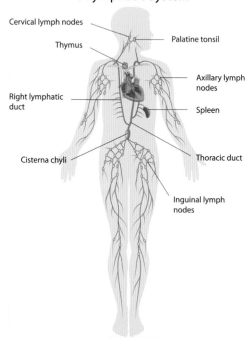

Lymphatic vessel

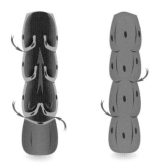

Propulsion of lymph through lymph vessel – the lymph is only able to move in one direction due to the valves

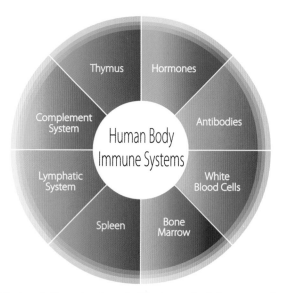

The lymphatic system is part of the human body immune system

Capillary Fluid Exchange

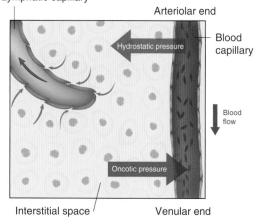

Hydrostatic pressure causes lymph to seep into the lymphatic capillary

Anatomy of a Lymph Node

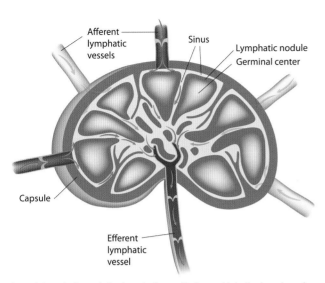

Lymph travels through the lymphatic capillaries and into the lymph nodes

Lymph Nodes of the Head and Neck

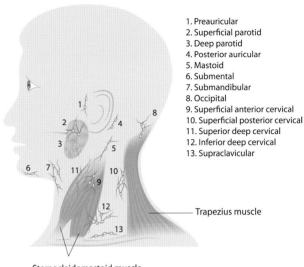

1. Preauricular
2. Superficial parotid
3. Deep parotid
4. Posterior auricular
5. Mastoid
6. Submental
7. Submandibular
8. Occipital
9. Superficial anterior cervical
10. Superficial posterior cervical
11. Superior deep cervical
12. Inferior deep cervical
13. Supraclavicular

Lymph nodes of the head and neck

Consultation prior to face massage

A successful face massage will always begin with the consultation. Here you must identify your client's requirements and their reasons for wanting a face massage. It is particularly important that you assess whether the client is suitable for the massage to go ahead.

During the consultation you should discuss the client's expectations with them and provide advice on the actual results that they can expect. Take the time to explain what is involved, especially if this is the client's first face massage.

It may help you to read Chapter 4, 'Client care for men' for more detailed information on consultation before reading this section.

Here are some important factors that you must consider before providing a face massage:

◆ Make sure you establish what the client wants.

◆ Ask why the client wants a face massage – what are his expectations?

◆ Does the client have a moustache, a beard or large sideburns? Clients with particularly long beards may not be suitable for face massage, as long beard hair is likely to pull during the massage and it is often difficult to perform the massage techniques effectively.

◆ Look for any signs of broken skin, abnormalities on the skin or any other contraindications to carrying out the massage. Remember that the contraindications may not always be obvious to the eye, so you should ask the client if he suffers from any skin disease or skin disorder, particularly allergies. Make sure you do this tactfully and confidentially, and take care not to embarrass the client.

◆ Examine the skin to determine whether its condition is normal, dry or greasy. Discuss your findings with your client and agree on the most suitable products to use.

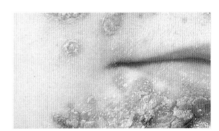

Impetigo

Contraindications

Your examination of the skin will ensure that you identify any adverse conditions that may be present. It is particularly important to establish whether a suspected infection or infestation is present – these are contraindications so if there is one, you must not carry out the face massage.

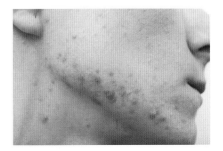

Acne

KEY DEFINITION

Contraindication: A condition that makes proceeding with a particular service inadvisable or impossible.

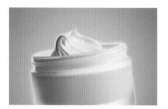

Massage cream

TIP ✓

Exfoliating products are available that help remove the dead cells from the outer layer of skin. These can be useful for preventing ingrown hairs especially on African-Caribbean men.

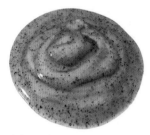

Exfoliating cream

KEY DEFINITION

Exfoliating: The removal of the oldest and dead skin cells from the skin's outermost surface, called the stratum corneum, so that new skin cells can replace them; thereby helping to maintain healthy skin.

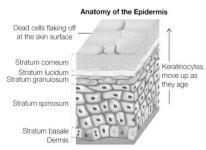

Anatomy of the Epidermis

Dead cells flaking off at the skin surface

Stratum corneum
Stratum lucidum
Stratum granulosum

Keratinocytes move up as they age

Stratum spinosum

Stratum basale
Dermis

The anatomy of the epidermis – exfoliation helps to remove the dead skin cells.

Here are the most common **contraindications** to face massage:

- Broken or bleeding skin.
- Bruising, inflammation or swelling.
- Skin disorders, such as severe acne.
- Eye disorders, such as conjunctivitis.
- Skin diseases, such as impetigo.

HEALTH & SAFETY

If you see any contraindications, especially any signs of broken skin, inflammation or disease, do not go ahead with the face massage. If you are unsure, seek help from a senior colleague and tactfully advise your client to see his doctor.

Products, tools and equipment

To provide face massage services you will need access to a range of products, tools and equipment.

Products

Cleansing creams are available for normal, dry and oily skin types. Massage creams are used as the massage 'medium', to lubricate the skin and to ensure that during the massage the hands can slide easily without dragging. There are many different kinds of massage cream available: choose the correct one for your client's skin type. Hypoallergenic products should be used where possible to avoid problems with clients who have allergies to ingredients, such as perfumes.

Finishing products include astringents, which, because of their alcohol content, have a bracing and cooling effect on the skin. The cooling effect is caused by the evaporation of the alcohol from the skin. This makes the pores of the skin close and so reduces the risk of infection. Talcum powder may be used to ensure the skin is dry. It has a soothing and smoothing effect and can help to reduce the effect of shiny, oily skin.

DON'T BE TEMPTED

Never place your fingers directly into the tub, as this would certainly contaminate the massage cream.

Tools

You will need a sterile spatula or applicator for removing the massage cream from the tub and applying it to the face.

Equipment

You will need hot and cool towels, which should be sterilized if they are not specially supplied pre-packed. A face steamer may be used in place of the hot towels if preferred. If you wish to provide mechanical massage you will need a vibro machine and its applicators: some clients enjoy the intense sensation that this technique produces.

An adjustable chair should be available, which can be positioned so that the client can recline comfortably whilst the face massage is being carried out. If the chair does not have a head-rest you must use some other suitable method of supporting the client's head. The height of the chair should be adjustable to avoid you having to bend uncomfortably.

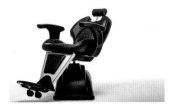
Adjustable chair

Preparation for face massage services

Before commencing face massage services the following tasks must be completed:

1   Carry out your consultation with the client. Look for signs of broken skin, abnormalities on the skin and any contraindications. Determine the condition of the skin.

2   Agree with your client the massage techniques and products that you will use.

3   Before you begin work, gather together all the materials, products, tools and equipment you will require. Place them on a trolley so that you can work efficiently.

4   Position the client in a reclining chair with support for their head, using a clean paper towel over the headrest.

5   Gown the client and place a clean towel across their chest, tucking it in at the neck.

6   Place a second towel around the head to protect the hair and keep it from falling onto the face during the massage. To apply this, first fold it in half lengthways and then in half again. Then place the folded towel around the client's head, following the hairline across the forehead. Fold the ends of the towel under and place them between the client's head and the headrest to keep the towel in place.

7   Your hands and nails should be clean. Let your client see that you have washed your hands – make it clear that you have a high standard of hygiene in your work.

8   Remove any rings, watches or bracelets that could scratch the client's skin before you commence the face massage.

Preparing the face for massage

Before the massage is carried out, you must ensure that the client's skin is cleaned of any visible signs of dirt and grease. It should be cleaned using a suitable cleansing cream.

1   Select a cleansing cream to meet the requirements of the client's skin.

2   Apply the cream using a circular motion. Start at the chin and work the cream up over the cheeks, then down the jawline and neck; follow up around the lips; go over the nose and around the eyes (taking extra care); and finally across the forehead.

3   Remove the cleansing cream with clean cotton wool or tissues. Use circular strokes in an upward and outward direction. If the client has a short beard or a moustache, ensure that it too is clean. (Remember that clients with longer beards may not be suitable for face massage.)

Applying hot towels

The facial muscles must now be relaxed and the skin pores opened. This is usually achieved by applying hot towels; a face steamer may be used if preferred.

Hot towels steam the face. In doing so, they help:

◆   To open the pores and remove dirt.

◆   To lubricate the face, by stimulating the oil-producing glands.

TIP

Remember to lock the chair before the client sits down to avoid accidents if the chair swivels.

HEALTH & SAFETY

Always ensure that the client's head is adequately supported throughout face massage services. Check that the client is comfortable, offer them breaks to change position and stretch if they need to, or harm may occur!

HEALTH & SAFETY

Make sure your nails are not too long or they will catch the client's skin. You should also remove any rings and bracelets or other jewelry that might catch the skin.

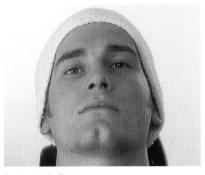
A prepared client

HEALTH & SAFETY

Always test the temperature of the towel on the client's chin before wrapping to ensure that it is not too hot.

Be sure that the client's nose is not covered completely with the towel, as this would obstruct their airway.

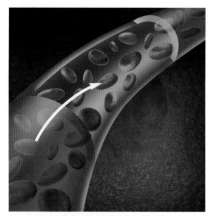

Blood flow is increased by massage

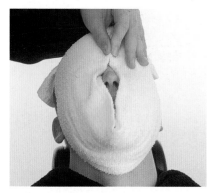

Hot towel applied to face

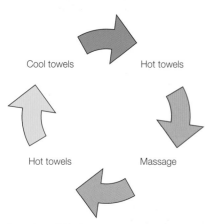

Overview of the face massage procedure

◆ To increase the flow of blood to the surface and relax the muscles, which makes massaging easier.

◆ To relax the client.

You must use *clean* towels. Some barbers use pre-packed towels, which are specially supplied ready-sterilized.

Hot towels are prepared in a steamer or by soaking them in hot water. Wring out the towel until it is nearly dry, and then roll up the towel so that it retains its heat while you carry it to the client.

Unroll the towel and wrap it around the client's face, being careful not to cover the nose, so that the client can breathe. Allow the towel to cool.

The cool towel should be replaced by a second, and if necessary a third.

When using hot towels, remember the following important points:

◆ Always use clean towels for each new client.

◆ Prepare and apply the towels as quickly as possible but be sure to work safely – the quicker you are the more effective they will be.

◆ Avoid covering the client's nose – make sure they can breathe easily at all times!

◆ The towels should not be too wet or they will drip and may wet the client's clothing – towels should be nearly dry when they are applied.

◆ Remove the last hot towel before it becomes too cold – face massage should be performed on a warm, relaxed face!

Face massage techniques

The face massage is performed using a variety of massage techniques, each of which produces a different effect. These techniques can be divided into two basic groups:

◆ Manual massage.

◆ Mechanical massage.

Manual massage techniques are performed with the hands and are used in virtually all face massage, and in most other massages too. Mechanical massage techniques require the use of a vibro machine: this imitates some of the manual massage movements, but its effect is often more intense. The vibro machine may be used on its own but is more often used in conjunction with manual massage techniques for clients who like the intense sensation that it creates.

All massage techniques should be adapted to suit the needs of the client and the area that is to be massaged. Both the speed of the technique and the depth of pressure applied may be adapted.

Remember that extra pressure should be applied only when working on the larger muscle areas.

Manual massage

Effleurage Effleurage is a circular, gliding stroking movement. Small or large circular or semi-circular movements are used depending on the area massaged. It is the foundation of all good massage and is used to induce relaxation, particularly at the start and the completion of the face massage. It is also used as a link between the different massage techniques, to maintain the sensation of continual massage for the client.

The depth of pressure that you apply must be adapted to take account of the thickness of the underlying tissues.

The movement should be light, slow and rhythmical, so as to promote a sense of relaxation.

The main effects of effleurage are:

◆ Relaxation of the muscles.

◆ Relaxation of the client.

◆ Increased circulation of the blood supply.

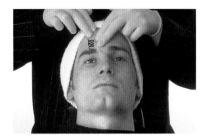
Effleurage

Petrissage Petrissage is performed through a mixture of *pinching*, *kneading* and *rolling* movements. It is applied with both hands, which often work together to gently lift the skin between the fingers and thumbs, where it is squeezed, rolled and pinched with a gentle but firm pressure. These movements are repeated around the fuller parts of the face in a rhythmical and systematic pattern.

The main effects of petrissage are:

◆ Toning of the muscles and the breakdown of fatty deposits in the tissues.

◆ Stimulation of the sebaceous glands.

◆ Increased circulation of the blood supply.

◆ Increased circulation of the lymphatic system.

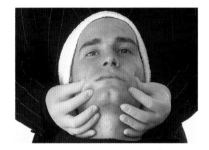
Petrissage

Tapotement Tapotement, or percussion, is the gentle *tapping* of the skin with the padded part of the fingertips. It is applied with both hands in a rhythmical manner to induce a pleasant and stimulating effect.

The main effects of tapotement are:

◆ Stimulation of the nerves, producing an invigorating sensation.

◆ Increased blood supply to the surface of the skin.

◆ Toning of the muscles and the breakdown of fatty deposits in the tissues.

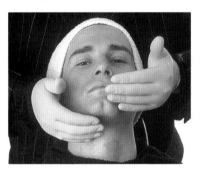
Tapotement

HEALTH & SAFETY

Great care is needed when applying tapotement in areas with little underlying tissue, such as the forehead, eyes and lip areas.

HEALTH & SAFETY

Make sure that your fingernails are not too long before performing manual face massage, particularly when using tapotement, as long fingernails would dig into the skin.

Friction Friction, or vibration, is applied to the site of the nerve endings or along the path of the nerves. It is performed by rapidly *vibrating* the fingers to produce a trembling movement, which is passed through the skin to the intended nerve.

Its main effect is:

◆ Stimulation of the nerves, producing an invigorating sensation.

Mechanical massage

The vibro massage is a mechanical massage technique that imitates the manual massage movements of tapotement and friction.

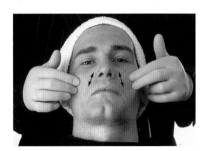
Friction

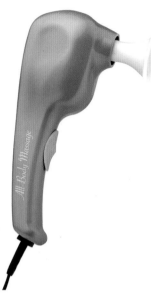

Vibro massager with cup applicator attached. Some machines include infrared lamps for applying direct heat.

HEALTH & SAFETY

Vibro massage must *never* be used directly over delicate areas, such as around the eyes, nose, throat or lips.

TIP   ✓

To check that your client likes the effect of the vibro massage, first apply the technique to their arm before using it on the face.

TIP   ✓

The face massage should be performed *before* the client's hair has been shampooed, cut or styled, otherwise the style will be ruined during the massage.

It may help you to read **CHAPTER 12**, 'Shaving services' for more detailed information on combining shaving and face massage before reading this section.

The massage is performed with a vibrating machine, which has a range of different applicators for use on the scalp, face or body. A spiky applicator is provided for use on the scalp, whilst a sponge applicator and a rubber cup-shaped applicator are mostly intended for use on the face. Other applicators may also be provided for use on the larger areas of the body.

The effect produced by a vibro massager can be much more intense than that of manual techniques, and is not enjoyed by every client.

The vibro machine can be used in conjunction with the manual massage techniques or on its own: often it is not used at all. It is operated with both hands, one directing the movements whilst the other holds the machine firmly. It is most suitable for the fleshier parts of the face.

The main effects of vibro massage are:

◆ Stimulation of the nerves, producing an invigorating sensation.

◆ Increased blood supply to the surface of the skin.

◆ Toning of the muscles and the breakdown of fatty deposits in the tissues.

Face massage routines

There are several different ways of performing a face massage. The starting place, the pattern of movements and the method of completion can all be tailored to suit the client and barber. Many barbers follow a preferred routine which they have developed through experience, and use their own creativity to make the massage more pleasurable and effective. With experience you too will begin to develop your own method of working.

A good face massage will always follow these simple rules:

◆ Each face massage must start and end with a relaxing massage movement, usually effleurage.

◆ The sequence of massage movements should flow logically so that the sensation created is one of continuous massage. For example, do not move your hands from one area to another, such as from the chin to the forehead, without linking the movement. Use broad, sweeping effleurage movements to link these areas together.

◆ Keep one or other of your hands in contact with the skin throughout the massage. Avoid any repeated stopping and starting, and try not to make jerky movements.

◆ Repeat each movement several times before moving on to the next area of the face.

◆ Ensure that you cover all areas of the face, unless your consultation has identified otherwise.

◆ Take your time. Your goal is to make the massage pleasant and relaxing: it is impossible to do this if you rush.

HEALTH & SAFETY

If the face massage follows on from a shave and there has been any blood spotting or the skin has been very lightly nicked during shaving, you must ensure that any bleeding has stopped before providing the face massage. Gloves should then be worn but they must be tight-fitting, surgical-type gloves or you will not be able to perform the massage techniques effectively. Try to use latex-free gloves to avoid problems with clients who have allergies.

DON'T BE TEMPTED   X

Never perform face massage if there is a visible cut on the client's face.

The following routine is one example of how a face massage may be performed.

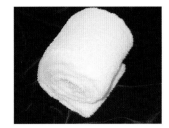

Remember a rolled-up towel retains the heat

A MANUAL FACE MASSAGE ROUTINE

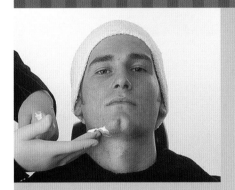

Step A

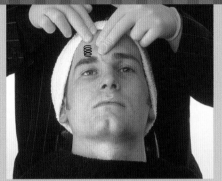

Step B

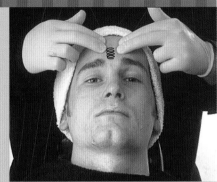

Step C

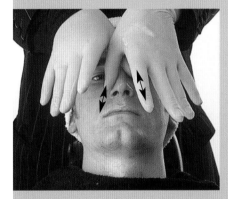

Step D

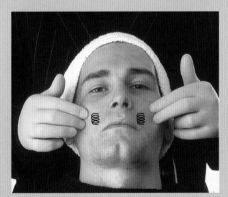

Step E

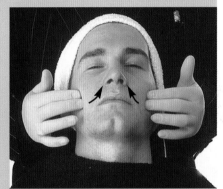

Step F

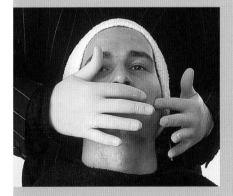

Step G

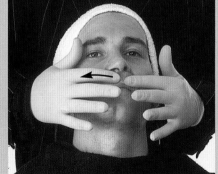

Step H

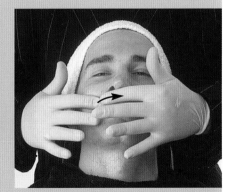

Step I

A MANUAL FACE MASSAGE ROUTINE (*Continued*)

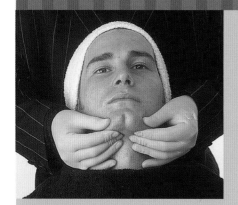

Step J

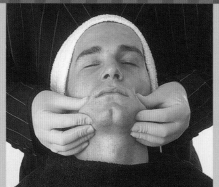

Step K

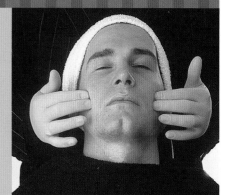

Step L

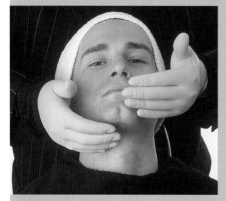

Step M

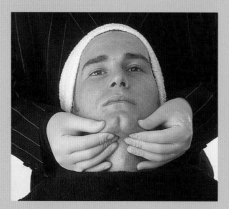

Step N

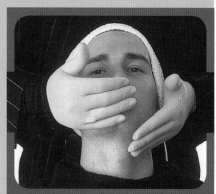

Step O

1. After the consultation ensure that your client is correctly gowned and protected.

2. Clean your client's face with cleansing cream.

3. Steam the face with two hot towels.

4. Apply sufficient massage cream to lubricate the face – do not apply too much or you will overload the skin. Starting at the chin, work the cream up over the cheeks, then down the jawline and neck (a).

5. Follow up around the lips, go over the nose and around the eyes (taking extra care), and finally go across the forehead.

6. Standing behind the client, gently lift their chin to position the head for the massage.

7. Start the massage by sliding your fingers from the client's chin up the sides of the face to the temples. Without removing your hands from the face, place the pads of the first and second fingers of each hand on the sides of the forehead. Now gently move your fingers up and down between the hairline and the eyebrows whilst moving across the forehead towards the centre (b).

8. Use light effleurage movements to relax the client, each hand moving in alternate directions (imagine you are drawing a zigzag pattern across the forehead). Work slowly and carefully to let the client become accustomed to the sensation.

9. Move the fingers back towards the temples, then make small circular effleurage strokes up and down between the eyebrows and the hairline, working towards the centre of the forehead (c). *Repeat this series of movements at least once.*

10. Slide the fingers of both hands down the forehead to the bridge of the nose. Slide the thumbs across the bridge of the nose and cross them so that the thumb on the right hand is situated on the left side of the nose and the thumb on the left hand is situated on the right side of the nose. Using gentle pressure, slide the thumbs down and then back up the nose (d).

11. Use slightly more pressure on the upward stroke. Take care not to depress the skin and actually block the nose. *Repeat this movement several times*, then uncross the thumbs at the top of the nose.

12. Slide your fingers down the sides of the nose and make spiralling effleurage movements across the cheeks, moving back up towards the temples (e). Slide your fingers gently under the eyes and back up to the top of the nose.

13. With each hand, place your middle finger on the eyebrow near the nose. Slide across the eyebrows towards the outer corners of the eyes. Slide down the sides of the cheeks to the corners of the mouth, and make spiralling movements back up the sides of the nose (f). *Repeat this series of movements at least once.*

14. Slide your fingers back down the sides of the nose to the top lip. Place the index finger of your right hand flat against the top lip: the fingertip should be level with the left corner of the mouth (g).

15. Gently slide the finger across the top lip keeping in contact with the skin (h).

16. When the tip of the finger reaches the right corner of the mouth, replace it with the index finger of the left hand and make the same sliding movement in the other direction (i). *Repeat this movement several times, first one hand then the other, in a gentle rhythm.*

17. Slide the fingers down to the bottom lip, and repeat the same movements there.

18. Place the fingers on the chin. Using light pinching and squeezing petrissage movements, work up along the line of the jaw to the earlobes (j, k).

19. Slide the fingers back down the cheeks and to the corners of the mouth; then work back up towards the top of the ear, using the pinching movements as before. Make sure you cover all of the cheeks, but *do not go too close to the eyes.*

20. Slide back down to the corners of the mouth. Using the middle fingers of each hand make two deep, rotating petrissage movements, then continue this movement up across the cheeks and to the temples. Slide back to the chin. *Repeat the movement,* but this time finishing at the earlobes.

21. Slide your fingers back to the chin. Using your fingertips, apply a very light tapping tapotement movement and work up across the cheeks to the earlobes and back to the corners of the mouth (l).

22. *Repeat these movements* from the mouth up towards the temples (m). Develop a gentle rhythm to make the movement enjoyable.

23. Slide your fingers down the jawline back to the chin. Start on the lower lip and apply gentle rotating petrissage movements over the chin and down the neck, avoiding the Adam's apple. Cover the rest of the neck, working out from the chin (n).

24. Complete the massage routine with gentle sweeping effleurage movements under the chin, across the neck and up over the cheeks (o).

25. Apply hot towels to remove all traces of the massage cream. Apply cool towels, an astringent, and talcum powder if required, and dry the face.

TIP ✓

As noted, sometimes it is *necessary* to wear gloves, but you may choose to wear them at all times when you are carrying out face massage. This conforms to the highest standards of hygiene. Make sure you wear tight-fitting, surgical-type gloves or you will not be able to perform the massage techniques correctly. Try to use latex-free gloves to avoid problems with clients who have allergies and to avoid such allergies yourself.

A face massage should be a relaxing experience for the client: it must not be rushed. A typical face massage will take about 15–30 minutes to complete.

HEALTH & SAFETY

Check that the client is comfortable at regular intervals, especially when commencing a new massage movement. Be alert to any non-verbal signs of discomfort shown by the client.

HEALTH & SAFETY

Never use a vibro massager on the nose or around the eyes.

A vibro massage routine

The face massage may be completed with a vibro massager, used either on its own or in conjunction with the manual massage techniques. Before using it, make sure your client desires this form of massage. Confirm this by first testing the effect it produces on the client's arm.

The vibro should be used following the same pattern of movements used when applying the manual massage techniques it replaces. However, extra care must be taken, especially on bony areas like the forehead and jaw. Do not use it on the nose or around the eyes.

The rubber cup applicator is used for most face massage movements. It can produce intense, stimulating effects which some clients will not like. The sponge applicator has a more gentle and relaxing effect, and should be used after the massage cream has been removed.

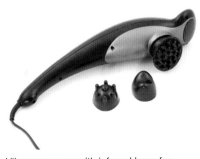

Vibro massager with infrared lamp for applying direct heat and attachments

TIP ✓

Little pressure is required when using a vibro massager on the face.

If the effects of a vibro massager are too strong, reduce them by placing your fingers on the client's face, and the cup on your fingers.

Finishing the face massage and aftercare

When the face massage is complete you should apply one or two final hot towels to remove all traces of the massage cream. Some clients enjoy the cooling and soothing effects of a cool towel: this is prepared and used just like a hot towel, but using cool water. Other clients even enjoy the bracing effects of a very cold towel, but you should ask before this is applied.

The effects of cool towels include:

◆ Closing the pores of the skin, thereby reducing the risk of infection.

◆ Making the skin contract, producing a stimulating, invigorating sensation.

A small amount of talcum powder may be applied to soothe and smooth the skin and to reduce any shiny effect that may have appeared. An astringent lotion may also be applied, if the client so desires. Astringent lotions have a bracing effect on the skin: as the alcohol in them evaporates, the skin cools, closing the pores of the face, and reducing the risk of infection.

When the face massage is complete, ask the client to sit up slowly and rest for a few moments. This is so that they can get used to sitting up after being reclined during the face massage.

DON'T BE TEMPTED ✗

You should ask the client to sit up slowly and rest for a few moments after the face massage. Don't be tempted to have them sit up too quickly as such a sudden movement can cause a fall in blood pressure and make the client feel dizzy.

The client's hair should be shampooed, cut (if required) and styled.

Remember to recommend another appointment and suitable facial products such as cleaners and exfoliators to your client from those you retail in your barber's shop – make sure you guide the client to follow the manufacturer's instructions!

Health and safety

It may help you to read CHAPTER 2, 'Health and safety in the barber's shop' for general information on working safely and hygienically in the barber's shop.

Anyone providing face massage services has a duty to work safely and hygienically. You must maintain high standards of hygiene in all aspects of your work to minimize the risk of cross-infection.

The following are some important factors to consider when carrying out face massage services.

Check for contraindications

◆ Do not go ahead with the face massage if you see any contraindications, especially any signs of broken skin, inflammation or disease. In these cases you should seek help from a senior colleague if necessary, and tactfully advise your client to see his doctor.

Use gloves as necessary

◆ If the face massage is following on from a shave and there has been blood spotting or the skin has been nicked during shaving, make sure that any bleeding

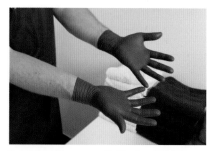

Remember to wear suitable gloves when providing face massage immediately after shaving

has stopped before providing the face massage. You must then wear tight-fitting, surgical-type gloves or you will not be able to perform the massage techniques effectively. Make sure you apply sufficient massage cream to lubricate the skin, as gloves can drag and pull the skin more easily. Try to use latex-free gloves to avoid problems with clients who have allergies. Do not attempt face massage it there is a visible cut or other injury on the client's face. Make sure you wear gloves if you have any cuts or abrasions on your own hands.

Do not harm the client!

◆ Take extra care when applying massaging techniques around the eyes, the nose, the temples, the throat and the lip areas. *Do not use tapotement or vibro techniques in these areas*, as the intense movement will be very uncomfortable and may cause harm.

◆ *Never apply massage techniques directly to the eyes.* Use only light pressure and movements on any sensitive area. Be alert to any non-verbal signs of discomfort shown by the client.

◆ Keep your fingernails short. If they are too long they may catch the client's skin.

◆ If the client feels dizzy during or after the face massage allow them to lie back and rest until the dizziness subsides. Should your client continue to feel unwell contact your first aider or call the emergency services if it appears to be an emergency.

Maintain a high standard of hygiene

◆ Use only clean towels, tools and equipment.

◆ Always pay special attention to hygiene when providing face massage: your hands will be working close to the client's mouth, eyes and nose. Always wash your hands thoroughly before you begin work, and make sure you are maintaining high standards of personal hygiene.

◆ Understand and maintain standards for sterilization and sanitization.

◆ You may wish to observe the highest standard of hygiene by always wearing gloves when providing face massage services. If so, they must always be tight-fitting, surgical-type gloves.

Be prepared for accidents

◆ Make sure that you know the whereabouts of your salon's first-aid kit.

◆ Keep yourself up-to-date with your salon's first-aid and accident procedures.

IMAGE GALLERY

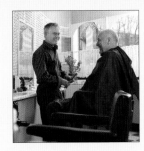

Visit the online gallery on this book's accompanying website to see ideas for the promotion of face massage services.

BRINGING IT ALL TOGETHER

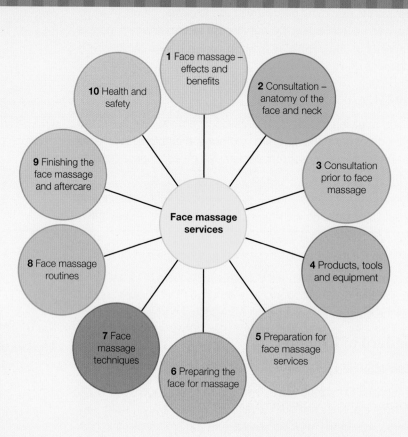

Summary

1   Face massage increases the circulation of the blood supply to bring oxygenated blood and nutrients to the skin. It also increases the flow of the lymphatic system, to help remove waste products and toxins from the skin. Face massage may be stimulating or relaxing for the client, both physically and psychologically, thereby helping to relieve tension.

2   The bones of particular interest in face massage are the maxillae, the mandible, the malar and the nasal bones. Most massage movements are made along the muscle, *towards the origin* and *away from the point of insertion*. If you apply massage in the wrong places or in the wrong directions, you may cause the client discomfort. The main nerves associated with the face are the fifth cranial nerve (the trigeminal nerve) and the seventh cranial nerve (the facial nerve). The main blood supply to the face and head is through the carotid arteries, which divide into smaller arteries (arterioles) and then into many capillaries. Massage can help to promote the flow of lymph from the face and towards the lymph nodes, thereby removing waste products and toxins from the facial tissues.

3   A successful face massage will always begin with the consultation. You must identify your client's requirements and their reasons for wanting a face massage. It is particularly important that you assess whether the client is suitable for the massage to go ahead by identifying any contraindications.

4   Hypoallergenic products should be used where possible when providing face massage services to avoid problems with clients who have allergies to ingredients, such as perfumes.

5   Remove any rings, watches or bracelets that could scratch the client's skin before you commence the face massage.

6   The facial muscles must be relaxed and the skin pores opened before the face massage. This is usually achieved by applying hot towels; a face steamer may be used if preferred.

7   Manual massage techniques are performed with the hands and are used in virtually all face massage, and in most other massages too. Mechanical massage techniques require the use of a vibro machine: this imitates some of the manual massage movements,

but its effect is often more intense. Vibro massage and tapotement must *never* be used directly over delicate areas, such as around the eyes, nose, throat or lips.

8   Each massage movement must link seamlessly to the next so that the sensation is of one continuous process.

9   Some clients enjoy the cooling and soothing effects of a cool towel after the face massage: this is prepared and used just like a hot towel, but using cool water. Other clients even enjoy the bracing effects of a very cold towel, but you should ask before this is applied! Don't be tempted to have the client sit up too quickly after the face massage, as such a sudden movement can cause a fall in blood pressure and make the client feel dizzy.

10   Do not go ahead with the face massage if you see any contraindications, especially any signs of broken skin, inflammation or disease. In these cases you should seek help from a senior colleague if necessary, and tactfully advise your client to see his doctor. If the face massage is following shaving services it is usually *necessary* to wear gloves, but you may choose to wear them at all times when you are carrying out face massage. This conforms to the highest standards of hygiene. Make sure you wear tight-fitting, surgical-type gloves or you will not be able to perform the massage techniques correctly.

Activities

1   Visit local barbers' shops and use the Internet to research how face massage services offered today compare to those offered in past times. Find out what type of clients request face massage services, the costs paid and whether shaving is also offered. Work out the reasons why the busiest salons are carrying out more face massage services. Consider whether your salon could do more to offer face massage and make recommendations to your manager. This activity may be combined with the activity in Chapter 12, 'Shaving services'.

2   Practise your face massage techniques on a colleague or mannequin head until the movements link together in a fluid, unbroken routine.

3   Draw and label a diagram of the head and face from memory after reading this chapter. Make sure you include the correct locations of the bones, muscles, circulation and lymphatic systems. Check how many you correctly included and not any omissions or corrections. Add this drawing to your revision materials.

Check your knowledge

1   List six effects of face massage.

2   List the main bones of the face affected by face massage.

3   What is the muscle's insertion?

4   Describe the position and function of the orbicularis oris.

5   What are the main function of nerves?

6   Describe how the blood supply is circulated to the face.

7   State two functions of the lymphatic system.

8   Which of the following most accurately describes how lymph is moved around the body?

   a. Lymph is pumped around the body by the heart
   b. Lymph is moved around the body by the movement of large muscles
   c. Lymph is pumped around the body by the air in the lungs
   d. Lymph is moved around the body by gravity.

9   List five contraindications to face massage.

10   What is the purpose of an astringent?

11   What piece of equipment is used to provide mechanical massage?

12   List four reasons for using hot towels prior to a face massage.

13   Why is a head rest important when providing face massage services?

14   List the main effects of the petrissage massage movement.

15   Which manual massage movement is used to stimulate the nerve endings?

16   State where mechanical massage techniques must not be applied.

17   Why must gloves be worn when providing face massage immediately after shaving services?

18   Describe how the barber's hands and nails should be prepared before providing face massage services.

19   Explain the course of action required if you suspect contraindications are present.

20   Why should latex-free gloves be used for face massage wherever possible?

14 Designing facial hair shapes

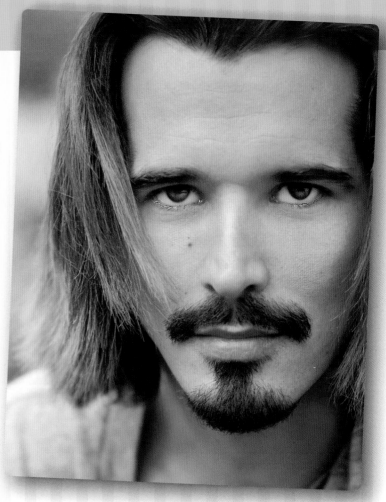

QUALIFICATION SIGNPOSTING

This chapter will help your studies of the following qualifications:

❖ Level 3 NVQ Diploma in Barbering.
❖ City & Guilds Level 3 VRQ Award in Cutting Facial Hair.
❖ City & Guilds Level 3 VRQ Diploma in Barbering.
❖ ITEC Level 3 VRQ Awards, Certificates and Diplomas in Barbering and Men's Hairdressing.
❖ VTCT Level 3 VRQ Certificates and Diplomas in Barbering.
❖ VTCT Level 3 VRQ Diploma in Barbering Studies.

LEARNING OBJECTIVES

In this chapter you will learn:

◆ The factors to be considered when designing a variety of facial hair shapes.

◆ The traditional, contemporary and emerging beard and moustache shapes.

◆ The procedures for cutting, finishing and aftercare.

◆ The health and safety requirements for creating facial hair shapes.

For further information on the qualifications covered by this chapter see the qualification mapping grid at the front of the book.

INTRODUCTION

Whilst longer beards and moustaches are now less often worn, the popularity of shorter beard and moustache shapes has continued to grow. Modern men are now often choosing to wear shorter facial hair shapes to suit their highly personalized short haircuts, which sometimes include patterns within the beard. But fashions often change and longer hairstyles could see longer beard and moustache shapes returning. The popularity of charity the 'Movember Foundation' that challenges men around the world to grow a moustache and raise funds and awareness for men's cancers and mental health has encouraged many more men to think of wearing facial hair as part of their look. The barber must be prepared for such events as the beard or moustache is again playing an important role in establishing an individual look for many men.

In this chapter we will be looking at the techniques used for designing and creating facial hair shapes and will be covering the following topics:

- Factors to be considered when designing a variety of facial hair shapes.
- Traditional, contemporary and emerging beard and moustache shapes.
- Cutting procedures.
- Finishing and aftercare.
- Notes on health and safety.

Before reading this chapter it may help you to read **CHAPTER 6**, 'Cutting facial hair using basic techniques'.

It may help you to read **CHAPTER 4**, 'Client care for men' for more detailed information on consultation before reading this section.

Factors to be considered when designing a variety of facial hair shapes

There are many similarities between maintaining an existing beard or moustache shape and designing and creating new shapes. The same cutting techniques can be used for most of the work required and, of course, the shapes produced often have styling features that are similar. Factors including the hairstyle, head and face shape, hair density and adverse hair and skin conditions still have to be fully considered. But differences do exist in the level of consultation required (establishing the factors is even more important when designing new facial hair shapes), and in the methods that are used to achieve the new shapes.

HEALTH & SAFETY

You must carry out a thorough consultation to ensure that you identify any adverse conditions of the hair or skin that may be present. It is particularly important to establish whether a suspected infection or infestation is present, as this would prevent you from cutting the facial hair.

The principles learnt earlier about shape and form in haircutting are also important when designing a new facial hair shape, as you are starting with what might be called a blank canvas. But, as with advanced haircutting, here too the principles are applied more loosely where required by the hairstyle, facial hair shape and overall look. The work undertaken regularly requires cutting techniques to be combined and adapted to take account of both the client's wishes and the many factors that affect the creation of the new shape. The client consultation is essential in designing and personalizing the right shape for each client.

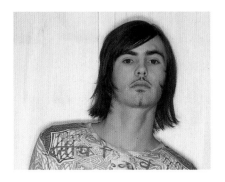

MK

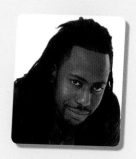

❝ Think of the haircut and facial hair shape as one design, they should normally work in harmony and follow the contours of the face. Make sure the client understands and agrees to the design, especially to any changes you feel are necessary whilst you work. Remember, outlining should complement the bone structure, especially the mandible and cheekbones. ❞

Consultation – designing the correct shape

Before you design a new beard or moustache shape you must carry out a thorough consultation to consider factors including the client's wishes, face shape and hairstyle. Here is a reminder of some of the critical factors that must be considered when designing and creating facial hair shapes:

◆ Accurately establish what the client wants.

◆ Determine why they wish to have a beard and/or moustache shape.

◆ Look for signs of broken skin, abnormalities on the skin or any unusual facial features or beard growth patterns – are there any contraindications?

◆ What is the facial hair type – type S1, W2, C3 or K4?

◆ What are the facial hair characteristics –

　◆ Is the beard hair fine, medium or coarse?

　◆ Is the beard growth dense or sparse?

　◆ Does the density of beard growth vary around the face?

◆ Determine the client's face shape.

◆ Determine the length and shape of his hairstyle.

See **CHAPTER 4** pages 60–62 for full details on hair types and classifications.

HEALTH & SAFETY

Take extra care when cutting very coarse or dense beards, as the hair is liable to fly in all directions while it is being cut. Make sure the client's eyes are well protected with clean cotton wool pads or tissues and keep your face well away from the work. If you find the hair is very strong and springy you may have to wear safety glasses to protect your eyes!

Face shape, facial features and hairstyle The client's face shape and facial features must be considered when choosing the most suitable shape for each client. The size and position of the mouth, width of the top lip, shape of the nose, jaw and chin and presence of any unusual features, such as moles, dimples, scarring or facial piercings must all be established.

Different face shapes require different beard and moustache shapes. Here are some examples:

Facial shape	Beard and moustache shape
A round face 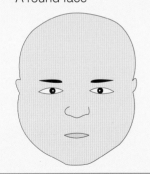	Choose a beard shape that is longer at the chin to make the face appear longer and less round. Keep the sides short and avoid bushy sideburns, as they will make the face appear more round. Partial beards, such as a goatee or full beards like a King Edward beard are often good shapes to choose
A large face 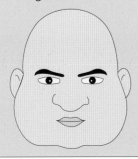	A larger moustache shape is usually more suitable, as a small moustache will appear lost and will make the face appear bigger. The width of the top lip must also be considered because a large moustache would appear too big on a narrow lip. Small, partial beards can also appear lost, so consider large partial or full beards

TIP ✓

Remember to look for variations in the density of growth when designing beard shapes. The hair may have to be left long in some areas to cover very sparse growth or a scar, while at other times sparse growth may mean that some shapes cannot be grown at all!

TIP ✓

Hair growth patterns must be identified because they determine both the shape that can be created and the techniques that you should use. Some clients have very strong hair growth patterns in their beard, such as hair whorls, which should be cut by following the direction of hair growth around the whorl.

TIP ✓

Remember, a *full beard* covers the whole area of beard and moustache growth on the face, though this may be outlined. A *partial beard* is any beard where part of the beard or moustache growth inside the natural outline is removed.

(continued)

Facial shape	Beard and moustache shape
A small face 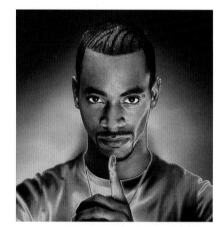	The smaller face is more suited to smaller beard and moustache shapes, such as a modern goatee. But be careful to consider other features such as a long chin which the goatee can make appear even longer.
A long face	Choose a beard shape that is fuller at the sides and shorter at the chin. This will help to make the face appear less long. Make sure any change in length is gradual so as not to be obvious
A square face	Full beard shapes are often more suitable, which should be shorter at the sides and longer towards the chin
An oval face shape	Almost any beard shape is suitable, but you must take into account the client's hairstyle

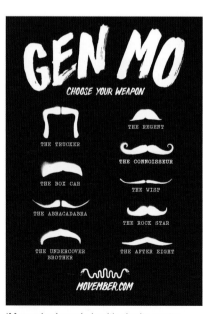

'Movember' men's health charity poster

The length and shape of the client's hairstyle are important factors affecting the design of the facial hair shape. Longer hairstyles tend to suit longer, fuller beard shapes as shorter shapes can appear unbalanced, but care must be taken not to 'overpower' the client's face, head and body shape with too much hair! Likewise, shorter beard shapes often work best with shorter hairstyles.

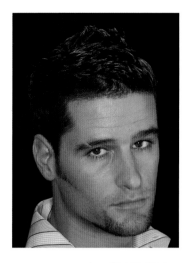

> ## TIP ✓
>
> If your client has male pattern baldness avoid longer and fuller shapes, especially if their hairstyle is cut short. Closer cut beards and moustaches usually work best as they are evenly balanced with such haircuts.

Cutting facial hair outlines

Most men have dense hair growth that grows outside the natural beard hairline. Shorter layered beard shapes should always be outlined and the unwanted hair from outside the outline removed or the beard will appear unfinished. In longer beards it can seem less important, as the longer hair may cover the outline, but unwanted hair outside the outline should still be removed for the result to appear professional. The outlines may be cut to give a natural appearance, or they may be created with lines that are more obvious.

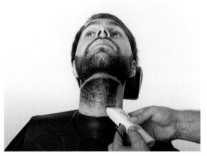

Cutting the neck outline

> ## TIP ✓
>
> Make sure that the neck outline is cut slightly higher in the centre than at the sides to compensate for the head being positioned back at an angle during cutting, or the outline will appear longer in the centre when the head returns to the normal position.

Strong, less natural outlines may be features of some shapes and in such cases the outlines can be cut to almost anywhere, or even incorporated into elaborate patterns and designs.

It may help you to read **CHAPTER 15**, 'Design and create patterns in hair' if you want to incorporate a pattern within your facial hair design.

> ## TIP ✓
>
> **Levelling outlines**
> To ensure that the outlines of the beard and moustache are cut level, place the thumb of one hand on the outline of one side of the face at the required position. Whilst looking in the mirror slide the other thumb down to the same position on the outline of the other side of the face until both thumbs appear level. Memorize the position of the thumbs; you can use a position on the face between the ear, eye and nose as a point of reference. Now cut each outline to the correct position and length. This method can be easily adapted to establish the width of the beard or moustache and so obtain symmetrical shapes, even in the most elaborate designs.

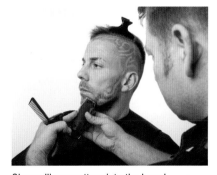

Channelling a pattern into the beard

Tramlines and **channelling** can be added to the beard and moustache design. These can range from simple 2D shapes to complex geometric designs and sometimes 3D effects are included. But most often it is simple tramlines that are used in facial hair designs.

Usually men want facial hair shapes that are less radical, with the emphasis on creating a natural balanced look that matches their haircut. In each case the face shape and hairstyle should be used to determine the correct choice of shape for each client. Here are some important things to remember about designing facial hair shapes:

> ## KEY DEFINITION
>
> Channelling: A technique used to make lines when creating patterns in hair. It is performed with electric clippers and trimmers.

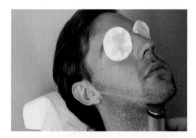

Creating a chin curtain beard

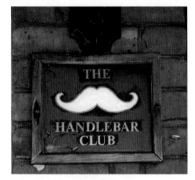

Plaque outside the handlebar
moustache club in London, England

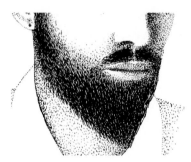

King Edward

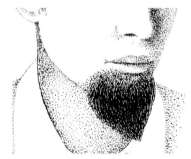

Norris Skipper

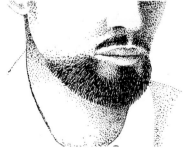

Balbo

◆ Many facial hair shapes are improved by having distinct outlines. Outlines help to define and balance the beard or moustache shape.

◆ Avoid cutting into the beard or moustache outline unless the look requires these more radical and less natural effects.

◆ Beard and moustache outlines should usually be cut level, unless the look is to be asymmetric. Do not use the ears or eyes to determine the level of the outlines, as they are not usually level themselves. (See Tip – Levelling outlines.)

◆ Pay particular attention to where the beard meets the haircut and ensure that they blend together, as required.

◆ Consider the sideburns when cutting moustache and partial beard shapes and ensure that they complement each other.

◆ Think of the haircut and moustache and/or beard as being integrated parts of one style.

Traditional and contemporary beard and moustache shapes

Many different traditional beard and moustache shapes have developed over the years. Many of these shapes were named after the men who wore them at different times, such as the King Edward, which means that similar shapes were sometimes known by different names around the world, e.g. the Van Dyke is similar to the King Edward. Some shapes were adopted by men in certain roles and acquired names to reflect this, such as the military moustache. Other shapes were popular with men in different social classes, e.g. in the early 1900s few working class men would wear a King Edward beard. Yet other shapes were popular in certain countries and were referred to by the country involved, e.g. the French Fork.

Some traditional shapes are still current or popular today and are usually referred to by their traditional name. Other newer, contemporary shapes do not often acquire specific names and are simply described by the shape formed, or by reference to a similar traditional shape. This can make identification of newer shapes difficult, so care must be taken to make sure the right shape has been chosen before commencing work. Reference to photographs or sketches is essential during the consultation for creating a new facial hair design.

Here is a selection of traditional and contemporary beard and moustache shapes to provide some ideas for your own designs and examples of some names used to describe them. Remember, any of the traditional shapes could become fashionable and some shapes appear to be 'in fashion' at all times. The men who wear them are often passionate about their facial hair look; indeed some shapes have even prompted those wearing them to form members clubs, such as the Handlebar Moustache Club in London.

Remember that traditional shapes which are 'in fashion' would then also be referred to as being current.

Traditional beard shapes

◆ King Edward

◆ Norris Skipper

◆ Balbo

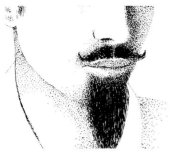

Goatee

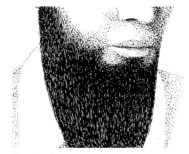

The Spade

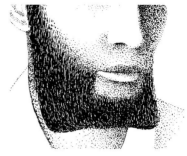

Old Dutch

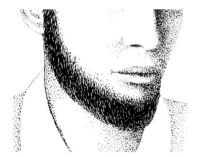

Chin Curtain

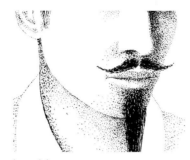

Imperial

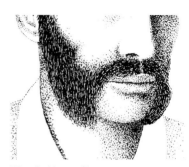

Friendly Mutton Chops

- ◆ Goatee
- ◆ The Spade
- ◆ Old Dutch
- ◆ Chin Curtain
- ◆ Imperial
- ◆ Friendly Mutton Chops
- ◆ French Fork

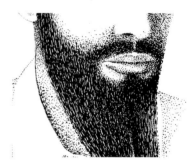

French Fork

Traditional moustache shapes

- ◆ Handlebar
- ◆ Major
- ◆ Regent
- ◆ Military

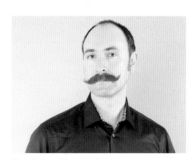

Handlebar Moustache

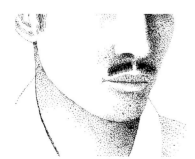

Major

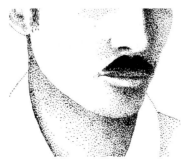

Regent

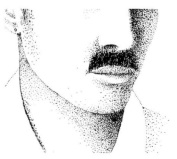

Military

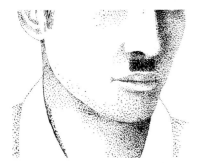

Chaplin or Square Button

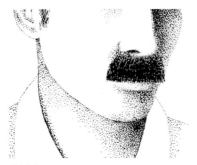

Old Bill

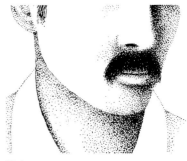

Walrus

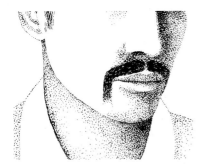

Mexican

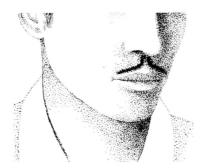

Pencil Line

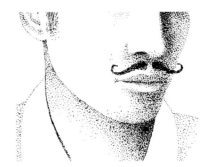

Howie

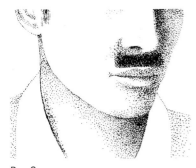

Box Car

- Chaplin or Square Button
- Old Bill
- Walrus
- Mexican
- Pencil Line
- Howie
- Box Car
- Horseshoe

Contemporary beard and moustache shapes

- Modern Balbo
- Cropped Modern Norris Skipper Beard
- Modern Goatee Beard
- Cropped Full Beard

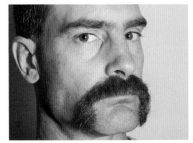

Horseshoe moustache

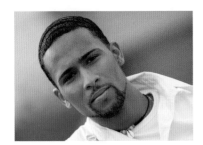

Modern Balbo

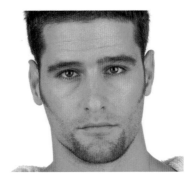

Cropped Modern Norris Skipper Beard

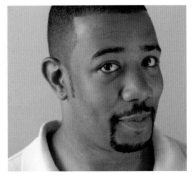

Modern Goatee Beard

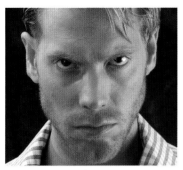

Cropped Full Beard – with blended outlines

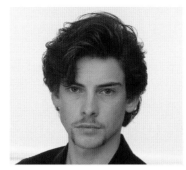

Thin Mexican Moustache

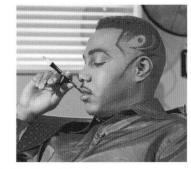

Modified Pencil Line Moustache

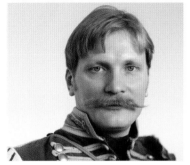

A versatile Handlebar Moustache – dressing the ends down would change it to a Colonel Moustache

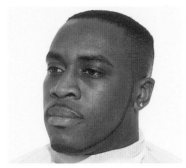

Pencil Line Chin Curtain and Moustache

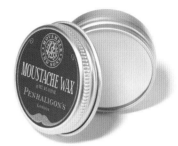

Dressing wax or pomade

- ◆ Thin Mexican Moustache
- ◆ Modified Pencil Line Moustache
- ◆ Colonel Moustache
- ◆ Pencil Line Chin Curtain and Moustache

Emerging beards and moustaches

Emerging beard and moustache shapes are developed as barbers consider the latest hairstyles and design beard and moustache shapes that complement the looks required. This often involves combining and adapting traditional and new beard shapes with traditional and new moustache shapes. These shapes are then amended and other newer ideas are added, such as tramlines, in order to create the unique looks required. Many emerging shapes and looks are first seen on celebrities and in magazines and at trade shows and exhibitions.

Competitions are also good places to see and develop ideas for emerging beard and moustache shapes, although often the looks are too extreme for most clients and are amended accordingly.

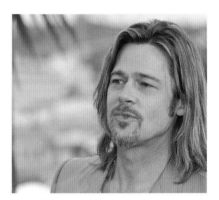

Brad Pitt – modern goatee

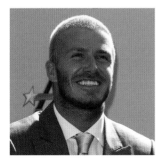

David Beckham natural '1 week growth look'

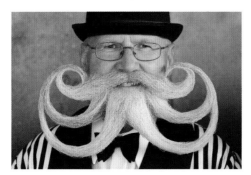

Moustache competition contestant

Cutting procedures

Current moustache and beard shapes

JORDAN – PENCIL LINE MODIFIED IMPERIAL MOUSTACHE AND BEARD

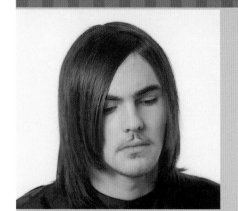

Step A

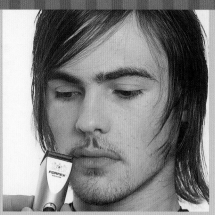

Step B

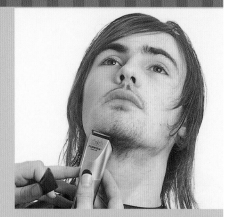

Step C

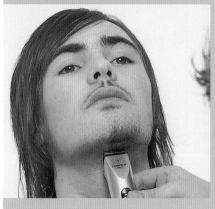

Step D

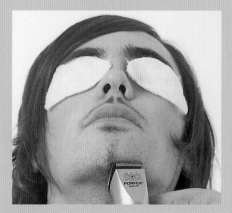

Step E

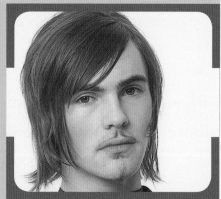

Step F

1. This client is an aspiring model who wants a distinctive contemporary look for his portfolio (a).
2. Start at one side of your client and begin cutting the beard hair to the correct length using the scissors- or clippers-over-comb technique.
3. Repeat this on the other side.
4. Move to the centre of the beard and blend the two sides together to create an even, continuous effect.
5. Move to one side of the moustache. Carefully outline the moustache along the top lip to create the required shape with the tips of your scissors or with the clippers (b).
6. Repeat this on the other side of the moustache.
7. Using your comb, lift small sections of the moustache hair and cut this to the required length.
8. Carefully establish the outline for the pencil line beard shape and cut the outline to the correct position (c).
9. Cut the other outlines on the cheeks, chin or above the moustache, as required. Refer to the mirror to keep the outlines symmetrical (d).
10. Remove unwanted hair from outside the outlines, as required. Eye protection is applied whilst removing main growth in case of flying hairs (e).
11. Shave the areas outside the outlines if required.
12. Comb the client's hair and show them the finished look (f).

HEALTH & SAFETY

Remove excess hair cuttings from the client's face and neck at regular intervals to ensure they are comfortable.

It may help you to read CHAPTER 12, 'Shaving services' to see how outlines should be shaved to achieve the closest finish.

ADAM – SHORT TRADITIONAL MEXICAN

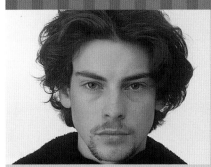
Step A

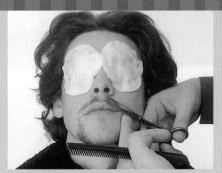
Step B

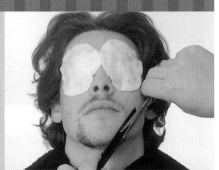
Step C

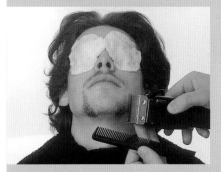
Step D

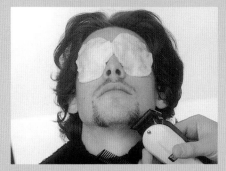
Step E

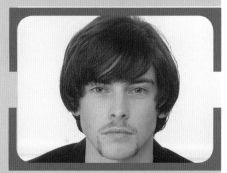
Step F

1. The client is a model who has grown a basic moustache shape for his role in a TV advertisement (a).
2. Move to one side of the moustache. Carefully outline the moustache along the top lip to create the required shape with the tips of your scissors or with the clippers (b).
3. Repeat this on the other side of the moustache.
4. Using your comb, lift small sections of the moustache hair and cut this to the required length (c).
5. Carefully establish the outline for the moustache shape and cut the outline to the correct position (d).
6. Cut the other outlines on the cheeks, chin and above the moustache, as required. Refer to the mirror to keep the outlines symmetrical.
7. Remove unwanted hair from outside the outlines, as required (e).
8. Shave the areas outside the outlines if required (see Chapter 12, Shaving services) (f).

TIP

Outlines can be achieved by cutting the hair with either close-cutting clippers, such as 'T blade' trimmers and balding blade clippers or an electric razor. The outline hair may also be removed completely by shaving with a razor, which should be used following the shaving procedure described in Chapter 12.

HEALTH & SAFETY

Protect the client's eyes from hairs, which may fly up during cutting, especially on very coarse beards. Keep your own face away from your work; wear safety glasses for protection if required.

KRIS – SHORT FULL BEARD WITH TRIBAL PATTERN

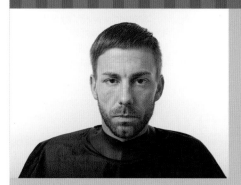

Step A

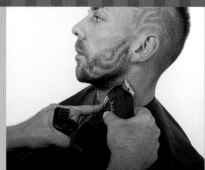

Step B

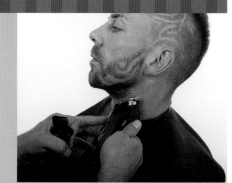

Step C

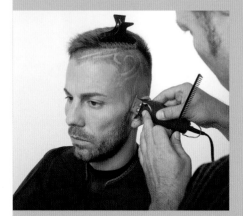

Step D

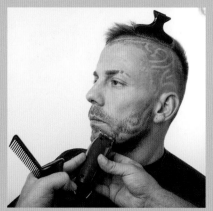

Step E

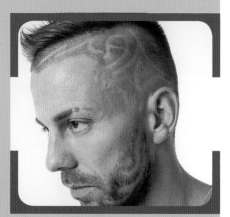

Step F

1. This client likes a strong look that will be noticed. He wants to keep a full beard with blended outlines except for the pattern (a).

2. Start at one side of your client and begin cutting the beard hair to the correct length using the scissors- or clippers-over-comb technique.

3. Repeat this on the other side and then move to the centre of the beard and blend the two sides together to create an even, continuous effect.

4. Repeat this across the moustache.

5. Cut the outlines on the neck, cheeks, and chin and above the moustache, as required. Refer to the mirror to keep the outlines symmetrical. Kris wants natural tapered outlines rather than obvious outlines so that the pattern stands out! (b).

6. Remove unwanted hair from outside the outlines, as required. A balding blade clipper can be used to get the closest clipper cut or the areas can be shaved, if required (see Chapter 12, Shaving services) (c).

7. The pattern is then channeled into the beard using a 'T blade' trimmer (d).

8. Notice how the design is worked down from the head for the best effect (e).

9. Dress the client's hair for the final look (f).

KEY DEFINITION

Pomade: A substance or ointment used to groom and fix the hair in place. Originally oil or wax based and shiny in appearance but now may be water based for easier removal.

Finishing and aftercare advice

Longer beard and moustache shapes may benefit from the application of a styling aid after cutting. **Pomade**, wax and creams will help to smooth the hair and retain more intricate shapes. Remember to comb the client's head hair into style.

You should advise your client on how to maintain their look at home. Here are some ways you can help them achieve good results:

◆ Products and how to use them – suggest which products will help them maintain and improve their facial skin and hair, including the benefits from using shampoo and conditioner rather than soap. This is a good opportunity to recommend retail products in your barber's shop. Show the client how the products should be used to achieve the best effects (you can highlight this to them as you style and finish their hair). Help them find and understand the manufacturer's instructions.

◆ How to maintain and style their facial hair look – show the client where to shave outside the outline shape. Discuss good grooming techniques – regular combing, cleaning, exfoliating and moisturising.

◆ When the next barber's shop appointment should be made – encourage the client to book their next visit before leaving if your barber's shop has an appointments system as facial hair will usually soon become untidy and the next cut will be required within 4 weeks.

It may help you to read CHAPTER 15, 'Design and create patterns in hair' to see how patterns can be incorporated into facial hair.

Read CHAPTER 13, 'Face massage services' for further information on good skincare routines.

Health and safety

Everyone in the salon has a duty to work safely and keep their environment safe. It is important to consider health and safety when cutting facial hair because of the risks associated with using electricity, the risk of cutting the skin and the risk of hair cuttings entering the eyes. Here are some important health and safety factors that you must consider when providing hair cutting services:

It may help you to read CHAPTER 2, 'Health and safety in the barber's shop' for general information on working safely in the barber's shop.

◆ If the client has any cuts or abrasions on their face, or you suspect that an infection or infestation is present, the work must not be carried out.

◆ Pay special attention to hygiene when cutting facial hair because of the risk of cross-infection through open cuts.

◆ Make sure the client's eyes are protected from any flying hairs with tissues or cotton wool pads. Keep your own face away from your work; wear safety glasses for protection.

◆ Open and safety razors have very sharp blades and must always be handled and used with great care.

◆ Always close the handle to protect the blade of an open razor when it is not being used or when it is being carried.

◆ *Never* place razors or other cutting tools in pockets.

◆ A fixed-blade razor must always be *sterilized* before each use.

◆ A new blade must always be used for each new client when using a detachable-blade open razor.

◆ Used razor blades, called sharps, must be disposed of correctly in accordance with your salon policy. Soiled disposable materials should be placed in sealed plastic bags for removal.

◆ Electrical equipment must always be handled and used with care in accordance with the manufacturer's instructions.

◆ *Never* use or place electric clippers or other electrical equipment near water.

◆ *Do not* go near electrical equipment that is lying in water – isolate the mains power first.

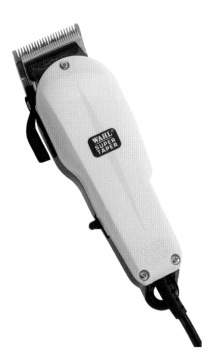

Wahl Super Taper Clipper

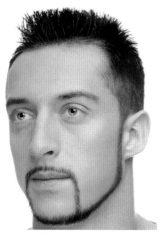

Chin curtain beard and Mexican moustache

- Visually check that electrical equipment is safe to use before commencing work – check that the cable has not frayed or been pulled and that the plug is not loose.

- Pay attention to the position of cables when using and storing electrical equipment.

- *Never* overload sockets by plugging too many items of electrical equipment into the same socket.

- Follow the manufacturer's instructions for the care of your clippers – ensure that you clean and lubricate the blades regularly to avoid damage.

- Only use clean tools and equipment.

- Make sure that you know the whereabouts of your salon's first-aid kit. Keep yourself up-to-date with your salon's first-aid and accident procedures.

- Electrical equipment must be regularly tested and given a certificate of testing to confirm that it is safe for use. Your salon owner will ensure that this is carried out, as required.

IMAGE GALLERY

Are you making the most of facial hair services in your work?

Visit the online gallery on this book's accompanying website to see other inspirational men's beard and moustache shapes.

BRINGING IT ALL TOGETHER

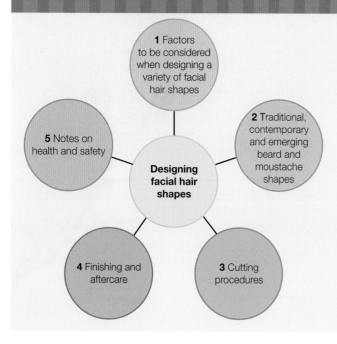

Summary

1   The principles learnt earlier about shape and form in haircutting are also important when designing a new facial hair shape, as you are starting with what might be called a blank canvas. Face shape is important to consider as certail beards and moustaches are suited to certain face shapes. Almost any beard shape is suitable, but you must take into account the client's hairstyle.

2   Many traditional beard and moustache shapes were named after the men who wore them at different times, such as the King Edward. Identification of modern beard and moustache shapes can be difficult by name alone. This can make identification of newer shapes difficult, so care must be taken to make sure

the right shape has been chosen before commencing work. Use visual aids to be sure you and the client know what each other expect! Emerging beard and moustache shapes are developed as barbers consider the latest hairstyles and design beard and moustache shapes that complement the looks required. This often involves combining and adapting traditional and new beard shapes with traditional and new moustache shapes.

3   Use the mirror regularly during cutting to ensure that the shape is centralized and symmetrical. A balding blade clipper can be used to get the closest clipper cut or the areas can be shaved, if required. Make sure you show the client how to maintain and style their facial hair look – show the client where to shave outside the outline shape and discuss good grooming techniques.

4   Never place razors or other cutting tools in your pockets. Remember to protect the client's eyes from hairs, which may fly up during cutting, especially on very coarse beards. Keep your own face away from your work; wear safety glasses for protection if required. Before commencing work, visually check that electrical equipment is safe to use – check that the cable has not frayed or been pulled, and that the plug is not loose. Always handle and use electrical equipment with care, and in accordance with the manufacturers' instructions.

Activity

1   Use the Internet and magazines to find images that show how men are currently wearing beards and moustaches and what new shapes are emerging. Use this information to design and create some new shapes. Photograph the created shapes – remember to get permission from your manager and clients before taking their photographs. Use all the images to produce a style book that can be used during consultation with clients in your salon. Remember to get permission from your manager before using the style book.

2   Collect together images of traditional beard and moustache shapes. Cut them out and label the back. Use them as flash cards for revision – see you can name them without turning them over.

Check your knowledge

1   When might you need to design a beard shape that is left longer in certain areas?

2   List techniques that can be used to incorporate patterns into beard and moustache designs.

3   How should the neck outline be cut to ensure that it appears level?

4   Why is it important to consider the hairstyle when designing a new beard and moustache shape?

5   Which of the following beard shapes is most suited to a client with a small face?

   a. King Edward
   b. Goatee
   c. Spade
   d. Mutton Chops

6   Why is it important to consider existing sideburns when designing a new moustache shape?

7   What differences would facial piercing make to the design and creation of a new beard shape?

8   Sketch a traditional military moustache shape.

9   Which of the following statements are correct?

   a. The handlebar is a traditional beard shape
   b. The Howie is a traditional moustache shape
   c. The Horseshoe is only a new shape
   d. The chin curtain is traditional shape

10   List two current beard and moustache shapes.

11   Describe how emerging beard and moustache shapes are developed.

12   What action should be taken if the client has an open cut on their face?

13   How should hair clippings be disposed of?

14   Why is it important to not plug too many items of electrical equipment into one socket?

15   What is Pomade?

15 Design and create patterns in hair

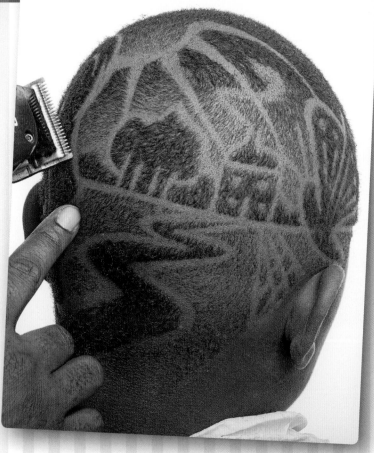

QUALIFICATION SIGNPOSTING

This chapter will help your studies of the following qualifications:

❖ Level 2 NVQ Diploma in Barbering.
❖ Level 3 NVQ Diploma in Barbering.
❖ City & Guilds Level 2 VRQ Award, Certificate and Diploma in Barbering.
❖ City & Guilds Level 3 VRQ Diploma in Barbering.
❖ ITEC Level 3 VRQ Certificate and Diplomas in Barbering and Men's Hairdressing.
❖ VTCT Level 3 VRQ Certificates and Diplomas in Barbering and Barbering Studies.

LEARNING OBJECTIVES

In this chapter you will learn:

◆ How to design 3D, pictorial, repeated and symmetrical patterns in hair.

◆ The factors that must be considered when creating complex patterns in hair.

◆ The cutting techniques used to create complex patterns in hair.

◆ How to work safely.

◆ Aftercare for advanced patterns in hair.

For further information on the qualifications covered by this chapter see the qualification mapping grid at the front of the book.

INTRODUCTION

At one time haircuts were occasionally personalized by the addition of simple lines and patterns, especially on African (Type K4) hair where partings would be channelled into the hair to make the haircut appear more interesting. Sometimes simple shapes or words were created, often representing a favourite sports team or club. More recently much more elaborate patterns are being created in both haircuts and facial hair. Two-dimensional (2D) and three-dimensional (3D) designs can be added and complex compositions produced that are perhaps better described as 'works of art'. In this chapter we will be looking at the techniques used for designing and creating advanced patterns in hair and will be covering the following topics:

❖ Factors to be considered when designing and creating patterns in hair.

❖ Principles of advanced design – including shape, form, perspective, scale, proportion and position.

❖ Cutting techniques – including channelling, tramlines and razoring.

❖ Cutting procedures.

❖ Aftercare.

❖ Notes on health and safety.

Factors to be considered when designing and creating patterns in hair

Before reading this chapter it may help you to read CHAPTER 7, 'Cutting men's hair using basic techniques' and CHAPTER 11, 'Advanced men's hair cutting'. You should also read CHAPTER 10, 'Cutting basic patterns in hair', as this will first introduce you to the requirements needed in basic pattern work.

The initial procedures used to create regular haircuts and create haircuts with patterns are often the same. The cutting techniques are the same and the head and face shape, hair characteristics, adverse hair and skin conditions and other factors all have to be fully considered. However, consultation for complex patterns does require special consideration, as the need to accurately establish the client's design wishes, or brief is especially important because patterns can make a strong statement about the client and can be very obvious.

The work involved requires great skill, vision and precise cutting techniques to be combined and adapted to take account of both the client's wishes and the many factors that affect the creation of the new pattern. The client consultation is essential in designing and personalizing the right pattern for each client.

HEALTH & SAFETY

Always carry out a thorough consultation to ensure that you identify any adverse conditions of the hair or skin that may be present. It is particularly important to establish whether a suspected infection or infestation is present, as these are contraindications that would prevent you from cutting the hair.

It may help you to read CHAPTER 4, 'Client care for men' for more detailed information on consultation before reading this section.

Consultation

You must carry out a thorough consultation to consider factors including the client's wishes, face shape and existing haircut. Here is a reminder of some of the critical factors that must be considered when designing and creating patterns in hair:

◆ Accurately establish what the client wants – called the client's design brief.

◆ Determine why they wish to have a pattern in their hair – does the client fully appreciate how the pattern will look and how long it will take to grow out?

◆ Look for signs of broken skin, abnormalities on the skin, or any unusual features or hair growth patterns – make sure there are no contraindications present.

◆ What is the hair type – type S1, W2, C3 or K4?

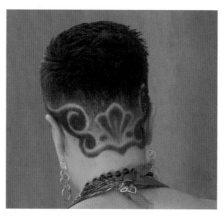

Symmetrical pattern

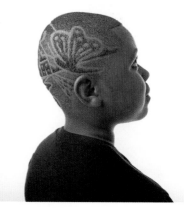

A pictorial pattern

- What are the hair characteristics –

  - Is the hair fine, medium or coarse?

  - Is the growth dense or sparse?

  - Does the density of growth vary around the head – does the client have male pattern alopecia, as this will significantly limit the extent of the pattern?

- Determine the client's face shape.

- Determine the existing and required length and shape of their hairstyle.

DON'T BE TEMPTED ✗

Don't be tempted to add anything to the pattern that was not agreed with the client as unexpected changes will soon be noticed and may not be welcomed!

TIP ✓

Include any variations in the density of growth into the pattern design. You may need to adapt the pattern significantly from the client's wishes to incorporate very sparse growth or a scar. Make sure the client understands this and agrees.

TIP ✓

The movement created by hair growth patterns should become features of the design. Incorporate strong growth movements into the pattern to create a particular effect, e.g. a whorl can make an interesting circular feature in the pattern.

Face shape, features and haircut length The client's face shape and features must be considered when choosing the most suitable haircut and pattern. The principles applied to choosing the right shape and length of haircut for different face shapes is explained fully in Chapter 7, 'Cutting men's hair using basic techniques' and they also apply here. The length of the client's existing haircut is a particularly important factor in advanced pattern design as some patterns cannot be achieved if the hair is too short, e.g. 3D effects cannot be created easily on hair layers shorter than 5 mm. Longer haircuts with layers beyond around 4 cm in length can of course be shortened to lengths suitable for creating patterns, but clients who wish to keep their hair layers longer than this should be discouraged from including patterns in these areas. Patterns may be included in other shorter areas though, such as in the back and sides and in disconnected cuts, even though the layers on the top are longer. Longer layers are generally less suitable for creating patterns because the hair tends to cover the pattern and the effect can appear unbalanced. Shorter, layered haircuts between 5 mm and 2 cm are usually best for 2D designs and geometrical shapes, but layers up to 4 cm often work better for 3D designs, as the thickness makes creating the 3D effect easier. Pictorial patterns too work well on hair this length. On hair shorter than 5 mm good pictorial, graphical or geometric shapes can be created.

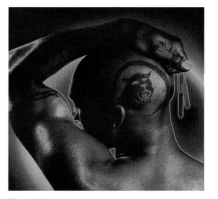

Pictorial pattern

MK

❝ Advanced pattern work is amongst the most creative and challenging that the modern barber carries out, but it is also amongst the most satisfying. Develop these high level skills and you will help to maximize your potential as a barber. ❞

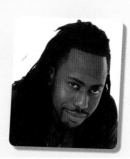

Principles of advanced design

The basic principles for creating linear patterns set out in Chapter 10 also apply to creating advanced pattern, but there are additional requirements and these are set out below in each of the key design areas:

◆ Shape, **form** and perspective.

◆ Scale.

◆ Proportion.

◆ Position.

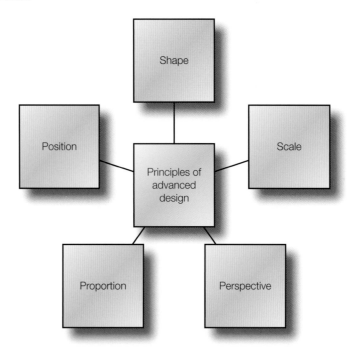

Shape, form and perspective

Shape describes a two-dimensional or 2D object. **Form** refers to the appearance of the 3D effect, or depth of an object. Shape and form both define the exterior outline shape of the overall pattern to be created and the outline shapes of each individual object within the pattern. **Perspective** refers to the skill of placing lines, shapes or objects into a design or picture in such a way that makes some objects appear to be nearer and others distant – creating a 3D effect. The main techniques used to create perspective in a design include:

◆ Using converging lines that move closer together in the distance.

◆ Making objects and shapes in the near ground larger and progressively smaller as they appear in the distance.

◆ Making objects in the distance less dark and less vibrant.

◆ Making objects in the distance less detailed.

The most important element of any shape or form is the line. Lines are used to determine the placing of the object and to create precise limits on the space between objects within the pattern. When creating complex designs any complicated shapes are usually broken down into simple geometric shapes that can be more easily created. They are then joined together when the composition is complete.

It may help you to read about the basic principles for designing patterns in hair in **CHAPTER 10**, 'Creating basic patterns in hair' before reading this section.

KEY DEFINITION

Form: The appearance of the 3D effect, or depth of an object.

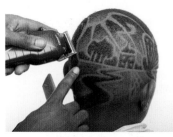

This pictorial pattern requires careful use of perspective

KEY DEFINITION

Shape: The outline of something, forming a two-dimensional or 2D object.

KEY DEFINITION

Perspective: How objects appear relative to each other according to their distance from the viewer, particularly the effects of this distance on their appearance which may create the illusion of depth.

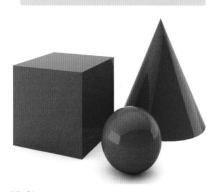

3D Shapes

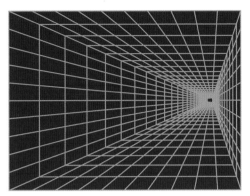

Perspective – converging lines

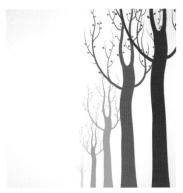

Perspective – smaller, lighter less detailed in the distance

Perspective in a hair pattern

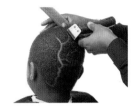

Freehand channeling is used to create lines according to scale, position, proportion and perspective

When creating advanced patterns in hair, the lines are created using a freehand technique with electric clippers, trimmers or scissors.

Scale

Objects that inspire designs are usually too big or too small for the size of pattern we wish to create. The object must be enlarged or reduced to fit into the design and scale is used to maintain the object's proportion. Scale uses ratios to establish the relative dimensions of objects to the design, e.g. an object measuring 1000 cm × 100 cm can be reduced to 1/10th its original size by dividing each measurement by 10, making the new size 100 cm × 10 cm. This design would be a 1:10 scale replica of the original object.

> **TIP** ✓
>
> 3D effects are enhanced by the illusion of light and dark within the pattern, representing highlights and shadows. These effects can be created by reducing the thickness of the hair in some area and leaving the hair longer in others, known as creating positive and negative effects. The colour of the scalp showing through from beneath helps to create the effect. Remember to establish the position of the light source for highlight and shadow effects (usually from the top of the head) and ensure the effects are created consistently with this light source throughout the design.

The barber must establish the dimensions of the area where the design is to be sited and use scale to design patterns that fit within these dimensions. This can be achieved when using freehand techniques by using estimation and imagining a grid across the area for the design. Features of the object to be replicated are estimated in size and reduced or enlarged to fit within each square of the imaginary grid until the design is complete. The tip on establishing accurate lines can help.

Proportion

Similar to scale, proportion describes the relative size of one shape or object within a design to the size of another shape or object. It is often referred to by ratios such as; the tree in the near ground is twice as big as the tree in the distance – a ratio of 2:1. Chapter 10 explains that artists try to make their compositions meet the rules of the 'Golden Ratio' in order to be especially appealing. This ratio is applied visually when arranging the composition through a technique known as the 'Fibonacci or Golden Spiral'.

> **TIP** ✓
>
> The relative scale of an object can be transferred practically to the pattern you are creating by using a technique developed by artists. Hold a comb at arm's length and look passed the comb to view the object that is being incorporated into the pattern. Slide your thumb along the comb to mark where the outside of the object is seen. Move your hand to view the hair pattern through the comb and memorize where the line of the object comes. Repeat this to transfer the scale of the object into your design.

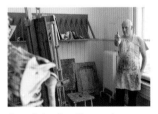

An artist estimating scale

It may help you to read about the basic principles of proportion in CHAPTER 10, 'Creating basic patterns in hair' before reading this next section.

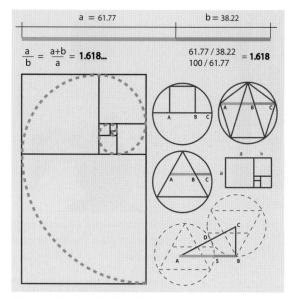

Fibonacci Spiral and Golden Ratio

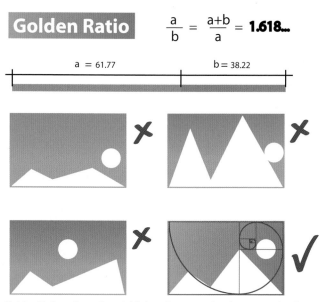

Golden Ratio – the ratio establishes the most pleasing proportion in this scene

This technique is particularly useful when composing pictorial patterns, as follows:

◆ Imagine that a grid of equal squares is placed over the area of the client's head where the pattern is to be placed.

◆ Decide where the central object in the pattern is to be placed within these squares.

◆ Imagine that the golden spiral connects the corner of this object and arcs across the grid of squares.

◆ Now consider where on this arc other objects you want in the pattern should be placed.

TIP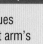

To ensure that the lines of the pattern are cut accurately when using freehand techniques place the thumb of one hand on the line of one object within the design. Stand back at arm's length, or by looking in the mirror, slide the other thumb to the position of the new line until both thumbs appear level. Memorize the position of the thumbs. Now cut the new line to the correct position and length. This method can be easily adapted to establish the width of lines and so obtain accurate shapes, even in the most elaborate designs.

Position

Position ensures that the pattern is placed or centred on the correct part of the head. Although the design might by symmetrical or asymmetric the correct position is still important. Many factors affect the positioning of patterns in hair, such as hair growth patterns, hair density and proportion. When using freehand techniques the correct position can be established by placing one thumb on the head at arm's length, or by looking in the mirror, and moving the thumb around until it appears to be in the correct place.

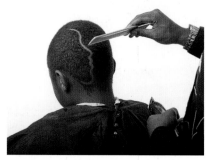

Determining the position – use a comb as a measuring guide

DON'T BE TEMPTED

Remember that as a professional barber your obligation is to ensure that your client's wishes or brief is achieved. Don't be tempted to suggest patterns that are not suitable for the client. Make sure that your consultation establishes all the factors and that your recommendations are suitable.

Here are some important things to remember about designing patterns in hair:

◆ Some patterns are improved by having no distinct outlines. They work best by simply fading out.

◆ Pay particular attention to where the haircut meets any beard and ensure that they blend together, as required.

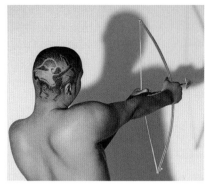

An award winning pictorial design

ACTIVITY: CASE STUDY – DANIEL

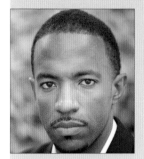

Daniel is attending a music festival next week. To mark the occasion he wants a pictorial pattern around the back and sides celebrating a famous album cover of one of his favorite bands, Pink Floyd, who are playing at the festival. He wants to keep length through the top but is happy to have a fade cut elsewhere. Suggest a design to meet Daniel's brief?

Cutting techniques

Cutting techniques, such as scissors-over-comb, clippers-over-comb and freehand are used when creating the foundation haircut for the pattern. These are explained fully in Chapter 7, 'Cutting men's hair using basic techniques' and for basic use in patterns in Chapter 10, 'Cutting basic patterns in hair'. Some of these techniques are used especially in creating more advanced patterns and are explained in the following sections.

Read CHAPTER 7, 'Cutting men's hair using basic techniques' for more information on techniques used in the foundation haircut for the pattern.

Channelling and tramlining

The channelling technique is used to create complex lines and shapes within the pattern. Channelling is performed with electric clippers, trimmers or T-liners with the edge of the blades placed end on to the scalp in order to remove the hair in narrow lines, or placed flat against the scalp to remove hair in the larger shapes. Close cutting fixed blades or the shortest setting on adjustable blades are usually used.

Tramlines are a form of channelling where simple lines are created.

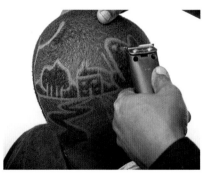

Channelling a shape within a pictorial design

HEALTH & SAFETY

Great care must be taken when using a razor. Always wear gloves and use light pressure and small movements, as the razor can quickly and easily cut the skin or remove too much hair if not used correctly. Balding blade clippers are recommended for removing hair within the pattern rather than shaving.

Razoring

Razoring (shaving) is sometimes used to create cleaner lines and shapes within the pattern and on the outlines. It is performed with a razor, which may be either an open razor or a safety razor. Disposable-blade razors should be used because they are more hygienic. Balding blade clippers are recommended for removing hair within the pattern rather than shaving. Electric razors are also sometimes used in larger areas; remember all razors must be sterilized before use on each client.

Accompanying video available for 'creating a negative effect'. Please scan this QR code.

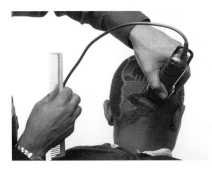

Creating a negative effect – the field next to the road

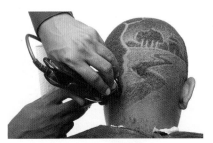

The road is the positive effect

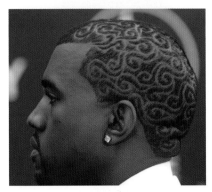

A repeated linear pattern

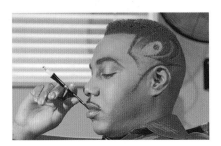

Channelling – a 3D graphical design

Techniques for creating negative and positive effects

Channelling and tramlining techniques can be used to create 3D effects that produce the illusion of light and dark within the pattern that represent the highlights and shadows we normally see. The effects are created by reducing the thickness of hair, or removing all the hair in some areas, (the **negative effect**) whilst leaving the hair longer in other areas (the **positive effect**).

MK

" The use of both negative and positive cutting techniques within the design will achieve the most realistic and interesting 3D effects. "

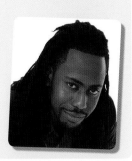

ACTIVITY: CASE STUDY – STEPHEN

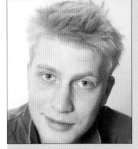

Stephen is a regular client in your barber's shop. He often has a simple 2D graphical design below his left temple but is getting married this weekend and wants something very special for the big day! He is very proud of his Celtic ancestry and culture but does not want anything associated with sports. He wants to keep length through the top but he's happy to be close cut elsewhere. He doesn't want a pictorial design. What design would meet Stephen's brief?

TIP

Remember, you should always follow your barber's shop policy for working on those under 16 years old, or on those who appear vulnerable. This is especially important when creating advanced patterns as the effects can be very obvious. Where necessary, confirm suitability before you start this work.

Cutting procedures

In this work it is the barber's creativity and individualism that comes to the fore, hence there are many different approaches to creating advanced patterns in hair. The following examples show how some advanced patterns can be achieved.

HEALTH & SAFETY

Always sanitize clipper and trimmer blades before use on each client. Use sanitizing cleansing wipes and sprays – the sprays also help to cool and lubricate the blades during use.

ORIENTAL DRAGON – A 2D PATTERN WITH REPEATED FEATURES

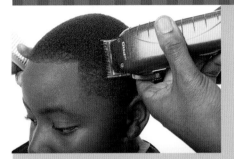

Step A

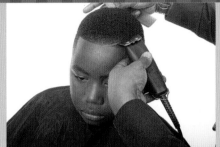

Step B

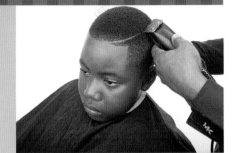

Step C

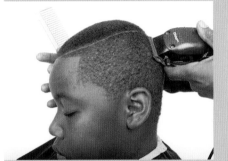

Step D

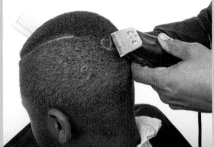

Step E

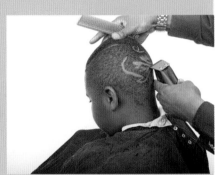

Step F

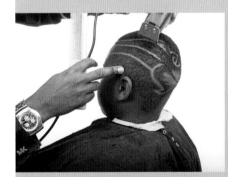

Step G

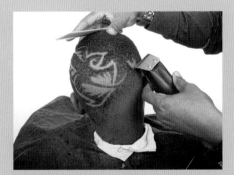

Step H

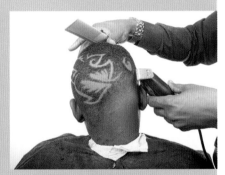

Step I

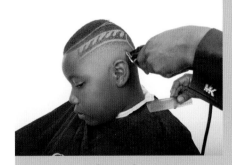

Step J

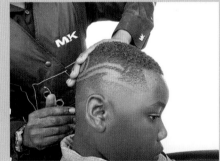

Step K

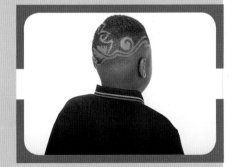

Step L

(continued)

ORIENTAL DRAGON – A 2D PATTERN WITH REPEATED FEATURES (*Continued*)

1. Cut the hair to the length required to create a foundation for the pattern (a).
2. Establish the position of the first line (b).
3. Channelling is used to extend the line to the centre of the pattern, according to the chosen scale and proportion (c).
4. Remove hair below the created line (d).
5. Create the centre of the pattern – this will be the dragon's face (e).
6. Add additional lines to build the pattern (f).
7. Lines are channelled back to the front from the centre to create the dragon's body (g).
8. Return to the centre and use channelling to create the dragon's fiery breath (h).
9. Stand back from the client or refer to the mirror regularly to check that the pattern is developing correctly.
10. Build up the dragon's breath by removing hair – creating a negative effect (i).
11. Notching is added to the dragon's body in a repeated pattern to create the illusion of scales. The area below the body is faded to emphasize the pattern (j).
12. Remove any unwanted hair from inside the lines, as required. Shave the areas inside the lines if required (see Chapter 12, 'Shaving services').
13. Remove all hair clippings from the pattern and client. Some clients enjoy the soothing effects of talcum powder or Aloe Vera based gels or cream on the skin within the pattern. Make sure that the client is not sensitive to such products before use. Always follow the manufacturer's instructions!
14. Styling gel or wax can be added to enhance definition, if required (k and l).

HEALTH & SAFETY

Razors have very sharp blades and must always be treated with care and respect. Keep the handle closed or cover the blade when not in use and especially when carrying or passing them. *Never* place a razor in your pocket and always keep them out of the reach of children.

HEALTH & SAFETY

Remove excess hair cuttings from the client's face and neck at regular intervals to ensure they are comfortable.

Accompanying video available for 'creating the Dragon Pattern'. Please scan this QR code.

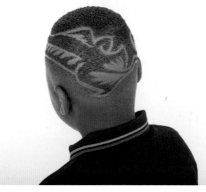

Dragon Pattern – the body

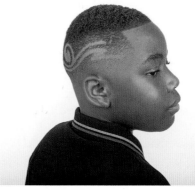

Dragon Pattern – breathing fire!

HOMEWARD BOUND – A 3D PICTORIAL PATTERN

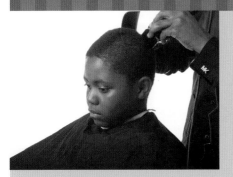

Step A

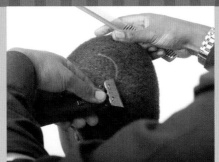

Step B

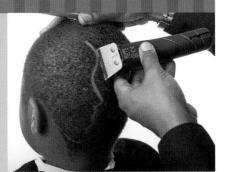

Step C

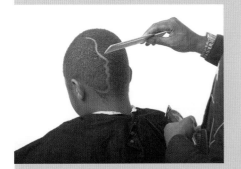

Step D

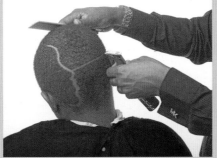

Step E

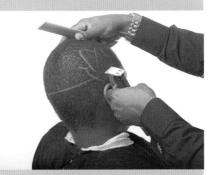

Step F

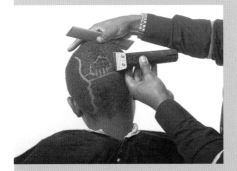

Step G

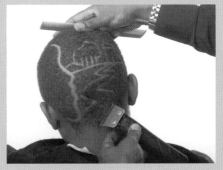

Step H

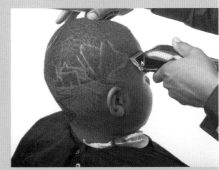

Step I

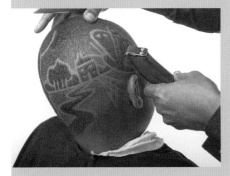

Step J

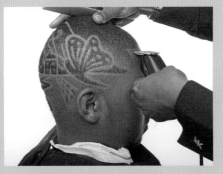

Step K

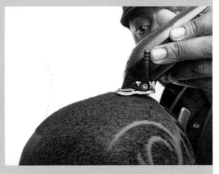

Step L

(continued)

HOMEWARD BOUND – A 3D PICTORIAL PATTERN (*Continued*)

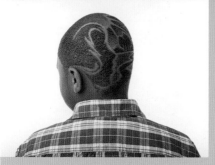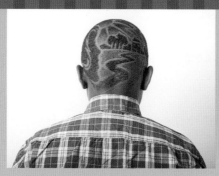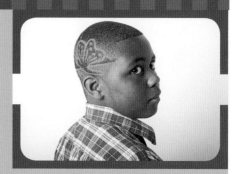

Step M

1. Before you begin work on the pattern, cut the area of the hair on which you wish to create a pattern using a number 1 clipper comb attachment (a).

2. Now blend the rest of the hair into this cut. This is to make sure that the pattern is clean and fits with the rest of the overall hairstyle.

3. Create the first line where the centre of the pattern will be (b).

4. When you want to mark straight lines in the pattern you can use your clippers as a basic line guide. Curved lines are made freehand by turning the clippers in an arc whilst keeping the wrist still. Keep working down – here the face in the composition begins to emerge (c).

5. Using your estimations of proportion and scale identify where the horizontal line, or plane will be in the pattern (d).

6. Extend the line across the composition to the right object – the butterfly (e).

7. Create the butterfly using delicate channelling movements with the corners of the trimmer blades (f).

8. Develop the pattern by adding the house and trees (g).

9. Adding the path and fence – notice how the path and fence lines converge towards the horizontal plane to create the perspective of distance (h).

10. Stand back from the client or refer to the mirror regularly to check that the pattern is developing correctly.

11. Fading is used to create 3D effects that enhance the illusion of distance (i).

12. Add finer details and clean up lines with T-liner trimmers – use the corner of the blades for the most precise work (j).

13. Remove hair outside the main haircut perimeter outlines (k).

14. Ensure the hair left longer to create the positive effect is level (l).

15. Shave the areas inside the pattern if necessary (see Chapter 12, 'Shaving services').

16. Brush away all the excess hair and brush a light dusting of talcum powder or apply Aloe Vera based gels or cream on the skin within the pattern, if your client agrees. Make sure that the client is not sensitive to such products before use and always follow the manufacturer's instructions!

17. Styling gel or wax can be added to enhance definition, if required (m).

Accompanying video available for 'creating the pictorial pattern'. Please scan this QR code.

TIP

Cleaner lines and shapes can be achieved by cutting the hair with either close-cutting balding blade clippers, T-liners or an electric razor. The outline hair may also be removed completely by shaving with a razor, which should be used following the shaving procedure described in Chapter 12, 'Shaving services'.

DON'T BE TEMPTED ✗

Remember that clippers and trimmers can become quite warm in use, especially during the more intricate work when creating pictorial patterns in hair. Don't be tempted to forget about the client's comfort whilst you are concentrating on creating the pattern. Use sanitizing spray to help cool, clean and lubricate the blades at intervals during the work.

TIP ✓

Remember: patterns work well on darker hair as it shows off the design better, particularly when creating 2D and 3D designs.

SKYLINE – RAJ – A 3D PICTORIAL PATTERN

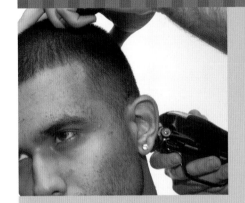

Step A

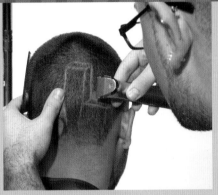

Step B

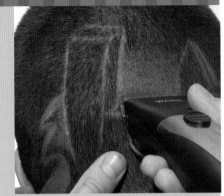

Step C

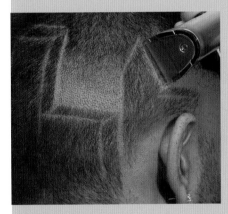

Step D

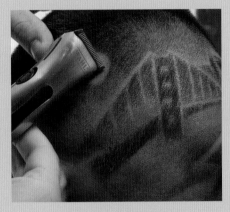

Step E

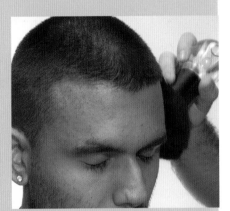

Step F

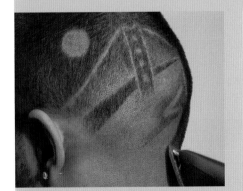

Step G

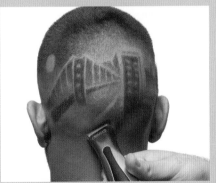

Step H

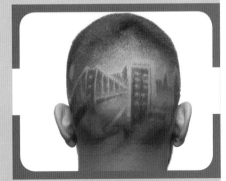

Step I

(continued)

SKYLINE – RAJ – A 3D PICTORIAL PATTERN (*Continued*)

1. Before you begin work on the pattern, think carefully about the placement and consider where your design will start and finish.

2. View the hair as a blank canvas. You need to take it down to a level no lower than grade 1 and no higher than grade 2; this is the best length to show off the full potential of the design (a).

3. The pattern is created using a trimmer. Get more detail out of your pattern by using the Detailer, the T Blade cuts really close for neat lines (b).

4. Remember to use your estimations of proportion and scale to identify where the horizontal plane will be in the pattern.

5. Use negative and positive effects to build up the 3D effects in the pattern. Fading into the outlines produces good 3D effects (c).

6. Use the full blade for straight lines; make sure the pattern flows with no disconnection (d).

7. Use the corners of the blade to create curved lines and round shapes (e).

8. Remember to keep the design simple, it shouldn't be over-complicated or the effects will blend together and won't be visible.

9. Use a brush and comb and constantly brush away the hair so your can see you design clearly (f).

10. Stand back from the client or refer to the mirror regularly to check that the pattern is developing correctly.

11. Fading is used to finish the neckline and further enhance the 3D effects that develop the illusion of distance (g).

12. Add finer details and clean up lines with trimmers – use the corner of the blades and T-liners for the most precise work (h).

13. Shave the areas inside the pattern if necessary (see Chapter 12, 'Shaving services').

14. Apply wax to enhance the pattern definition, if required (i).

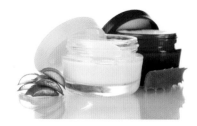

Soothing Aloe Vera cream

Aftercare

Your client will need to know how to look after their new pattern and haircut before they leave. Make sure you provide this aftercare advice and remember; this is an opportunity to recommend retail products and make the client a further appointment. Aftercare advice should include the following:

◆ Recommend when the client should book the next appointment – remember that in shorter styles the haircut will need restyling sooner as the new hair growth is likely to quickly equal the length of the actual haircut. This would soon be noticeable. Unwanted hair outside the haircut perimeter would also soon be visible and will need removing. In shorter styles appointments should generally be for every 2 to 4 weeks. However, where the haircut includes a pattern the client will need to visit sooner if they wish the pattern to remain distinct, as over time the pattern will fade. If the pattern is no longer wanted it can be removed by cutting but close cut patterns may need to grow for 1–2 weeks first, otherwise faint traces might still be visible unless a balding blade or shaving is used.

◆ The client should shampoo and cleanse their hair according to the hair length, hair and scalp condition and their lifestyle.

◆ Which products can help the client maintain the overall style; particularly those such as gel and wax that can help define the pattern by smoothing the hair outside the pattern lines. Some clients also enjoy the soothing effects of gel or cream, such as Aloe Vera gel on the skin within the pattern. Consider retailing such products in your barber's shop!

Health and safety

Health and safety is particularly important when creating patterns in hair because of the risks associated with using electricity and the risk of cutting the skin. Here are some important health and safety factors that you must consider when providing hair cutting services:

◆ If the client has any cuts or abrasions on his face or head, or you suspect that an infection or infestation is present, the work must not be carried out.

◆ Pay special attention to hygiene when cutting hair because of the risk of cross-infection through open cuts.

◆ Always protect the client's eyes from hairs with tissues or cotton wool pads when cutting facial hair. Keep your own face away from your work; wear safety glasses for protection.

◆ Open and safety razors have very sharp blades and must always be handled and used with great care.

◆ Always close the handle to protect the blade of an open razor when it is not being used or when it is being carried.

◆ *Never* place razors or other cutting tools in pockets.

◆ A fixed-blade razor must always be *sterilized* before each use.

◆ A new blade must always be used for each new client when using a detachable-blade open razor.

◆ Used razor blades, called sharps, must be disposed of correctly in accordance with your salon policy. Soiled disposable materials should be placed in sealed plastic bags for removal.

◆ Electrical equipment must always be handled and used with care in accordance with the manufacturer's instructions.

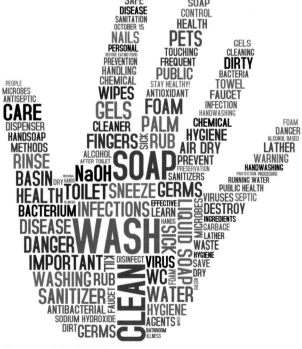

Always work hygienically

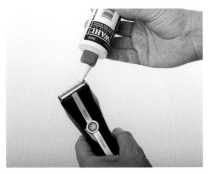

Oiling blades

◆ *Never* use or place electric clippers or other electrical equipment near water.

◆ *Do not* go near electrical equipment that is lying in water – isolate the mains power first.

◆ Visually check that electrical equipment is safe to use before commencing work – check that the cable has not frayed or been pulled and that the plug is not loose.

◆ Pay attention to the position of cables when using and storing electrical equipment.

◆ *Never* overload sockets by plugging too many items of electrical equipment into the same socket.

◆ Follow the manufacturer's instructions for the care of your clippers – ensure that you clean and lubricate the blades regularly to avoid damage.

◆ Only use clean tools and equipment.

◆ Make sure that you know the whereabouts of your salon's first-aid kit. Keep yourself up-to-date with your salon's first-aid and accident procedures.

◆ Electrical equipment must be regularly tested and given a certificate of testing to confirm that it is safe for use. Your salon owner will ensure that this is carried out, as required.

IMAGE GALLERY

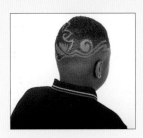

Visit the online image gallery on this book's accompanying website to see other inspirational advanced hair patterns.

BRINGING IT ALL TOGETHER

Summary

1 Two-dimensional (2D) and three-dimensional (3D) designs can be added together within patterns to produce complex compositions that are better described as 'works of art'.

2 Always carry out a thorough consultation to ensure that you identify any adverse conditions of the hair or skin that may be present.

3 3D effects cannot be created easily on hair layers shorter than 5 mm.

4 Perspective refers to the skill of placing lines, shapes or objects into a design or picture in such a way that makes some objects appear to be nearer and others distant.

5 When creating complex designs any complicated shapes are usually broken down into simple geometric shapes that can be more easily created.

6 Scale uses ratios to establish the relative dimensions of objects to the design. Proportion determines the size of objects with other objects in the composition. The golden spiral helps to establish proportion.

7 Negative and positive effects are created by reducing the thickness of hair, or removing it all in some areas, (the negative effect) whilst leaving the hair longer in other areas (the positive effect).

8 Razoring (shaving) is sometimes used to create cleaner lines and shapes within the pattern.

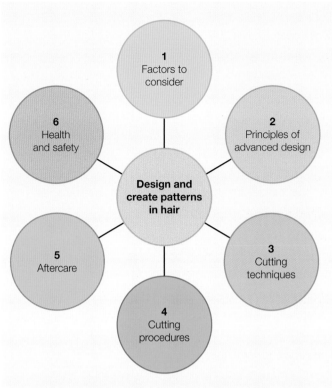

9   Follow the manufacturer's instructions for the care of your clippers – ensure that you clean and lubricate the blades regularly to avoid damage. Clean the blades and use sanitizing wipes and spray before using clippers and trimmers on each new client. Use sanitizing spray to clean, cool and lubricate the blades during use.

10   Never use or place electric clippers or other electrical equipment near water.

Activities

1   Take photographs of your best work and produce a style book from the resulting images to help show clients designs they can have. You might also be able to use them to publicize your salon or even to submit them to magazines and competitions for wider coverage and recognition of your work. Remember to get permission from your manager and the client first, expesially if the client is under 18 years old.

2   Research the types of 3D, pictorial, repeated and symmetrical patterns that are currently popular. Consider how you could develop these into patterns for your barber's shop and produce sketches to illustrate your ideas for sharing with your manager and colleagues.

Check your knowledge

1   Describe the principle of form.

2   Which of the following statements is correct:

   a.   Describing one object compared to another as being on a scale of 2:1 is the same as saying one object is twice as large as the other.
   b.   Scale is used to transfer a larger shape into smaller design.

3   Describe how 3D effects are created in a pattern.

4   Describe the channelling technique.

5   When might razoring be used to create a pattern?

6   Describe how to maintain high standards of hygiene for using razors.

7   Which of the following are techniques used to create perspective:

   a.   Converging lines
   b.   Objects are lighter in the foreground
   c.   Objects are less detailed in the distance
   d.   Objects are larger as they near the foreground

8   What are negative areas within a pattern?

9   What are positive areas within a pattern?

10   Describe the tip for ensuring the correct location of a pattern.

11   Which of the following correctly describe what T-liners are best used for?

   a.   Fading
   b.   Removing hair from within large shapes in the design
   c.   Channelling
   d.   Detailed work

12   Which of the following statements is correct?

   a.   In shorter style patterns appointments should generally be for every 2 to 4 weeks.
   b.   Close cut patterns may need to grow out for 1–2 weeks before they can be completely removed without using a balding blade.

Glossary

accelerator a machine that produces radiant heat (infrared radiation); it can be used to speed up processes such as colouring or conditioning

acid a substance that gives off hydrogen ions in water, and produces a solution with a pH below 7

acid mantle the natural protective coating on the skin's surface made from sweat and sebum

acne a skin disorder, characterized by spots and pustules resulting from inflammation of the sebaceous glands

activators chemicals used in bleaches or some perm lotions to start or boost their action

adipose tissue body fat or loose connective tissue

adverse conditions conditions that may affect what services can be provided or change how the service should be provided

aesthetically an artistic composition that is visually appealing

Afro-Caribbean hair (sometimes known as **African-Caribbean hair, African hair, Black hair or Curly Hair**) the very curly hair (sometimes called 'tight curly', or 'kinky' hair, and now known as 'Type VC4 or K4') typical of people of African descent

aftercare advice providing information on products and their use and tips on grooming and styling to help the client maintain his style at home

AIDS acquired immunodeficiency syndrome; a condition in which the immune system is damaged and the body becomes vulnerable to infections

albinism an inherited condition in which there is virtually no colour pigment in the hair or skin

albino hair a condition where the hair contains little or no pigment so that it appears nearly white or very light yellow; the condition is usually present at birth

alkali a substance that gives off hydroxide ions in water, and produces a solution with a pH above 7

alopecia baldness or hair loss resulting in areas where there is no hair growth so that the scalp is visible

alpha keratin the hair in an un-stretched state

alternating current (AC) an interrupted electrical current that causes the flow of electrons to reverse direction

alum powder see styptic liquid

amino acids simple organic compounds that form the basic ingredients of proteins

anagen the active growing stage of the hair growth cycle

androgen the male hormone

aniline a colourless oily liquid present in coal tar or crude oil that is used in manufacturing dyes

anterior towards the front

antioxidant a substance that slows down or prevents deterioration due to oxidation

antiseptic a substance that kills disease-causing micro-organisms or prevents them from growing

appraisal see **performance appraisal**

arrector pili the small muscles that raise the hairs when they contract

arteriole a very small artery

artery a blood vessel that carries oxygenated blood away from the heart

assignment a set task or a practical activity

astringent a finishing product that may be used in shaving and face massage. It has a bracing affect on the skin causing the pores to close when the alcohol they contain evaporates

asymmetrical something lacking in symmetry which creates an uneven balance

athlete's foot see **tinea pedis**

attributes a quality or characteristic inherent in or ascribed to someone or something

autoclave a device that uses high-temperature steam to sterilize items

azo dyes they are synthetic dyes in temporary colours that coat the surface of the hair

bacteria a large group of different microorganisms, many live on or in the human body and some cause diseases

bactericide a substance that kills bacteria

baldness hair loss resulting in areas where there is no hair growth so that the scalp is visible

barba a Latin word meaning 'beard' from which the term 'barber' is derived

barber a person who specializes in providing hairdressing services to men

barbering the art of providing specialist hairdressing services to men incorporating barbering principles; includes cutting and shaping men's facial hair, cutting, shaping and styling men's hair, shaving, face massage and scalp massage

barbering principles a system of rules that should always be followed when cutting and styling men's hair to incorporate typical male features, such as head and face shape, facial hair and neck hair and produce the most suitable masculine looks

barber's hand the feel or touch that has to be developed by a barber to perfect the art of shaving

barber's shop the premises where the barber provides barbering services

barber-surgeons the term used to describe barbers in the middle ages who performed barbering and simply surgery

barrier cream a waterproof cream used to protect the skin or scalp when using chemicals

beta keratin the hair in a stretched state

bleach a substance that removes natural colour

bleaching the removal of natural colour

bloodletting a technique used by barber-surgeons in times past to remove blood via a client's vein. The blood was thought to be affected by evil spirits and its removal would alleviate illness caused by this 'bad blood'

blow-waving creating temporary waves in the hair while blow-drying

blue beard a very dense beard growth that makes the skin appear tinged blue even when newly shaved

body language communication using body actions and/or posture instead of speech

boosters substances that add additional oxygen to speed up a chemical process

boston a rounded neckline

buzz-cut a style where the hair is cut in a uniform layer about 10 mm long over the whole head, sometimes called a crew cut

bylaws rules made by local councils that have legal status and must be followed. Some bylaws set out in detail the minimum standards of hygiene and practices that barber's shops must meet and in some cases the bylaw will prohibit certain services from being offered

canities hair with no pigment that appears grey or white

capillary a very fine tube; used to refer to a very small blood vessel

capilliary action the movement of liquid through absorption

catagen the hair growth stage when the hair stops growing, but the hair still active

caucasian hair the wavy or straight hair typical of a European, also known as Type S1 or W2 hair

channelling a cutting technique used to cut lines and shapes into the hair to create patterns

circumspect being discreet when dealing with people

characteristics physical features of the hair, skin and head, such as the density of the hair and face shape

clear layer also known as the stratum lucidum, is a clear layer of skin found in the epidermis between the horny layer and the granular layer

client a customer or patron of a business

client care looking after customers, making sure that they are comfortable and that they will be satisfied with the service they receive

club cutting or **clubbing** cutting hair straight across to produce level ends

cold permanent waving a perming process that does not rely on heat for activation

colonies large groups of microorganisms forming a physically connected structure

colourants colouring substances that are used on the hair

colouring the process of adding artificial to hair

comb attachments guard attachments that fit onto clippers to give a preset cutting depth

communication providing and receiving information in order to establish understanding

compatibility two or more substances that work well when mixed together; they mix harmoniously and do not react badly

compensation a payment made to make good for poor service, loss, damage, etc.

composition combining different shapes, parts or elements to form a whole piece of work

compound colourings a mixture of vegetable and mineral dyes

compound henna vegetable henna and metallic salts mixed to create colour for hair; it is incompatible with chemicals in modern hairdressing products so it is not used in salons

conditioners a range of products used to improve or correct the state of the hair

confidentiality keeping information secret; maintaining the salon's or an individual's privacy

connective tissue tissues in the body that provide structure and support

consultation the process of interviewing a client to establish what he wants; it involves selecting the best options to meet his request, if possible, or finding suitable alternatives, providing advice and establishing the best products and techniques to use. Determines whether the client is suitable for the requested service

contact dermatitis a rash and irritation of the skin caused by contact with irritant substances and frequent wet and damp conditions. It can be a serious condition and in the worst cases the sufferer may have to leave the barbering profession to prevent the condition recurring

contagious a disease or condition that can be transmitted between people through physical contact

contraindication a sign that the treatment or service is inadvisable or could be harmful, which makes proceeding with a particular service inadvisable or impossible

contamination when an item or substance is polluted by some other potentially harmful substance

contemporary modern or up-to-date

continuous professional development (CPD) completing further training, qualifications and development activities determined by your personal development plan to make sure your skills and knowledge are updated and suitable for current work, sometimes called 'lifelong learning'

contract of employment a legally binding agreement between the barber and the employer based on the employment conditions, roles and responsibilities, often making reference to the job description, that were agreed when the barber first started work

cortex the middle part of the hair shaft made up of many long strands of fibres that resemble springs twisted together

cowlick a hair growth pattern at the front hairline where the hair grows up and then apart forming a natural parting

crew cut a style where the hair is cut in a uniform layer about 10 mm long over the whole head, sometimes called a buzz-cut

cross-infection the passing of an infection from one individual to another

cross selling recommending an additional product or service that might be beneficial to the product or service being requested

crown a circular hair growth pattern on top of the head, the hair appears to radiate out from this point

current look a look that is currently fashionable

cuticle the outermost transparent layer of the hair shaft that resembles scales or the tiles on a roof

cut-throat razor a traditional open fixed-blade razor

cutting angle the angle at which the hair is held and then cut

cutting collar a collar used to form a good seal around the client's neck to prevent hairs from falling down their collar

cutting comb a flexible comb specifically designed to be used when cutting

cutting guideline the line made by the ends of the previous cut hair section when held against the section of uncut hair

cutting method a sequence of cutting techniques to achieve a specific haircut

cutting technique a special cutting skill aimed at producing a specific result

cysteine an amino acid containing sulphur that occurs in proteins such as keratincystine; two cysteine atoms when joined together (oxidized) make a cystine molecule

damaged cuticle the outer layer of the hair when broken or torn

dandruff a scalp disorder where scales of dry dead skin build up and flake from the scalp

Data Protection Act legislation in the UK designed to protect an individual's right to privacy

density describes the amount of hair growing in a given area

density of hair the amount of hair in a specific area

depth of colour a measurement of how light or dark a colour is

dermatitis inflammation of the skin, *see* **contact dermatitis**

dermis the thickest layer of the skin directly below the epidermis

detergent an cleansing agent that reduces the surface tension of water to improve its wetting ability and is able to attract and hold onto dirt particles so that they become suspended within the liquid, called an emulsion

development time the time required by some hairdressing products to achieve their effect such as in tinting

diagnosis establishing symptoms in order to identify a disease or disorder

direct current an electrical current where the electrons flow constantly in one direction

disconnected haircut where the layers between two areas of the head are not blended together in order to produce a clear contrast in hair length

disinfectant a substance that kills disease-causing micro-organisms

disposable razor a razor designed to be disposed of after a few uses

disuiphide bridges the links between different keratin bonds in the hair structure

distilled water water that has had many of its impurities removed through distillation, which involves boiling the water and then condensing the steam back into water. Used in water heaters to prevent limescale deposits

double crown two crowns instead of one that may grow towards each other and cause the hair to stick up, especially if cut too short

dry cutting cutting the hair whilst it is dry

dry shaving shaving the skin whilst dry using and electric shaver

eczema an inflammation of the skin identified by redness and irritation

effleurage a light, soothing, stroking massage movement

elasticity the ability of a material to stretch and then return to its original length

electrical circuit the flow of electrons from an electrical supply to an electric appliance

electrode the term used to describe applicators used in high frequency treatments

emollient a substance used in some conditioners to soften and enhance the hair

emulsion where the molecules in one liquid or substance are suspended within a second liquid or substance even though normally they do not mix well (e.g. oil in water)

emulsify the process used to make different liquids or substances that normally do not mix to come together into an emulsion

end paper a small paper wrap used to secure the hair ends during perm winding

epidermis the outermost layers of the skin

erythema reddening of the skin caused by increased blood flow

essence the most important quality, feature or nature of something that identifies it, defines it or simply makes it what it is

eumelanin the black and brown pigment in the skin and hair

exfoliating the removal of the oldest and dead skin cells from the skin's outermost surface, called the stratum corneum, so that new skin cells can replace them; thereby helping to maintain healthy skin

facial a service or treatment involving the cleansing of the face followed by face massage

facial hair any hair growing on the face, including eyebrows, sideburns, beards and moustaches

finger (hand) drying using the fingers as a brush or comb when drying the hair

finishing the process of completing a service by dressing and styling and applying products as required in order to achieve and maintain the desired effect

fixed-blade razor an open style razor with a permanent blade that must be honed and stropped before use

folliculitis inflammation of the hair follicles probably caused by bacterial infection

form an object's three-dimensional affect, depth

fragilitas crinium the splitting of the hairs at their ends

fraudulent actions or claims that are dishonest, false or deceitful

freehand cutting the technique of cutting hair without holding it in place or forcing it out of its natural position

friction a stimulating massage technique using the pads of the fingers in a vigorous movement

fringe hair that covers the forehead from one side to the other

fungicide a substance that kills a fungus

fungus a group of living organisms that are plant-like and may cause disease

furunculosis boils and abscesses

geometry mathematics concerned with the shape, size and positions of different objects

germinal matrix the living cell reproducing part of the hair

germinating layer the deepest layer of the epidermis where the regeneration of cells takes place

gift voucher a prepaid voucher that can be used as part of a payment, or as full payment

gown a protective wrap placed around the client during services

graduation an increase or decrease in the length of layers of hair across the head

granular layer the layer of the epidermis between the soft living cells and the harder dead cells

greasy hair (seborrhoea) a condition caused by an over-production of the natural oil sebum

guideline a feature or previously cut section of hair that is used to indicate where the next cut should be made

hair bulb the base of the hair follicle containing actively growing cells where new hair forms

hair characteristics the physical properties of the hair, for example: hair density, hair texture, hair elasticity, hair porosity, hair condition and hair growth patterns

hair follicle the thin tube-like space in the dermis in which the hair develops and grows

hair friction scalp massage a traditional barber's shop scalp massage that uses friction massage techniques to apply a spirit based hair and scalp tonic, which creates an invigorating sensation when the alcohol evaporates during the massage

hair growth patterns the way in which individual hairs in a section of the skin naturally grow in particular directions

hair muscle (arrector pili) a small muscle attached to the hair follicle and the epidermis that causes the hair to stand up when contracted, trapping a warm layer of air around the skin

hair papillae it connects the bottom of the follicle with the epidermis and nourishes cellular activity

hair shaper a razor-like cutting tool that usually includes a safety guard

hair texture the breadth of the hair; fine, medium or coarse

hair type the classification of hair according to the structure of the hair and traditionally by reference to its racial and geographical related features, including: Type 1 – Straight Hair (Caucasian, European and Mongoloid hair was usually in this category); Type 2 – Wavy Hair (Caucasian or European hair is usually in this category); Type 3 – Curly Hair (Caucasian, European and Black hair can all be found in this category); Type 4 – Very Curly Hair (Black or African-Caribbean hair would typically be in this category)

hair whorls a hair growth pattern where the hair grows in a circle, similarly to the crown, often occurring in the nape or beard hairline

hairpiece see postiche

hamilton pattern the typical pattern of hair loss found in men with male-pattern alopecia

hard water water that contains calcium and/or magnesium salts; it produces scum with soap and is likely to leave deposits in water heaters, such as kettles and steamers

hazard an item, substance, action or circumstances that have the potential to cause harm

henna (lawsonia inermis) a tropical shrub with small pink, red or white flowers used as an ingredient is some hair colourants

hepatitis a disease causing inflammation of the liver

hereditary a condition or feature that passes from a parent to a child, such as the colour of the eyes or hair that is naturally passed on from parents to their children

herpes simplex a viral skin infection, commonly called 'cold sores'

high frequency a treatment that uses a high frequency electrical current to stimulate the tissues of the skin

highlighting lightening, shading or colouring selected parts of the hair to enhance the style

HIV human immunodeficiency virus, thought to lead to the condition of AIDS

hone a rectangular block of abrasive material used to set, or sharpen fixed-blade razors

horny layer the surface layer of the epidermis consisting of dead, hard, flat, cells

humectant a substance that attracts and holds moisture

humidity the amount of moisture held in the air

hydrogen bonds bonds in the hair structure that are easily broken when styling

hydrogen peroxide an oxidizing agent used in neutralizing and colouring

hydrolysis the chemical breakdown of a compound due to reaction with water

hydrophilic a substance that is attracted to water and is easily dissolved in water

hydrophobic a substance that is repelled by water and is difficult or impossible to dissolve in water

hygiene performing procedures that maintain cleanliness and good health

hygroscopic absorbing moisture from the atmosphere

hyperaemia redness and flushing of the skin due to improved blood flow

immune system the body's defence system against disease

impetigo a bacterial infection of the epidermis

incompatibility two or more substances that do not work well when mixed together; they sometimes react badly, *see* **compatibility**

infection the presence of microorganisms in the skin or underlying structures, which may multiply and result in injury and disease

infectious a condition that is capable of being transmitted or passed to another person so that they then become affected by the same condition. Sometimes such conditions are also said to be contagious

infestation a condition where the hair and/or skin is infested with parasites such as scabies or head lice

ingrowing hairs hairs that grow into the skin rather than out of the hair follicle, sometimes caused by shaving too close

international colour chart a chart that codes and defines hair colour by depth and tone

itch mite an animal parasite that causes scabies

job description a written summary of the barber's role within the barber's shop and the responsibilities that this role includes

keloids bumps in the skin caused a build-up of skin cells, a form of over-developed scarring due to overgrowths of fibrous skin tissue

keratin the main protein in hair, nails and the skin. Keratin has elastic properties which allow it to stretch and return to its original length without damage. This makes the hair flexible and allows it to be stretched and curled without breaking

lanolin an emollient extracted from wool fat

lanugo hair the soft downy hair on an unborn child

lather a creamy substance applied to the area to be shaved prior to shaving. It helps clean the skin and hair, soften the hair and lubricate the skin

lathering lubricating and softening the beard before shaving

layering cutting hair at various angles to produce different degrees of graduation

leeching the medical practice of using leeches to help stimulate the movement of blood through the veins

legislation laws that are approved and written down by Parliament – usually the most important laws that are superior to all others. They are sometimes referred to as an 'Act of Parliament', 'Statute' or as 'Statutory Law'

lightening the process of lifting the base shade of hair, *see* **bleaching**

lighting the effect created by natural or artificial light

limescale hard deposits of calcium carbonate that separate from hard water when it is heated

linear design a one-dimensional design that only uses lines

litmus papers *see* (pH papers)

lowlighting shading or colouring parts of the hair to enhance the style

lymph the pale yellow fluid of the lymphatic system

lymphatic system a network of lymph vessels, lymph nodes and lymph glands that closely follow the veins to remove bacteria, foreign matter and excess fluids from the body's tissues

macrofibrils slender fibres that make up the cells in the cortex of the hair

massage moving the skin and muscles by rubbing and kneading in order to improve blood flow, lymph flow and to promote relaxing or stimulating sensations as required

medulla the central core of the hair shaft

melanin naturally occurring pigments found in the skin and hair that determine the skin or hair colour

mesh the sections within a haircut, sometimes referred to as meshes

metallic dyes dyes that are derived from metal or have a metallic sheen

microfibrils fibres that group together to form the macrofibrils in the cortex

microorganism a minute life form, such as bacteria that may be seen only with a microscope

mixed layer the layer of the epidermis found immediately below the granular layer

moisturiser a substance that attracts and holds moisture

mongoloid hair straight hair typical of Asian or Amerindian people, also now known as Type S1 hair

monilethrix beaded hair

muscle insertion the point at which a muscle is attached to a movable bone or to another muscle

muscle origin the point at which a muscle is attached to a static bone

natural colour the hair's colour produced from the natural hair pigment, melanin

neck strip a long and thin paper tissue placed around and between the client's neck and the gown to prevent hairs from falling down their collar

neckline the perimeter of the haircut across the nape of the neck

neutral a substance that has a pH close to 7

neutralizer a product used to return the hair to its normal condition after cold perming

nit an egg of the head louse, **pediculosis capitis**

nitro dyes semi-permanent colours that penetrate to just below the cuticle

normalizer *see* neutralizer

open razor a traditionally styled type of razor where the blade closes into the handle for protection when not in use

one-dimensional shape a shape consisting only of a line

outlines the perimeter of a haircut, beard, moustache or pattern, e.g. neckline, beard outline, etc.

outlining the process of marking out the perimeter of the haircut, beard, moustache or pattern

over-processing leaving a chemical product on the hair longer than required or recommended

oxidant an oxidizing agent

oxidation the second chemical stage of the perming process where the addition of oxygen combines with hydrogen in the perm lotion to form water, allowing the hair's disulphide bridges to reform in their new positions

oxidizing agent a substance that reacts with other chemicals to release oxygen, such as hydrogen peroxide

ozone a gas produced during high frequency treatment that has a germicidal action on the surface of the skin

papilliary layer the uppermost layer of the dermis that connects with the lowest layer of the epidermis

parasite an organism that lives on another organism, which may cause symptoms of disease

partings selected divisions in the hair

pathogen a microorganism or virus that produces harmful effects and disease

portable appliance testing (PAT) the requirement for electrical appliances used by employees or the public, or if appliances are repaired or serviced to be regularly tested and given a certificate of testing to confirm that they are safe for use

pediculosis capitis an infestation of the head by the head louse

performance appraisal a time where you and your manager consider whether you have met the requirements stated in your job description and employment contract. They help to establish the strengths and weaknesses in your work, so that you can recognize them and make improvements where required. Called performance reviews where they are completed more often

perm lotion a reducing agent used to break the disulphide bonds in the cortex

permeable allows other substances or materials to penetrate or pass through

perming or permanent waving a process that changes the structure of the hair so that straight hair permanently holds waves or curls

perspective the skill of placing lines, shapes or objects into a design or picture in such a way that makes some objects appear to be nearer and others distant – creating a 3D effect

pétrissage a deep, kneading massage movement

pH papers a paper that changes colour when in contact with a liquid to indicate whether it is acid or alkaline

pH scale a method of measuring acidity or alkalinity

pheomelanin the red and yellow pigment found in the skin and hair

pigments give the hair its natural colour and found in the hair cortex

pityriasis capitis *see* **dandruff**

polishing colouring parts of the hair to enhance the style

polypeptides a polymer consisting of amino acids which form all or part of a protein molecule

pomade a substance or ointment used to groom and fix the hair in place. Originally oil or wax based and shiny in appearance but now may be water based for easier removal

porosity (of hair) the hair's ability to absorb moisture or liquids

porous a property of materials constructed of small holes through which liquid or air may pass

post-damping applying perm lotion after the hair has been wound onto rods

posterior towards the back

postiche hairpieces that are added for ornamentation or to disguise hair loss

pre-damping applying perm lotion before or during the winding of perm rods into the hair

pre-lightening bleaching hair to a shade that is lighter before colouring

pre-pigmentation adding a colour to porous hair before re-colouring to allow the colour to adhere to the hair and prevents patchy or greenish results

pre-softening technique used to soften the hair cuticle before applying a permanent colour

prickle cells cells in the mixed layer of the epidermis between the granular layer and the basal layer

primary colours of light: blue, green and red; of pigments: blue, yellow and red

proactive anticipating an event or problem then making a change or offering help before the event or problem occurs

processing time the amount of time it takes for a chemical product to work on the hair

productivity the rate at which services and retail sales are completed

proportion describes the relative size of one shape or object within a design to the size of another shape or object in the design

proteins long chains of amino acids

protofibrils fibres in the cortex that determine the strength, elasticity, thickness and curl of the hair

psoriasis a condition that produces inflammation, irritation and scaling of the skin

quasi-permanent colour a hair colour that is long-lasting as it fades gradually over time and through shampooing

reactive responding to an event or problem after it has occurred and then making a change or offering help

reception area an area of the salon where clients are received

reducing agent ammonium hydroxide. In perming it releases hydrogen in the hair, and is then oxidized to stabilize the hair structure in neutralizing

reduction the first chemical stage of the perming process where the hair's disulphide bridges are split apart by the addition of hydrogen

regrowth application colouring hair that has grown since the last colour or bleach

relaxing the process of removing curl or waves from the hair

resistant hair hair that typically has tightly closed cuticles and a reflective surface and consequently resists the penetration of products into the cortex

restyle to change the hair shape and style to a new shape and style

reticular layer the lowest layer of the dermis, immediately above the subcutaneous layer

retouching colouring or relaxing regrowth hair

risk how likely it is that a hazard will cause harm

root the bottom of the hair where it lies in the scalp

rotary a circular massage movement used in shampooing where the pads of the fingers move over the surface of the scalp

safety razor a razor with a guard that covers and protects the blade when in use

salt bonds bonds found in the hair structure that can be easily broken to give a new temporary shape when styling the hair

sanitation the destruction of most, but not all microorganisms

scabies an animal parasite that burrows under the skin causing a rash

scale using ratios to establish the relative dimensions of objects in a design

scalp the skin and tissue that covers the top of the head

scrunch drying a technique used in blow-drying where the fingers gripe and squeeze the hair to produce fuller effects, producing softer curls and used less often on men

sebaceous cyst a swollen sebaceous gland

sebaceous gland a natural oil gland in the skin that produces sebum

seborrhoea over-production of the natural oil sebum by the sebaceous glands that leads to greasy skin

sebum the natural oily secretion of a sebaceous gland

second-time-over shaving shaving a second time against the hair growth to produce a closer shave

secondary colours of light: yellow, cyan and magenta; of pigments: violet, green and orange

sections the divisions of hair for the purpose of cutting, perming, etc.

semi-permanent colouring a hair colourant that lasts through several shampoos

shades a numbered coding system used to refer to different shades of hair colour

shampoos products used for cleaning hair, some include conditioning ingredients

shape the outline or profile of an object

sharps used or contaminated blades, needles, etc.

sideburns the name used to describe the facial hair on men adjacent to the ears but not connected through to the other side of the face

silicones a durable synthetic resin found in hairspray

singeing using either a lighted wax taper or electrical singeing equipment to singe the ends of the hair after cutting

skin fade a cutting effect where longer hair is graduated so that it appears to blend into the skin without any visible outline

soft water water that does not contain calcium and magnesium salts; thereby less likely to leave deposits in water heaters, such as kettles and steamers

softened beard facial hair that has been steamed with hot towels so that the cuticles open and moisture and lather enter to increase the elasticity of the hair in preparation for shaving

sparking a technique used in high frequency treatments to produce an intense tingling sensation as the electrical current jumps the gap between the applicator and the client's skin

spectrum the colours contained in light that we see as white unless split apart by a prism. Most people can recognize red, orange, yellow, blue, green, indigo and violet

split ends see fragilitas crinium

sponge shave a shaving technique where a small sterile sponge is drawn across the face directly in front of the razor's path so that the hairs stand up and a closer shave is achieved, replicated in modern safety razors by a band of rubber strips immediately before the blades

stabilizer a chemical added to bleach to prevent deterioration

static electricity electrical charges on the hair that produce a 'flyaway' behaviour

steamer a machine used to supply moist heat for treatments

sterilization the process of killing all microorganisms on an item

stock rotation a procedure used to ensure that old stock is used up before newer stock

strand colour test used in colouring to check that the colour has developed

stratum aculeatum found in the mixed layer of the epidermis

stratum malpighi found in the mixed layer of the epidermis

stratum spinosum found in the mixed layer of the epidermis

strop a canvas and leather covered strap or block, (canvas to clean and leather to polish fixed-blade razors)

styptic liquid/powder a coagulant, helps promote clotting of the blood

subcutaneous layer the tissue lying immediately below the skin, also known as the fatty layer

surface tension a natural electrical force that acts at the surface of water or a liquid to make it come together to form a rounded shape

sycosis barbae a bacterial infection of the hair follicles

symmetrical an evenly balanced effect that is the same shape on both sides

symptom a specific sensation or change in the body which may enable a disease to be identified

synthetic a man-made substance or material

tactful thinking about the rights and feelings of other people, maintaining their privacy and dealing with their needs sensitively

tapering (taper cutting) cutting a hair section to a tapered point

tapotement a tapping or patting massage movement

telogen the hair growth stage where a hair ceases to grow before it is shed

temporary colours hair colourants that are washed away by shampooing

terminal hair the longer, coarser hair of the head and of facial hair in men

test curl a test made on a curl to determine the required perm lotion, rod size and processing time

texture the thickness of individual hairs, may be fine, medium or coarse

texturizing removing specific amounts of hair to break up solid shapes, producing a more broken effect without reducing the overall length

thinning reducing the bulk of hair without reducing its length

threading a technique used to remove hair, usually around the eyebrows, similar to plucking hair with tweezers

tinea capitis ringworm of the head

tipping colouring parts of the hair to enhance the style

tone the overall visual effect given by a colour

toning adding tint or colour to hair after bleaching

tonsor a Latin word meaning 'barber'; the barber is sometimes referred to as a tonsorial artist, also used to describe the practice in some religions of shaving a circular area of the crown

top-notch something of the highest quality, sometimes called first-rate or excellent

toupee a small piece of postiche designed to cover the area of hair loss in the Hamilton pattern and be blended with the remaining hair growth

traditional look a look that was popular over many years in the past

tramlining see **channelling**; a simpler form of channelling

translucent allows light to pass through

trichologist a person specializing in the scientific treatment of diseases and disorders affecting the hair and scalp

trichorrhexis nodosa nodules appearing on the hair that often lead to splitting

trim removing just the excess growth by cutting and clipping – to make neat and tidy

trimming removing small amounts of hair in order to recreate the original style, sometimes called having a '**trim**'

two-dimensional shape a shape with a flat plane, such as a circle or rectangle

under-processing not allowing a chemical sufficient time to develop to meet the recommended or required development time

unhygienic unclean and risking harm to health

uniform layering a haircut when all sections of the hair are cut to the same length

vaccination treatment with a vaccine, usually a modified mild version of a specific virus, that triggers the body's immune system to produce antibodies that help to protect the body if it is attacked by a real infection

vapours a method of sterilization

vasodilation dilation or expansion of a vessel such as the capillaries and lymph nodes during high frequency treatments

vein a small blood vessel that carries oxygen depleted blood towards the heart

vellus hair very fine hair that covers the skin, usually visible on the face

venule a very small vein

vibro massager a mechanical massage machine

virgin hair natural hair that has never been treated by any chemical process

virus a minute life form that can only be seen with an electron microscope. It lives in the cells of other organisms, is able to reproduce itself and often causes diseases

wart a viral infection of the skin

wet cutting cutting the hair while it is wet

wet shaving shaving the skin after lathering

wetting agents substances that reduce the surface tension of water and other liquids and allow them to spread easily over the hair and scalp

whetted edge the name given to the edge of a fixed-blade razor when the correct cutting edge has been achieved through honing and stropping

widows peak a hair growth pattern at the front hairline where the hair grows up and forwards into a peak

Index